D1369290

INTRO

A Guide to Communication Sciences and Disorders

Second Edition

INTRO

A Guide to Communication Sciences and Disorders

Second Edition

Michael P. Robb, PhD

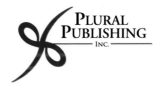

PLURAL
PUBLISHING
INC.

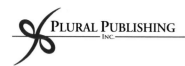

5521 Ruffin Road
San Diego, CA 92123

e-mail: info@pluralpublishing.com
Website: http://www.pluralpublishing.com

Typeset in 11/13 Palatino by Flanagan's Publishing Services, Inc.
Printed in the United States of America by Bang Printing
17 16 15   2 3 4 5

For permission to use material from this text, contact us by
Telephone: (866) 758-7251
Fax: (888) 758-7255
e-mail: permissions@pluralpublishing.com

*Every attempt has been made to contact the copyright holders for material originally
printed in another source. If any have been inadvertently overlooked, the publishers will
gladly make the necessary arrangements at the first opportunity.*

Library of Congress Cataloging-in-Publication Data

Robb, Michael P., author.
  INTRO : a guide to communication sciences and disorders / Michael P. Robb.—
Second edition.
       p. ; cm.
  Guide to communication sciences and disorders
  Includes bibliographical references and index.
  ISBN-13: 978-1-59756-542-4 (alk. paper)
  ISBN-10: 1-59756-542-3 (alk. paper)
  I. Title. II. Title: Guide to communication sciences and disorders.
  [DNLM: 1. Communication Disorders. 2. Hearing Disorders. WL 340.2]
  RC423
  362.196'855—dc23
                                                        2013033491

CONTENTS

SECTION 4: AUDITION   **335**

Introductory courses in communication sciences and disorders typically serve several purposes and audiences. The course is an introduction to the professions of speech and language pathology and audiology and the underlying discipline on which they are based, communication sciences and disorders. Fundamentally, it is a first course laying the foundation for more advanced study in the professions. Its focus is broad, and students are provided with the beginnings of a working vocabulary in the field. Students are familiarized with basic concepts and issues encountered in research and in practice in speech and language pathology. In addition to serving as a first course for students entering the field, the vocabulary and basic concepts of communication disorders are useful to students from related professional fields of education, health care, and psychology who often take the introductory course. An effective textbook for an introductory course aims to accomplish a number of objectives. It must be accurate, reflect contemporary knowledge and thought, and be sufficiently engaging to sustain the interest of the neophyte. Professor Robb's *INTRO* clearly hits the target.

When writing the foreword to the first edition of this introductory level textbook by Professor Robb, I wrote from the perspective of someone with a number of years of experience teaching an introductory course in communicative disorders for which this book is intended and from having, over those years, used a number of other introductory textbooks. I had read *INTRO* and was impressed with the clarity of the writing style and appropriate level of presentation for the beginning student. Several other distinguishing features were appealing such as the inclusion of historical referents within each chapter, the global-multicultural emphasis, and discussion of current theory and research within the wide scope of disorders encompassed by the field. My view that it would be an excellent text to help accomplish the objectives of an introductory survey course in communication sciences and disorders has subsequently been validated. I wrote this foreword to the second edition from the enhanced perspective informed by having used *INTRO* for four years in my course and by the overwhelmingly positive student responses to the text conveyed in their course evaluations and comments. *INTRO* is a wonderful medium to help beginning students become familiar with the variety of communication disorders that can occur across the life span and to understand the influences of genomics, human development, neurophysiology, and social-cultural factors on communication disorders and their treatment.

INTRO is both student friendly and instructor friendly, made even more so in this second edition with the inclusion of the instructor CD, learning objectives, and study questions.

John H. Saxman, PhD
Professor Emeritus, Speech and
     Language Pathology
Teachers College, Columbia
     University

Four years have passed since the first edition of **INTRO**. The response to the original edition exceeded my expectations. I was pleased with the positive comments about the format and writing style of the book. I have retained this approach for the second edition. **INTRO** is designed for the beginning university-level student who has an interest in entering the field of communication sciences and disorders, or for a student who may be interested in entering one of the companion health professions. As is the case for any book claiming to be introductory, the aim is to paint a picture for the student using broad strokes. This book provides straightforward and essential information concerning a wide range of communication disorders found in children and adults.

The second edition, like the first edition, is organized into four sections. Section 1 provides background information related to communication disorders. The chapters in this section cover the topics of communication science, the professions of audiology and speech-language pathology, and anatomy and physiology. Section 2 is concerned with developmental communication disorders, and includes chapters on child language disorders, child phonological disorders, fluency disorders, and cleft lip and palate. Section 3 covers acquired and genetic communication disorders. The chapters in this section describe voice disorders, neurogenic communication disorders, dysphagia,

and genetic-based communication disorders. Section 4 addresses audition and contains chapters on hearing disorders and aural rehabilitation.

Unique aspects of the book include its use of an identical structure for each chapter to assist beginning students in grasping new vocabulary and concepts. Each chapter also provides a focus on "past and present." An introduction to each of the various disorders would not be complete without knowing some of the fascinating historical background surrounding each disorder, as well as current theories and research. In the years that have passed since the first edition, there have been exciting research advancements in communication sciences and disorders. Each chapter highlights some of the very latest research findings. The book holds worldwide appeal and is written for an international audience.

A portion of each chapter is dedicated to cultural aspects of communication disorders, as well as prevalence information about various communication disorders as found in English-speaking countries around the world, including Australia, Canada, the United Kingdom, the United States, and New Zealand. The chapters include a series of FYIs (for your information), which present interesting and novel information about the particular topic area. A number of websites are listed at the end of the chapters that to provide students with an opportunity to learn more about each topic. Many of these websites provide up-to-date links to streaming video examples.

The sole authorship of the book ensures a balanced writing style that is missing from existing introductory texts. *INTRO* is a clear and concise primer for students wishing to obtain fundamental information about the myriad of communication disorders that occur across the life span. For some, this information will serve as a springboard for pursuit of a professional career in audiology and speech-language pathology. For others, my hope is that you will acquire an appreciation of the gift of communication that we so often take for granted.

Students and instructors alike should be pleased with this new edition of *INTRO*. I wish to thank Ray Kent who encouraged me to write a book of this kind and provided valuable oversight throughout its creation. Several colleagues provided reviews on various chapters of the book: Kenn Appel, Maggie Lee Huckabee, Emily Lin, Greg, O'Beirne, and Natalie Rickard. All of the book illustrations were made possible by the tireless work of Chia Pan. Finally, my initial exposure to the field of communication sciences and disorders was provided by my mother, Mary Jo Robb, whose professional career was spent educating children. During my first year of university study, she introduced me to a school speech-language pathologist. Little did I know this meeting would set the stage for a life-long career that has proved to be more rewarding than I could have imagined. Thanks Mum.

M. P. R.

To Jenne

SECTION 1

Background to Communication Disorders

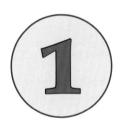

COMMUNICATION
SCIENCE

After reading this chapter, the student should be able to:

- Recognize the different forms and types of human communication.
- Recognize the importance of effective communication in various situations.
- Recognize that communication is a multifaceted process.
- Recognize that speech is an important tool for thinking, learning, and communicating.
- Recognize listening as an active, constructive process.
- Recognize that communication is an interactive process between sender and receiver.
- Recognize the role of culture in communication.
- Recognize the need for formal and informal oral communication.
- Recognize how theories of normal communication serve as a basis for the diagnosis and remediation of communication disorders.

INTRODUCTION

Communication involves the transfer of information between two living organisms. As humans, we are born with the physical attributes to communicate. Our earliest forms of communication are quite basic and revolve around fundamental needs and wants. The transfer of information is between infant and caregiver. As we grow, we learn to communicate more effectively by observing other people communicating. We model our communication on what we see, hear, and experience. Our communication skills grow in complexity and sophistication through formal education, and by practicing those skills and having them evaluated.

Communication science is an academic field of study that examines how people communicate as individuals, within a society, and in various cultures. Communication science is a field that has grown rapidly in large part due to advances in technology. Some of the greatest technological advances that have occurred over the past decades are directly related to improvements in the way we communicate. Contemporary students of communication science draw on theories and practices common in the fields of linguistics, mass communication, political science, journalism, psychology, sociology, anthropology, and animal behavior. There are a variety of careers that can be pursued with a background in communication science. A listing of some of the many possible career choices is provided in Table 1–1. According to the U.S. Bureau of Labor, the majority of these fields are expected to grow over the next 10 years.

The primary focus of this book concerns situations when the transfer of information between humans is somehow impaired. When communication fails, misunderstandings occur and sometimes people become frustrated, worried, or even angry. Some communication impairments are minor and can be easily corrected, whereas others are more severe and may require an extensive period of treatment. As a prerequisite to understanding various communication disorders, it is important to first have a grasp of normal communication. Knowledge concerning the normal process of communication serves as foundation for the identification and management of communication disorders. The aim of this chapter is to introduce concepts of normal communication that subsequently will serve as a platform for learning about various disorders presented in later chapters.

TERMINOLOGY AND DEFINITIONS

The word *communicate* is related to the word *common*. The word has its origin in the Latin verb *communicare*, which means "to share" or "to make common." When we communicate, we make things common. Communication is one of those activities that we take for granted. It seems to occur naturally, and we spend the majority of our living hours engaged in some form of communication. Although we tend to think of communication as talking to someone, communication also occurs in other ways, like when we watch television or surf the Internet. We communicate to others by the way we dress, the style of

Table 1–1. Possible Career Options in the Various Fields of Communication Science

Field of Study	Career Choices
Advertising	marketing specialist, sales manager
Communication Education	speech teacher, coach, professor
Journalism	reporter, editor, script writer
Radio/Television Broadcasting	disc jockey, announcer, news anchor
Public Relations	press agent, lobbyist, public opinion poller
Theatre/Performing Arts	actor, director, producer, model
Business	sales rep, negotiator, human resources manager
Education	college recruiter, teacher, researcher
Government/Politics	speech writer, press secretary, elected official
Health Careers	health care counselor, hospital administrator
International Relations and Negotiations	diplomat, foreign correspondent, foreign relations officer
Law	public defender, district attorney, legal secretary
Social and Human Services	social worker, recreational supervisor, human rights officer

our hair, and the tattoos we choose (or do not choose) to wear. At a fundamental level, communication can be defined as a two-way process in which a message is sent and received. The sender's role in the process of communication is to generate (or **encode**) a message. The receiver's role is to translate (or **decode**) this message. Communication is never a one-way process. Both the sender and the receiver need to participate. If the sender is unable to clearly encode a message, then a breakdown in communication occurs. Similarly, if the receiver is unable to successfully decode a message, then communication is likely to fail. Excellent communicators are those who have mastered the process of both sending and receiving messages.

Communication is a phenomenon that is common to all living beings. All communication takes place by means of signs. A sign is something that stands for something else. These signs can take a variety of forms such as vocalizations, nonverbal gestures, physical movements, vibrations, smells, pictures, and letters. All of these signs serve the same purpose: to help with the exchange of information between the sender and receiver. A branch of communication sciences that is concerned with the various types of signs used in communication is called **semiotics**. People who study semiotics are interested in how signs and symbols create meaning and how this meaning is communicated.

It is estimated that 75% of a person's day is spent communicating in some way. Most of our daily communication involves speaking and listening to others. The remaining portion of the day is spent communicating via reading and writing. The face-to-face communication that occurs between people, usually in a private setting, is called **interpersonal communication**. For most of us, this is the type of communication where we feel most comfortable and at ease. **Group communication** relates to the exchange of information that takes place among a small collection of people. **Public communication** occurs on a larger scale than group communication and includes settings such as university lectures or formal presentations. **Organizational communication** takes place in environments such as workplace offices and corporations. Finally, **mass communication** is related to the exchange of information to a large public audience through some sort of medium, such as radio, television, or the Internet.

ANIMAL COMMUNICATION

Ethology is the study of animal behavior. The term is derived from the Greek word *ethos* meaning "character." Scientists, called ethologists, observe, record, and analyze how animals behave and interact with others. Ethologists are particularly interested in the way animals communicate. Two well-known ethologists are Charles Darwin and Jane Goodall (Figure 1–1). **Charles Dar-**

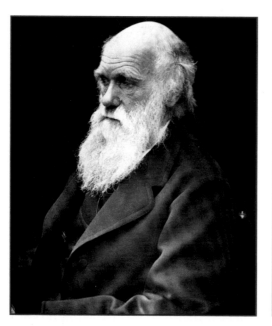 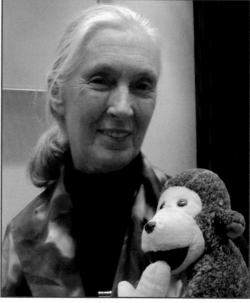

FIGURE 1–1. Famous ethologists Charles Darwin and Jane Goodall. Images from Jeekc at Wikimedia Commons. Permission granted through Creative Commons Attribution 2.5 License.

win (1809–1882) is considered the first modern ethologist because of his extensive work examining the evolution of animal behavior and the expression of emotion. **Jane Goodall** (b. 1934) is a world-renowned ethologist and conservationist who has studied the vocalizations produced by chimpanzees at Gombe National Park in Tanzania since the 1960s.

The ability to communicate is not unique to humans. Many species of nonhuman animals and even insects communicate with each other. Examples of the wide range of communication that occurs among nonhumans are provided in Table 1–2. Animals regularly send signals to each other, and most of this communication is intraspecific (occurring between animals of the same species). The type of messages that are communicated within a species usually relate to basic matters such as signaling danger, marking territory, and sexual mating. The signals may be instinctive or learned. The mode of animal communication is quite varied and

---

FYI

Before the development of speech, the most primitive form of mass communication was likely to have been shouting. A group of primates would construe loud sounds as associated with danger.

Table 1–2. Some Forms of Communication Displayed by Nonhuman Species

Animal	Form of Communication
Bees	dance when they have found nectar
Chimpanzees	touch hands as a form of greeting
Dogs	stretch their front legs out in front of them and lower their bodies when they want to play
Dolphins	use vocalization and echolocation to communicate and navigate
Elephants	entwine their trunks as a show of affection
Fiddler Crabs	wave their single giant claw to attract female fiddler crabs
Giraffes	press their necks together as a show of affection
Gorillas	express anger by sticking out their tongues
Horses	rub noses as a sign of affection
Kangaroos	thump their hind legs to warn others of danger
Swans	entwine their long necks when courting as well as fighting
Whales	breach (leap out of the water) repeatedly to send messages to other whales
White-Tailed Deer	show alarm by flicking their tail upward

may include: (1) auditory, (2) visual, (3) tactile, or (4) chemical transmission. **Auditory communication** involves use of a variety of sounds for communication. A sound is uttered by one animal, which is then heard and interpreted by other members of the same species. Animals make many different sounds to communicate. From the roar of a lion to the mew of a cat, sound is a way for animals to send messages to other animals. Another form of auditory communication used by animals is **echolocation**, which involves bouncing sound off objects to provide information about size, location, and movement of those objects. Echolocation is used at night or in environments that are perpetually dark, such as inside caves or deep in the ocean. **Visual communication** involves two types of signals: (1) badges and (2) displays. **Badges** are the color and shape of the animal used to send a message to animals of the same species. For example, the size of male deer antlers sends a message to other males regarding its dominance (Figure 1–2). Badges can also help females pick a mate. The sex of many species of birds is often differentiated by color, with males being the more colorful. Male birds with the brightest color are perceived by female birds as being most healthy. **Displays** are related to animal body language and can be used to attract a mate or to warn off a predator. A dog will place its tail between its legs to display submission. A cat will arch its back to present a threatening profile. **Tactile communication** differs from other forms of communication because the sender of the message must be in physical contact with the receiver. Baboons are known to groom each other, which is a behavior pattern that serves to lessen tension between one another. **Chemical communication** is used by animals that have particularly keen senses of smell or taste. Depending on the type of chemical, either the sender or the receiver benefits from the message. Dogs and cats rely primarily upon the sense of smell for an awareness of events occurring around them. Many insects use chemical signals as well. Some animals release an odor containing **pheromones** (airborne chemicals) to send messages to others. The female gypsy moth produces a potent pheromone that can attract male moths from several miles away. The unique trail displayed by marching ants is a result of a pheromone laid down by ants that have gone ahead of others (see Figure 1–2).

HISTORY OF HUMAN COMMUNICATION

The ability to speak in a clear, eloquent, and effective manner has long been considered to be the hallmark of an educated person. Under the rubric (or label) of **rhetoric**, the study of the theory and practice of communication dates back to the time of the ancient Greeks. **Plato** (428–347 BC) was a critic of rhetoric and suggested that it was simply a style of speaking and did not reflect substance or breadth of knowledge. He believed that one's speaking style is often used to deceive others because it does not distinguish between conviction and knowledge. **Aristotle** (384–322 BC) wrote extensively on the topic of rhetoric (Figure 1–3). He believed that good rhetoricians (i.e., good communicators) needed to develop five essential skills: (1) invention, which is the ability to generate ideas, (2) disposition, which is the ability to organize ideas, (3) style, which is use of appropriate language,

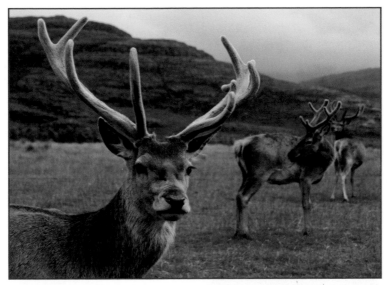

A

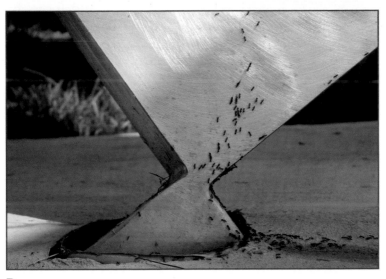

B

FIGURE 1–2. **A.** Deer antlers provide a form of visual communication. From M. Karatay at Wikimedia Commons. **B.** A trail of ants reflects a form of chemical communication. From R. Whittle at Wikimedia Commons. Permission granted through Creative Commons Attribution 3.0 License.

(4) memory, which is the ability to recall facts and ideas, and (5) delivery, which is the use of voice and gestures. When a person poses a rhetorical question, they are not seeking an answer. Rather, they are using a style of speaking that is designed to make a point.

Major advancements in the study of human communication occurred in England during the 18th century in what

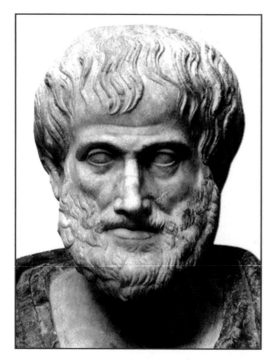

FIGURE 1–3. Aristotle wrote extensively on the topic of rhetoric.

was termed the **Elocutionary Movement**. Elocutio was the Latin word for style, but it literally means "speaking out." Its English derivative *elocution* was adapted as a term for reading aloud. This movement was concerned with the skill of communication in public settings, such as poetry readings, speeches, or plays. Correct elocution stressed the importance of vocal quality and inflection, force and projection, articulation and pronunciation, and gestures and facial expression. The movement also had a considerable influence on English education in the latter half of the century. The third U.S. president, **Thomas Jefferson** (1743–1826) was influenced by the elocutionary movement in his pursuit of the establishment of a democratic and free society in early America. The early 20th century saw a general melding of the concepts of rhetoric and

elocution into what was called **speech communication**. This term was used to describe the discipline concerned with the act of speaking and making speeches. Use of the term communication or communication sciences has since become the preferred term because this encompasses the many forms of communication that are not exclusive to making public speeches.

A number of advancements have occurred in human communication over the centuries. They are too numerous to discuss here, but a listing of some of the more significant advancements are provided in a time line format in Table 1–3. As new forms of communication have emerged, the old forms have become more specifically designed but not completely abandoned. For example, the radio did not vanish once the television was invented. Rather, these older forms of communication have become specialized. In regard to modern human communication, major advancements have occurred in media communications, or the methods used for communication. The history of these various methods of communication can be broadly categorized into two areas: (1) written communication and (2) telegraphy.

Written Communication

The earliest evidence of written communication dates back to our ancestors who lived in caves. As long ago as 25,000 BC, early humans painted pictures on cave walls that depicted events that happened in daily life such as hunting or planting. The earliest of these pictures were found in caves of southern France and Spain (Figure 1–4). It took primitive man thousands of years to create a written form of communication.

Table 1–3. Some Highlights in the Evolution of Communication

Date	Event
BC	
10,000:	An engraved antler exists, with animals and plants portrayed (discovered in France).
2600:	The Egyptian Book of the Dead exists.
2200:	Writing on papyrus paper exists—the oldest written document ever found.
1400:	Chinese write on bones.
400:	Chinese write on wood, bamboo, and silk.
AD	
600:	Books are printed in China.
1200:	European monasteries create a letter system for communication.
1450:	Johann Gutenberg creates a printing press.
1565:	The pencil is invented in England.
1609:	The first regularly published newspaper is produced in Germany.
1639:	The first printing press is created in the American colonies.
1755:	A regular mail ship sails between England and the American colonies.
1785:	Stagecoaches carry mail between towns in the United States.
1804:	The lithograph is invented in Germany.
1815:	There are 3,000 post offices in the United States.
1831:	The electric telegraph is invented in the United States.
1835:	Morse code is created for electronic communication.
1868:	The first modern-style typewriter was invented.
1876:	Alexander Graham Bell invents the telephone.
1893:	The electric typewriter is invented, called the Blickensderfer.
1901:	Guglielmo Marconi transmits a radio signal across the Atlantic Ocean.
1904:	A photograph is transmitted by wire in Germany.
1905:	The postage meter is introduced in New Zealand.
1919:	People are able to directly dial telephone numbers.
1933:	Phonograph records are created with stereo sound.
1938:	Allen DuMont markets a television for the home.
1948:	Long-playing (LP) records are created on vinyl disks.
1951:	Computers are sold commercially.
1952:	Bell Laboratories builds a primitive speech recognition system.
1959:	Xerox manufactures a copying machine.
1961:	FM stereo broadcasting begins.
1965:	First communications satellite begins orbiting the earth.
1966:	FAX machines are distributed commercially.
1976:	The Apple microcomputer is created.
1979:	Japan creates the first cellular phone network.
1980:	CNN, the 24-hour news channel, is created.
1984:	The first portable compact disk player is created.
1989:	Timothy Berners-Lee creates the framework for the World Wide Web.
1991:	Video cassette recorders are found in 75% of U.S. homes.
1996:	Over 9 million people use the Internet.
2000:	AT&T develops the "How May I Help You" speech recognition system.
2010:	Facebook reaches 400 million active users.

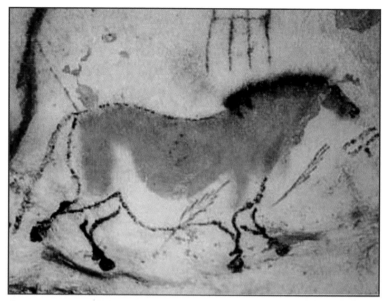

A

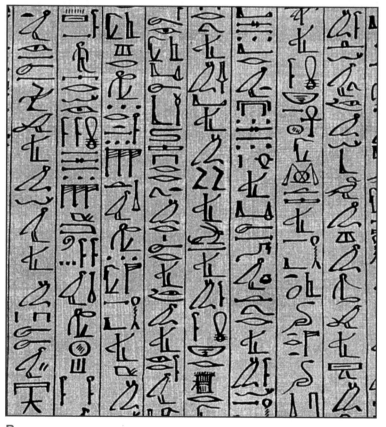

B

FIGURE 1–4. Two forms of early written communication. **A.** A cave painting discovered in Lascaux, France, ca. 15,000–10,000 BC. **B.** An example of abbreviated hieroglyphic writing known as hieratic. ca. 2000 BC.

Those civilizations that had written communication were the ones that developed most rapidly. Around 2000 BC, the Egyptians developed a writing system that used **hieroglyphics**, which means, "the words of God," and is a form of writing in which the various symbols stood for certain sounds and words. It was used primarily by scribes, doctors, and priests to decorate the walls of temples and tombs. An abbreviated form of hieroglyphics, called **hieratic**, was used for more informal communication. This was a type of handwriting in which the symbols were abbreviated to the point of abstraction (see Figure 1–4).

Somewhere between 1700 and 1500 BC, the **alphabet** was established as a form of written communication. The word is derived from the Latin, *alfabetum*, which combines the first two symbols of the Greek alphabet, "alpha" and "beta." The use of alphabetic symbols was easier and faster to draw than pictures and was more universally recognized for their meaning. The use of an alphabet allowed for the creation of words and sentences. The Greek and Hebrew alphabets were established around 100 BC. The Greek alphabet became the source for the Latin alphabet created in 7 BC, which in turn became the source of the present-day English alphabet. The Hebrew alphabet that is used today dates back to 600 BC. The Greek and Latin alphabets were designed to be written from left to right. These early alphabetic systems only used uppercase letters with lowercase letters introduced during the first century (Figure 1–5).

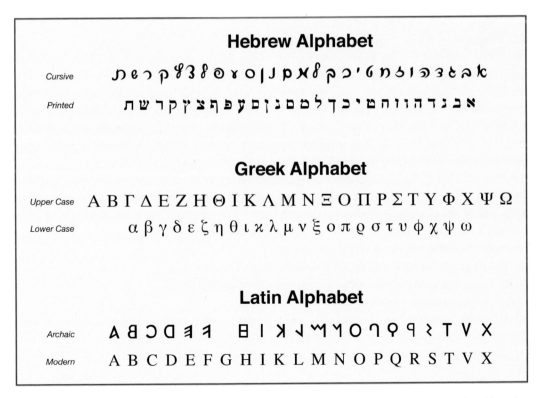

FIGURE 1–5. The Hebrew, Greek, and Latin alphabets and the two forms of writing for each alphabet.

The invention of paper and writing instruments also played an important role in the development of written communication. A form of writing paper known as **papyrus** was developed by the Egyptians around 3000 BC. The raw material of papyrus paper came from the plant *cyperus papyrus* that grew along the banks of the Nile, which was used to create rope, baskets, and boats. The method of paper production was kept secret by the Egyptians. The first widely used writing instrument that was predominant was the quill pen that was introduced around 700 AD. The quill is a pen made from a bird feather, and some of the strongest quills were those that were taken from living birds. Usually quill pens only lasted about a week before it was necessary to replace them.

Throughout the subsequent centuries, the written word became more accessible to large groups of people, but the process of writing was very laborious. The earliest books were primarily religious in nature, containing prayers and songs. To reproduce any written material, an individual needed to completely rewrite the document. A great deal of this work was completed by monks who spent long hours in monasteries making copies by hand of religious books and manuscripts. This approach to document reproduction came to an abrupt halt in 1450 with the invention of the movable-type printing press. **Johann Gutenberg's** (1398–1468) printing press was revolutionary, allowing for easier and faster reproduction of written material (Figure 1–6). The invention contributed to the creation of mass media communication and the free spread of ideas in an unprecedented fashion. The use of newspapers as a form of written communication became widespread with the introduc-

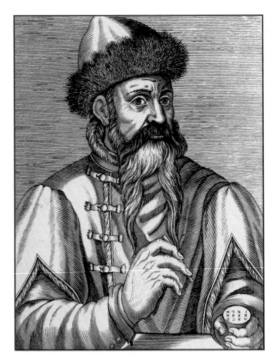

FIGURE 1–6. Johann Gutenberg, inventor of the movable-type printing press.

tion of the printing press. The essential features of the Gutenberg printing press remained unchanged until the 19th century, when in the early 1800s a steam-powered printing press using continuous rolls of paper and iron (instead of wooden) machinery was created. This technologic advancement in printing made it possible for daily newspapers to be distributed at a fraction of the previous cost.

Telegraphy

Telegraphy refers to the long-distance transmission of written messages without the need to physically transport the message. Forms of telegraphy that have had a historical impact on human communication include the: (1) telegraph, (2) telephone, (3) television, and

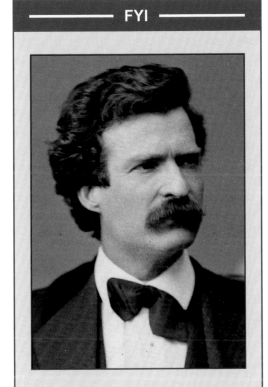

The famous American novelist **Mark Twain** (1835–1910) enjoyed and made use of new inventions during his lifetime. He was the first author to discard his pen and submit a typewritten manuscript to his publisher.

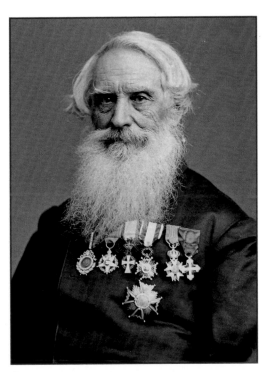

A

Morse Code Alphabet		
A .-	**N** -.	**0** -----
B -...	**O** ---	**1** .----
C -.-.	**P** .--.	**2** ..---
D -..	**Q** --.-	**3** ...--
E .	**R** .-.	**4** ....-
F ..-.	**S** ...	**5** .....
G --.	**T** -	**6** -....
H	**U** ..-	**7** --...
I ..	**W** .--	**9** ----.
K -.-	**X** -..-	**Fullstop** .-.-.-
L .-..	**Y** -.--	**Comma** --..--
M --	**Z** --..	**Query** ..--..

B

(4) Internet. **Joseph Henry** (1797–1878) was an important American scientist of the 18th century. One of his discoveries occurred in 1830 when he demonstrated that an electrical signal could be transmitted over a wire that spanned the distance of one mile.

    This discovery led to the creation of the electric **telegraph**. Five years later, in 1835, **Samuel Morse** (1791–1872) formulated the **Morse code**, which is an alphabetic system that uses a combination of short and long clicks to create words (Figure 1–7). The combination

FIGURE 1–7. A. Samuel Morse. **B.** His coded alphabet used for the telegraph.

of the electric telegraph, along with a simple to use alphabet system transformed the way we communicate. With the invention of the telegraph, it became possible to transmit a message without the need for physical movement. This electric message traveled faster than people, horses, or trains. To this day, Morse code remains a viable means of providing reliable communication during difficult communication conditions.

The telegraph had been established for over 30 years before the development of another wire-based electrical communication system, the **telephone**. The telegraph was limited to sending a series of single electrical sounds along a wire. **Alexander Graham Bell** (1847–1922) determined a way to convert voice into a combination of electrical sounds and send these sounds along a wire (Figure 1–8). In 1876, Bell's famous first words to his assistant on the telephone, "Mr. Watson come here I want to see you," ushered in a new form of communication, and signaled a demise in popularity of the telegraph. Since then, the telephone has become an integral part of our society, even leading to the establishment of an industry known as **telecommunications**. The invention of the telegraph and the telephone led to the eventual development of the **radio**. In 1901, an Italian inventor **Gugliemo Marconi** (1874–1937) sent and received the first radio signal, thus marking a new age of wireless communication (Figure 1–9). This wireless technology has now been applied to devices such as telephones, global positioning systems (or GPS), garage door openers, and of course the Internet.

The **television** has become a device that the majority of people cannot live

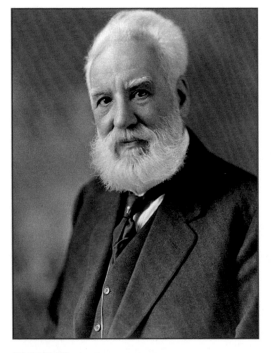

FIGURE 1–8. Alexander Graham Bell, inventor of the telephone.

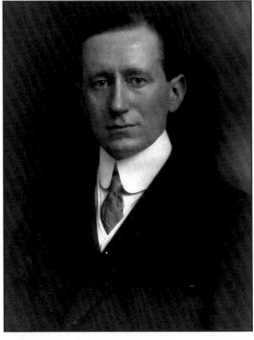

FIGURE 1–9. Gugliemo Marconi, inventor of the radio.

without. Television is the transmission and reception of moving images by use of electrical signals. Around 1908, an English inventor by the name of **Alan Archibald Campbell-Swinton** (1863–1930) conceived the idea for an electrical method of scanning, or collecting an image, although it was not until the 1930s that the actual method using electron (or cathode) rays was developed by an American electrical engineer, **Allen B. DuMont** (1901–1965; Figure 1–10). DuMont has been called the "Father of Television," and his invention of the picture tube still serves as the basic

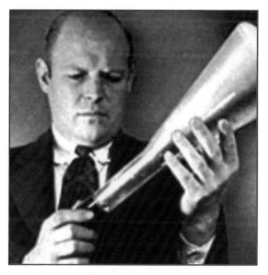

FIGURE 1–10. Allen B. DuMont, known as the "Father of Television."

foundation for the type of televisions used today. Television is a mode of communication where television viewers serve as decoders of information; its use has become the primary mode of communication to the mass media. For example, presidential elections today would be entirely different without the use of television.

Finally, the manner in which we communicate in this modern world has undoubtedly been transformed by computers. Two features of computer-based communication that have had wide-sweeping influence are the **Internet** and **speech recognition**. The Internet is a worldwide network of thousands of computers and computer networks. The Internet began in the early 1970s as a computer network that linked computers at several universities and research laboratories in the United States. As more and more universities began linking to the network, a software system was developed that allowed for anyone to roam, browse, or contribute to the Internet. This software was developed in 1989 by English computer scientist **Timothy Berners-Lee** (b. 1955; Figure 1–11) for the European Organization for Nuclear Research and became known as the **World Wide Web**. He is known as the "Father of the Internet." The Internet has dramatically changed our world, allowing people to share

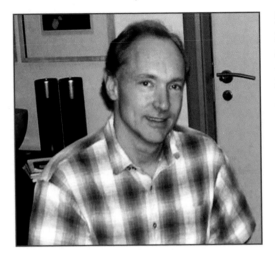

FIGURE 1–11. Timothy Berners-Lee, known as the "Father of the Internet." From U. Bojars at Wikimedia Commons. Permission granted through Creative Commons Attribution 2.5 License.

information in spite of geographic barriers. By the early 1990s, there were around 600 websites and 2 million computers connected to the network. The use of e-mails had replaced paper letters as the most common form of telegraphy. New forms of Internet communication have developed rapidly with unique names to these various forms of communication such as **blogging**, **instant messaging**, and **microblogging** (e.g., **Twitter**). A description of forms of Internet communication is provided in Table 1–4.

Speech recognition (also known as automatic speech recognition or computer speech recognition) is a process whereby the computer learns to understand discrete words and phrases. The

Table 1–4. Some of the Currently Used Forms of Internet Communication	
Electronic Mail (E-mail)	The process of typing a message and sending this message electronically across a computer network.
Internet Relay Chat (IRC)	A communications system that permits people from across the world to conduct online, text-based communication with one or more other users. IRC users normally see the text conversations of all users on the network.
Instant Messaging (IM)	A form of electronic communication that involves immediate correspondence between users who are all online simultaneously. IM tends to differ from IRC because the communication is typically only between two users.
Blogging	A blog is an online journal (a shortened form of Web log). Blogging is writing in one's blog for users on the Internet to openly view.
Skype	A software program that allows users to make telephone calls over the Internet.
Social Networks	A website, such as Facebook, that offers its viewer members the ability to share messages, media, and other information with each other.
Twitter	A social networking service that allows users to send one another a short message (or *tweets*, text-based posts, up to 140 characters long) to a person's personal website. Twitter is a form of microblogging.

earliest computer-based speech recognition systems were developed in the 1950s at Bell Telephone Laboratories in the United States. The challenge in developing such a system is that the computer must be able to decipher the wide degree of variability in the manner of speaking demonstrated from one person to the next. These differences encompass features such as age, sex, accent, and rate of speaking. Early systems were only able to recognize individual vowel or consonant sounds. This technology is rapidly evolving and is now entering the service industry. A current example is the automatic flight information system used by United Airlines. The system is referred to as "How May I Help You?" and is used for call routing of consumer help line calls. Although automatic speech recognition and speech understanding systems are far from perfect in terms of the word or task accuracy, they are becoming yet another form of communication used in society today.

FYI

Millions of people send text messages daily. So it is not surprising to find this has led to the development of a unique shorthand form of written communication that makes sending messages quicker and easier. Examples of this shorthand include:

Phrase	Shorthand
Laughing out loud	LOL
How are you?	HRU
See you later	CUL
Talk to you later	TTYL
Best of luck	BOL
You are a star	URA*
Please call me	PCM
I love you	143

FYI

The classic 1968 movie *2001: A Space Odyssey* was possibly the first movie to introduce speech recognition technology into mainstream culture. One of the stars of the movie was an intelligent computer named *HAL* who spoke in a naturally sounding voice and was able to recognize and comprehend speech.

MODELS OF COMMUNICATION

The term **model** has a wide range of uses. It can refer to a type of product, a person who poses for photographers, or a miniature version of an object. From an academic standpoint, a model refers to an abstract idea. The **transmission model** of communication is an idea regarding the way in which humans communicate. This classic model was proposed by Claude Shannon and Warren Weaver (1949) who were electrical engineers working for Bell Telephone Laboratories in the United States. The essence of the model is that the successful transmission of a message requires both a sender and a receiver. A simplified version of the transmission model is shown in Figure 1–12. The model depicts the process of communication as one in which a person affects the behavior

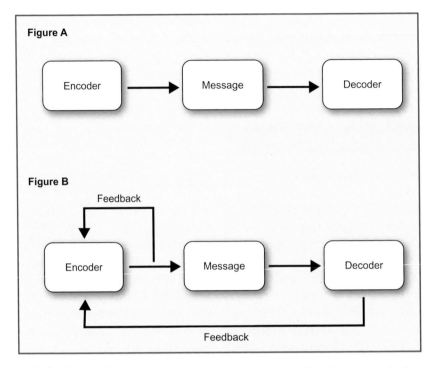

FIGURE 1–12. Models of communication. **A.** Classic transmission model of communication. **B.** Revised transmission model that includes feedback loops.

or state of mind of another person. If the effect was smaller or different from what was originally intended, than a failure in communication takes place. A criticism of the model is that communication is viewed as a discrete event in which there is a simple beginning and end to the delivery and reception of a message. However, we know that communication is a much more complicated and sophisticated process that does not simply start and stop. Rather, communication is an ongoing and dynamically changing activity. Another criticism of the transmission model is that the model does not deal with the *meaning* associated with sending messages from the speaker to the listener, simply the transmission of a message from one point to the other. Too often the message sent is not the message received,

and the speaker's meaning does not come across to the listener.

A modification of the transmission model was proposed by Wilbur Schramm in 1954 through the inclusion of **feedback loops**. Feedback refers to the activity whereby information is sent back to the source from where the message came. As a reaction to this information, the speaker adjusts his or her message by strengthening, de-emphasizing, or changing the content or form of the original message. The feedback can come from either the speaker or the listener. As speakers, we are constantly monitoring and evaluating our personal communication behavior. During the encoding of a message, we may revise our message mentally before actually speaking, or we may even choose to revise our message midstream to ensure the message is clearly presented. Feedback from the listener can take many shapes and forms. The listener may send nonverbal body language cues (e.g., eye contact, head nod) indicating that the message was understood, or the listener might simply state back to the original speaker that the message was not understood. The use of feedback is critical to the successful communication of messages. An example of the modified transmission model that includes feedback is shown in Figure 1–12.

The transmission model of communication is based on a single speaker and listener. This concept of communication is like a ball being tossed back and forth between two individuals. In reality, communication may involve more than two people. By simply introducing a third person into the communication setting, it becomes apparent that communication involves many balls being tossed in both directions at the same time. The term **coregulation** is used to describe the exchange of information that occurs between individuals in a conversational setting. The manner in which each member of a conversational setting adjusts their speaking and listening behavior serves to affect the transfer of messages. These adjustments can help to improve overall communication among the group or lead to possible breakdowns in communication. An example of transfer of information that can occur among a group of three people is displayed in Figure 1–13. In this particular setting, there are at least five different communication interactions that can take place among the group (Brown & Van Riper, 1966). The arrows represent who can talk to whom and who can listen. If we were to assume that the three people were working together to solve a particular problem, such as determining the best driving route from Sydney to Melbourne, the following conclusions might be drawn:

- Condition 1 solves the problem with the greatest accuracy.
- Condition 5 solves the problem least accurately.
- Condition 5 gets the message through in the shortest time.
- Listeners are more confident in the two-way means of communication.
- Speakers are surer of themselves in the one-way means of communication.
- The group morale in Condition 1 is likely to be the highest.
- Creativity is likely to be greatest in Condition 1.
- Condition 1 is the noisiest and least orderly.

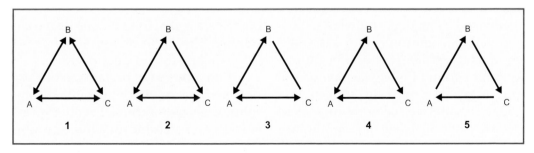

FIGURE 1–13. Communication nets composed of three people. The point of each arrow indicates the direction of communication.

FORMS OF COMMUNICATION

The term **form** is defined as the shape and structure of anything, giving it individuality or distinctive character. This term can be applied to communication through two primary forms of communication: (1) verbal communication and (2) nonverbal communication. **Verbal communication** is at the core of what most of us do; it is the expression of language using spoken words. Our verbal communication varies depending on the particular communication act, as well as the formality of communication. Acts of verbal communication include: (1) discussion, (2) dialogue, and (3) debate. **Discussion** is an act of verbal communication to make decisions. Discussions are likely to involve the exchange of facts and opinions between communicating partners. **Dialogue** refers to the free-flowing conversational exchange of ideas. These ideas involve the sharing of perspectives and understandings. The act of **debate** differs from discussion and dialogue because this form of verbal communication is used to achieve agreement on a topic, which other participants of the communication may not share. We often think of debate as the verbal communication found in the political arena. One person states a point of view, which is subsequently challenged by an opposing view.

Verbal communication also varies in its formality. The level of formality can be found in the vocabulary and grammar characterizing spoken language. Formal verbal communication follows a specific code of communicating that might be found in settings such as classrooms, courtrooms, job interviews, or formal parties. Alternatively, informal communication also has a specific code of communication but allows for a much varied manner of speaking. Situations such as hanging out with friends and informal parties are likely to reflect a markedly different form of verbal speaking, compared with more formal settings.

Nonverbal communication refers to the features of communication that occur aside from what is actually spoken or heard. There are at least six different types of nonverbal communication that we use and experience on a daily basis. These include: (1) paralanguage, (2) sign language, (3) body language, (4) tactile communication, (5) proxemics, and (6) appearance. **Paralanguage** refers to factors such as tone of voice, loudness, inflection, and pitch. By altering these various parameters of voice, the message conveyed is likewise altered. A simple example would be to communicate an identically worded message, such as, "Watch your step" in a soft comforting voice, versus a loud, alarming voice. A listener of this same message would likely interpret these messages quite differently.

Sign language is a form of expressive communication where words are replaced by gestures. Commonly used gestures include waving, pointing, and using fingers to indicate number amounts. There are also fully developed language systems that rely exclusively on signs, as often found in the deaf community. This form of sign language is discussed further in Chapter 13.

Body language pertains to our use of facial expressions or postures to communicate information. Facial expressions are responsible for a huge proportion of nonverbal communication. One need simply smile or frown to communicate a clear nonverbal message. One way of concealing our communication via body language would be to put on a poker face, which is a face that shows no emotion or change in expression. Expert card players are masters in the use of body language to prevent other card players from knowing the strength of their card hand.

Tactile communication refers to communication that occurs via touch. The use of touch can play a comforting role when paired with verbal communication such as consoling a grieving spouse. Use of touch between parent and child during the infancy period has also been shown to play an integral part in establishing social interaction. **Proxemics** concerns how space and time are used to communicate. A common example is our need for interpersonal space when communicating with others. The amount of personal space needed when having a casual conversation with another person usually varies between 18 inches to four feet. On the other hand, the personal distance needed when speaking to a crowd of people is around 10 to 12 feet. Finally, our **physical appearance** plays an important role in communication. Physical appearance such as clothes and hairstyle serves to convey a message regarding a person's attitude, mood, wealth, and cultural background, which subsequently affects the judgment and interpretations of others.

LEVELS OF COMMUNICATION

We communicate to people at a variety of personal levels, ranging from very superficial to deeply intimate. Powell (1969) identified five levels of communication that humans use to talk

(or not to talk) to each other based on their familiarity with the other individual (Figure 1–14). His research was prompted by the view that most people are initially hesitant about communicating openly with another person for fear of the other individual judging them negatively. The first or lowest level is the **cliché level**. This level of communication involves speaking to others with no real forethought or genuine intent. We use typical or routine questions (e.g., "How's it going?") and give automatic answers (e.g., "Fine") that may not be truthful. In reality, we would not expect an unfamiliar person to provide an elaborate and thoughtful response. The next level is the **fact level**, and involves communication concerning information or statistics about the weather, workplace, the news, and personal activities, such as, "How do you think Manchester United will perform this year?" This level of communication requires no in-depth thinking or feeling and does not reveal anything personal about ourselves.

The third level of communication is the **opinion level**. This is a level of communication that occurs between two people on a more personal level and includes comments, concerns, expectations, and personal goals. A question such as, "Do you think the war will ever end?" would likely result in communication occurring at the opinion level of familiarity. The fourth level of communication is the **feelings level** and usually occurs between two people who know each other well and do not worry about communicating openly. Both individuals feel safe to share openly personal emotions. The highest level of communication is the **needs level**. This level of communication occurs between two people who know one another

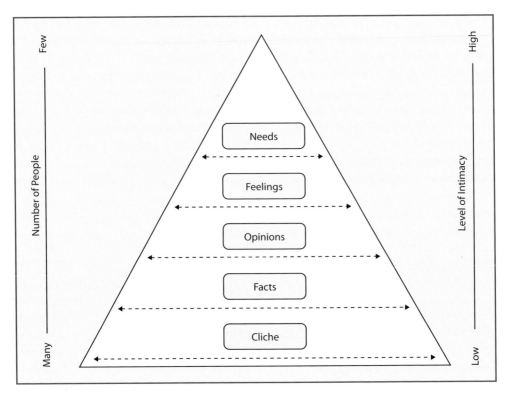

FIGURE 1–14. Five levels of communication according to the number of people and level of intimacy.

intimately. We feel completely safe to reveal our unique needs with another person. We also may seem to know intuitively what the other person thinks.

CURRENT RESEARCH IN COMMUNICATION SCIENCE

The field of communication sciences has grown enormously in recent decades and continues to evolve. The current areas of research in communication sciences can be summarized into three major themes: (1) technology, (2) culture, and (3) social media.

Communication Technology

The **technology** encompassing communication is undeniably a rapidly evolving area of research. Advancements in computing technology are closely linked to the manner in which we communicate. There are several research journals dedicated to the topic of communication technology. Announcements concerning new innovative developments in communication and information technology are being made regularly. Less than 20 years ago, the telephone and television were two very distinct forms of technology used for communication. These two forms are rapidly merging and are evident in the mass marketing of handheld computers and smart phones. We are likely to be further exposed to a wide array of telecommunication devices that are an amalgamation of *listening* and *viewing* aspects of communication. In particular, the development of **apps** (an abbreviation for application) is changing the way we communicate with one another. An app is a piece of software that can run on electronic devices such as mobile phones. Apps work much like user-installed software on a computer and allow the phone to perform specific tasks that the user needs. In January 2011, the American Dialect Society named app as the word of the year for 2010.

Communication Culture

Communication and **culture** are intricately related. Communicative interaction is the means by which cultures are created and learned. As the notion of global communication and global interdependence becomes a reality, advances in communication are likely to impact one's culture. For example, access to the Internet now allows for information transfer to some of the most remote and isolated parts of the world, although we know little about how this information influences various cultures. Currently, some countries strictly filter and ban various aspects of Internet communication, whereas other countries are much less restrictive. The way in which communication technology converges with culture raises important questions about the effects of communication on the maintenance of cultural diversity.

Social Media

Another area of research that is being explored in communication science is related to growth and impact of **social media** networks. Social media is now used extensively for advertising, political lobbying, as well as for match making. Some forms of communication practice that take place in this unique social environment may cross moral and ethical boundaries, such as cyber bullying. Cyber bullying includes threatening text messages or e-mails, or spreading rumors and embarrassing photographs on social media networks. Current research indicates that an alarming number (approximately 20%) of high school children are affected by

---

FYI

Communications satellites have a quiet, yet profound, effect on our daily lives. If you used your cell phone today, listened to the radio, or watched television, you accessed a communications satellite either directly or indirectly. These objects serve to link remote areas of the earth. A signal (such as a television program) is sent from earth to the satellite, which then amplifies the signal and sends it to another point on earth. In this way, millions of people can watch an event, such as the Olympics, with only the smallest time difference in delay. There are over 1,000 satellites in space, and the United States owns more than one-half of these, followed by China and Russia.

cyber bullying. The use of social media networks may not necessarily provide the most intimate and secure mode of communicating; however, they provide researchers with insight as to how people use social media networks in their everyday lives.

COMMUNICATION SCIENCES ON THE WORLD WIDE WEB

Listed below are websites that provide further information on the topic of communication sciences. At the time of publication, each website was freely accessible.

Animal Communication Videos
http://www.pbs.org/saf/1201/video/watchonline.htm

http://video.nhpt.org/video/1491134392/

Evolution of Communication Video
http://www.archive.org/details/ChiuShienZangRolandEvolved Communication

Exploring Nonverbal Communication Video
http://nonverbal.ucsc.edu/

History of Communication Video
http://www.historyworld.net/wrld his/PlainTextHistories.asp?history id=aa93

Human Communication Video
http://highered.mcgraw-hill.com/sites/0072560053/student_view0/new video_series.html#

STUDY QUESTIONS

1. What are some of the career options available to graduates with a degree in communication?
2. Describe the process of communication.
3. List and describe the various modes of animal communication.
4. What are some of the landmark inventions in the areas of written communication and telegraphy?
5. List and describe the verbal and nonverbal forms of communication.

REFERENCES

Brown, C., & Van Riper, C. (1966). *Speech and man.* Inglewood Cliffs, NJ: Prentice-Hall.

Powell, J. (1969). *Why am I afraid to tell you who I am?* Niles, IL: Argus Communications.

Shannon, C., & Weaver, W. (1949). *Mathematical theory of communication.* Urbana: University of Illinois Press.

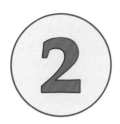

COMMUNICATION DISORDERS AND THE PROFESSIONS

OBJECTIVES

After reading this chapter, the student should be able to:

- Demonstrate an understanding of the audiology and speech-language pathology professions.

- Describe the various work settings for audiologists and speech-language pathologists.

- Demonstrate an understanding of developmental and acquired communication disorders.

- Demonstrate an understanding of organic and functional communication disorders.

- Demonstrate an understanding of epidemiology, including prevalence and incidence.

- Demonstrate an understanding of evidence-based practice.

- Demonstrate an understanding of the Code of Ethics.

- Describe sociocultural influences on normal and disordered communication.

INTRODUCTION

Communication is the process of speaking and listening. Most of us take communication for granted. We tacitly assume that when we speak, we will be understood, or when someone speaks to us, we will understand them. Only when a breakdown in communication occurs do we realize how special and vital this act is to our daily lives. A communication disorder is one of the most common types of disabilities found throughout the world. Recall from Chapter 1 that the transmission model provides a useful way to conceptualize the act of communication, involving a speaker and a listener. A more detailed version of this model was proposed by Denes and Pinson (1973) with particular reference to the linguistic and physiological contributions to speaking and listening. They referred to this model as the speech chain (Figure 2–1).

According to the speech chain model, the process of encoding a message is organized across three levels: (1) linguistic (2) physiological, and (3) acoustic. The linguistic level is the first step in the speech chain, whereby the message is organized in the brain. It is the point in the chain where we think about speaking. Once we determine the message to be spoken, various motor nerves required to produce the sounds and words of the message send impulses from the brain to the speech musculature. Structures such as the lips, tongue, and jaw are set into motion. This physiological process represents the next link in the speech chain. Once these words leave our mouth, they become an airborne acoustic signal, thus representing the third and final link in the process

(chain) of speech encoding. There is also a side, or *feedback*, link in the process of speech encoding. We naturally listen to our own voices when talking. By doing so, the message spoken is compared with what was originally intended to be spoken. An example of this type of feedback is evident when we produce a **spoonerism** (or slip-of-the-tongue). The phrase, "mix up your words" spoken as, "wix up your mords," is one such example. If we judge the message to be incorrectly spoken, the message can be modified. The remaining links of the speech chain are related to the process of decoding.

The steps involved in decoding the message occur in the reverse order of those just described for speech encoding. When listening to a message, our ears are exposed to the acoustic signal after it leaves the mouth of the speaker. At a physiological level, the muscles, bones, and nerves of the ear transform this acoustic signal into electrical impulses along auditory (sensory) pathways leading to the brain. Once the sensory impulses reach the brain, they are deciphered into individual sounds, words, and sentences. This deciphering of the acoustic signal into a linguistic message represents the final link in the speech chain.

The speech chain model is useful to illustrate communication disorders. Any breakdown or disruption in the process of encoding that occurs along the pathway from the brain to the actual execution of speech can result in a communication disorder. Similarly, any breakdown in the decoding process between the ear and the brain can result in a communication disorder.

The focus of this chapter is to introduce the nature and type of communication disorders found in children and

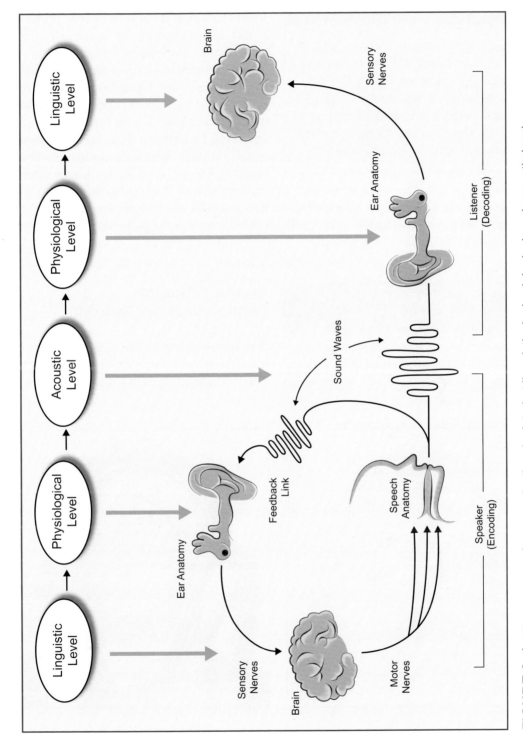

FIGURE 2–1. The process of communication depicted at linguistical, physiological, and acoustic levels.

adults. As well, the professions dedicated to helping individuals with communication disorders are profiled.

TERMINOLOGY AND DEFINITIONS

A **communication disorder** is a diagnosed condition in which a person is unable to say correctly what she or he wants to say, and/or is unable to understand some or most of what is being said. Some individuals may have an isolated impairment in speech or hearing; others may have impairment in both domains. Simply stated, a communication disorder is any impairment in speaking or hearing that deviates from what might be considered normal. The nature of the disorder may range from mild to severe. However, the impact of the disorder upon a person's ability to communicate may be profound, regardless of the severity.

Classification of Communication Disorders

Communication disorders can be grouped into two general categories (Figure 2–2). The first grouping is in regard to the tim-

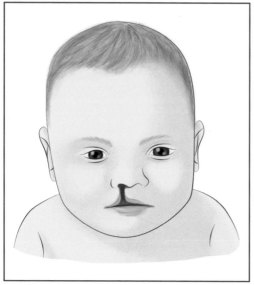

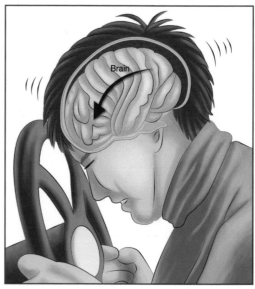

A   B

FIGURE 2–2. Examples of developmental and acquired communication disorders. **A.** Shows a child born with a cleft lip and palate. **B.** Depicts an individual with a head injury resulting from a motor vehicle accident.

ing of when the disorder first occurred. Specifically, did the disorder occur before or after birth? Any medical or health condition, including a communication disorder that occurs prior to birth, during birth, or shortly after birth, is referred to as a **developmental** or **congenital disorder**. An example of a developmental communication disorder is a child who is born with a cleft of the lip or palate (see Figure 2–2). This cleft, if left unrepaired, can greatly impair speech production. The second grouping of communication disorders pertains to whether the medical or health condition is found to occur later in life (i.e., after birth); if so, the disorder is referred to as an **acquired disorder**. Most often, an individual with an acquired communication disorder was demonstrating normal communication prior to experiencing the disorder. An example of an acquired communication disorder is an individual who suffers a traumatic brain injury following a motor vehicle accident (see Figure 2–2). As a result of this accident, the individual may experience a marked impairment in the ability to produce or understand speech. Prior to the accident, the person's communication most likely was normal.

Communication disorders can also be classified in regard to the cause (i.e., **etiology**) of the disorder. A medical or health condition with a known physical cause is called an **organic disorder**. In most cases, the physical condition is visible to the naked eye. Such is the case in a typical seven-year-old child who has lost her two front (central incisor) teeth. This condition is likely to pose a problem for the correct articulation of speech sounds that involve these physical structures (e.g., /s/ and /th/ sounds; Figure 2–3). An organic disorder can also be invisible to the naked

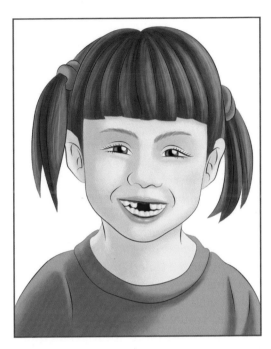

FIGURE 2–3. Example of an organic communication disorder found in most normally developing children. The absence of upper central incisors is likely to affect speech sound production but only temporarily.

eye such as impairments resulting from brain abnormalities such as a stroke. If there is no known anatomical, physiological, or neurological basis for the observed disorder, the term **functional disorder** is used. A closely related term is **idiopathic**, which denotes a condition that has an unknown cause. School-age children who mispronounce speech sounds, such as "wabbit" for "rabbit," who show no apparent physical problems would be classified as showing a functional communication disorder. A number of communication disorders have no readily identifiable cause. Although we may not know the precise cause of these functional disorders, they still can be successfully treated. An illustration of the overlap of developmental and acquired disorders that have a functional or organic basis is shown in Figure 2–4. These terms can be used collectively to refer to communication disorders. The ensuing chapters categorize each type of communication disorder according to both the timing and cause of the disorder.

A final comment about classifying communication disorders relates to the label we may place on a person who is demonstrating a disorder. In the past, it was common to place the disorder (or label) first and the person second. We might have referred to an individual as being a "cleft palate child." In other instances, an individual was simply labeled by the disorder, where we referred to the person as a "stutterer." These days, the more appropriate manner of referring to a communication disorder is to place the individual first and the disorder second. So as professionals in the field of communication disorders, we may encounter a child *with* a cleft palate or a person *who* stutters. Clearly, this form of labeling is not unique to communication disorders. In practice, placing the individual first should be applied when referring to any medical or health-related condition.

Occurrence of Communication Disorders

Epidemiology refers to the study of how often diseases and conditions occur in people and why. A common way of charting the occurrence of a disorder or disease is in reference to the overall population. **Prevalence** is a frequently used epidemiological measure of how commonly a disease or condition occurs in a population at a particular point in time. The prevalence is calculated by dividing the number of persons with the disease or condition at a particular time by the number of individuals examined. Prevalence often is expressed as a percentage. The **incidence** of a disease is another epidemiological measure. Incidence measures the rate of occurrence of new cases of a disease or condition, and is likewise expressed as a percentage. Incidence is calculated as the number of new cases of a disease or condition in a specified time period (usually one year) divided by the size of the population. So prevalence is a measure of all the cases of a disease at a point of time, and incidence is the measure of new cases of disease in a time period. In the

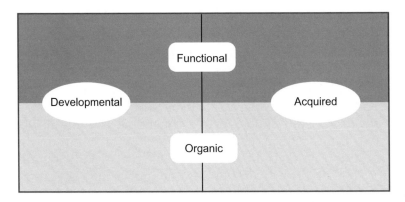

FIGURE 2–4. Categorization of communication disorders according to when the disorder occurred (developmental versus acquired), and how the disorder occurred (functional versus organic).

context of communication disorders, prevalence would refer to the estimated population of people who are managing communication disorders at any given time, whereas incidence would refer to the annual diagnosis rate of new cases of communication disorders.

The majority of epidemiology information on communication disorders relates to prevalence. Approximately one out of every seven individuals, or 12% of the population, has some form of a communication disorder. This percentage encompasses disorders of either speech or hearing, ranging in severity from mild to profound. The prevalence of communication disorders in the United States is around 46 million people. Approximately 2.7 million Australians have a communication disorder. There are also prevalence data regarding certain types of communication disorders, as well as age groups. Specific prevalence information for various communication disorders is presented in the following chapters. Some types of communication disorders occur more often than others. For example, there are estimates that 2.5 million people in the United Kingdom have speech and language disorders. Of this number, 800,000 have a disorder so severe that it is difficult for most people to understand them. The worldwide prevalence of communication disorders in children is approximately 25% of the population but lowers with increasing age. This lowering in prevalence presumably reflects a large number of children outgrowing or receiving treatment to alleviate the disorder.

Boys and Girls

A well-known fact is that boys tend to be more susceptible than girls for a large number of childhood diseases. This vulnerability is evident early in life with male infants showing significantly higher rates of premature birth and congenital abnormalities than female infants. In the first year of life, boys get sick and die more often than girls. **Infant mortality** refers to deaths that occur prior to one year of age. Infant mortality is often used as an index of the general well-being of a population. Around the world, the number of deaths for boys is greater than for girls. In 2012, the infant mortality rate (deaths per 1,000 live births) in the United States was 6.6 for boys and 5.3 for girls. A similar pattern was found in Australia with a mortality rate of 4.8 for boys and 3.4 for girls. Developmental disorders such as autism are three to four times more common in infant boys than girls, and behavioral disorders are at least twice as common. The same is true for communication disorders. Take, for example, the condition of stuttering—boys are three times more likely to develop a stuttering disorder than girls. The precise reason as to why males are more prone to various health disorders remains unknown. Some genetics experts believe there probably is a biological difference that gives females a health advantage over males. One suggestion is that males are disadvantaged by not having the second "X" (sex) chromosome found in women. Having two "X" chromosomes may help to protect women against disease. This vulnerability is apparent in male mammals of all species, indicating a likely evolutionary explanation. It could well be that nature provides a health advantage to females because the survival of the species depends on them. Males simply may be more expendable than females!

THE PROFESSIONS

Speech-language pathology and audiology are health professions that collectively contribute to the field of human communication sciences and disorders. The profession of **speech-language pathology**, also referred to as speech-language therapy, encompasses the study of human communication, swallowing, speech and language development, and their disorders. The profession of **audiology** encompasses the study of human communication, normal processes of hearing, and hearing loss. A **speech-language pathologist** is a professional educated in the study of human communication, swallowing, speech-language development, and its disorders. By evaluating the speech, language, and swallowing skills of children and adults, the speech-language pathologist determines what communication or swallowing problems exist and the best way to treat them. An **audiologist** is a professional educated in the study of human communication, normal hearing processes, and hearing loss. The audiologist determines if a person has a hearing loss, the type of loss, and the best way to treat the loss.

Speech-language pathology and audiology are distinct disciplines, but they have considerable overlap. To be fully skilled in either discipline, one should be familiar with both. Each discipline deals with impairments that disrupt the ability of the individual to communicate normally.

The audiology and speech-language pathology professions are found worldwide but are not uniform across nations. A listing of some of the professional associations for audiologists and speech-language pathologists found around the world is shown in Table 2–1. There are approximately 140,000 speech-language pathologists and 13,000 audiologists currently working in the United States. Approximately 4,000 speech-language pathologists and 1,600 audiologists work in Australia, and approximately 900 speech-language pathologists and 180 audiologists are found in New Zealand. There are around 12,000 speech-language pathologists and 3,000 audiologists currently practicing in the United Kingdom. The combined number of speech-language pathologists and audiologists in India is approximately 2,000 and rapidly growing. Both speech-language pathologists and audiologists are in high demand, and there are an insufficient number to meet the demand, which is likely to increase because the number of people with communication disorders is predicted to grow. Members of the baby boomer generation are now well into their middle age years, and this large population is likely to contribute to an increase in the number of communication disorders that accompany old age. In addition, medical advances are resulting in improved survival rate for premature infants, as well as elderly stroke victims. The increase in survival rate will undoubtedly increase the num-

---

FYI

Most audiologists and speech-language pathologists engage in clinical practice. They often are referred to as *clinicians*. The people with communication disorders seen by these professionals are referred to as *clients*.

Table 2–1. Some of the Professional Associations in Audiology and Speech-Language Pathology

Australia	Audiological Society of Australia (ASA)
	Speech Pathology Australia (SPA)
United Kingdom	British Academy of Audiology (BAA)
	British Society of Audiology (BSA)
	Royal College of Speech and Language Therapists (RCSLT)
Canada	Canadian Academy of Audiology (CAA)
	Canadian Association of Speech-Language Pathologists and Audiologists (CASLPA)
India	Indo-International Society of Communication and Hearing Sciences (IISCHS)
	Indian Speech and Hearing Association (ISHA)
Ireland	Irish Society of Audiology (ISA)
	Irish Association of Speech and Language Therapists (IASLT)
New Zealand	New Zealand Audiological Society (NZAS)
	New Zealand Speech-Language Therapists Association (NZSTA)
Singapore	Speech-Language and Hearing Association, Singapore (SHAS)
South Africa	South African Association of Audiologists (SAAA)
	South African Speech-Language-Hearing Association (SASLHA)
United States	American Academy of Audiologists (AAA)
	American Speech-Language and Hearing Association (ASHA)

ber of individuals likely to require the services of a speech-language pathologist or audiologist.

HISTORY OF THE PROFESSIONS

The field of communication sciences and disorders has evolved over time. The first audiologists and speech-language pathologists were not given formal professional titles. They were researchers and teachers who took an interest in helping individuals with speaking and hearing difficulties. The foundation of the audiologist and speech-language pathologist professions was influenced by many disciplines including biology, psychology, medicine, physics, linguistics, rhetoric, and education. A number of individuals contributed to the field, and some of the more noteworthy contributions are highlighted below.

John Thelwall (1764–1834) is recognized as a pioneering speech scientist and therapist in the United Kingdom (Figure 2–5). Thelwall was part of the Elocutionary Movement in the early 1800s that stressed high standards of education and high standards in the use

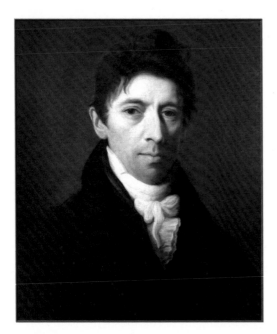

FIGURE 2–5. John Thelwall, a pioneering speech scientist and orator.

of language. Thelwall was well known for giving radical political speeches. In addition to his oratory skills, he also published a number of works dealing with elocution, the acquisition of language, the anatomy of the speech organs, and the link between speech and mental illness. Thelwall noted that some children with speech defects respond better in therapy with a female, compared with a male. He also was the first to classify speech disorders as being either natural (organic) or habitual (functional).

Alexander Melville Bell (1819–1905) and **Alexander Graham Bell** (1847–1922) were father and son who were both eminent English scientists and inventors. The family eventually settled in Canada and the United States. Although most know of the contribution made by Graham Bell to the development of the first practical telephone, few know of the contributions made by his father. Melville spent the majority of his life assisting others with their speech, whether it was formal elocution lessons or correction of speech disorders (Figure 2–6). His wife Eliza was severely hearing impaired, which influenced his own work, as well as that of his son. Melville Bell developed a transcriptional system known as *visible speech* that included drawings of the head and neck showing the physical movements behind the articulation of individual speech sounds. Following his father's death, Graham published the transcription system and taught it to teachers of the deaf.

Henry Sweet (1845–1912) was a pioneer in modern transcriptional phonetics (Figure 2–7). He was an Oxford graduate and studied speech through an interest in the English language. He developed the Broad Romic symbol system that eventually led to the International Phonetic Alphabet. He established England as the birthplace of the science of phonetics. The 1913 play *Pygmalion,* written by George Bernard Shaw (which later became the theatrical musical, *My Fair Lady*), is thought to be based loosely on the life of Henry Sweet (aka Henry Higgins).

One person who contributed to the development of the professions in Germany was **Hermann Gutzmann** (1865–1922). He helped to establish the field of **logopedics**, which is the science and study of dealing with speech defects in children. Gutzmann studied speech disorders from a medical point of view. He went on to create the Berlin School for Speech and Voice Therapy. The services provided by the Berlin School attained worldwide acclaim.

Wilhelm Wundt (1832–1920) was a German medical doctor, psychologist, physiologist, and professor who attended the Leipzig School in Germany (Figure 2–8). The Leipzig School was a

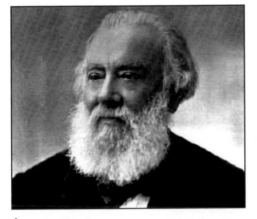

FIGURE 2–6. A. A photo of Alexander Melville Bell. **B.** A copy of Bell's business (professional) card as published in his textbook *Visible Speech* in 1867.

A

PROFESSIONAL CARD.

Mr A. MELVILLE BELL, Author of 'Visible Speech' may be consulted in all Cases of Impediment or Defect of Speech, Vocal Weakness, Monotony, Oratorical Ineffectiveness, &c.

STAMMERING AND STUTTERING.

The experience of upwards of Twenty-five years' Practice enables Mr A. MELVILLE BELL to undertake the permanent, and, in most cases, the speedy Removal of Stammering and other forms of Vocal Impediment.

References of the highest class are furnished to inquirers.

A limited number of Pupils can be accommodated as Boarders; but residence in the Establishment is not required in order to effect a Cure.

DEFECTS OF ARTICULATION.

In cases of Lisping, Burring, and other Single Elementary Defects, the entire Removal of the Faculty Habit rarely needs more than from Six to Twelve Lessons.

Children who are backward in acquiring the power of Speech are trained to the perfect use of their Vocal Organs. Parents or Governesses are invited to be present at the Lessons, and are directed in the means of carrying on the improvement, which is always rapidly commenced.

ELOCUTION.—PRONUNCIATION, READING, DELIVERY AND ACTION.

Clergymen, Barristers, Members of Parliament, and other Public Readers and Speakers, are Privately Instructed in the Principles and Practice of Effective Delivery, Oratorical Composition, &c.

Ladies and Non-professional Pupils, receive Special Lessons in the art of Reading, &c., according to individual requirements.

VISIBLE SPEECH—UNIVERSAL ALPHABETICS.

Pupils are practically initiated in the Physiology of Speech, and in the use of the Universal Alphabet, so as to be enabled to produce, and to record, all varieties of Native or Foreign Sounds.

Dialectic peculiarities are corrected; and Foreigners are taught to pronounce English with the characteristics of vernacular utterance;

TERMS.

Single Lessons in any Department, - - - - -		One Guinea.
Cure of Stammering, Stuttering, &c., -	(Twelve Lessons,) -	Ten Guineas.
Removal of Lisping, Burring, &c., - -	(Six Lessons,) -	Four Guineas.
Elocution, Reading, Delivery, &c., -	(Six Lessons,) -	Three Guineas.
Visible Speech,—Vocal Physiology, &c.,	(Six Lessons,) -	Three Guineas.

The following additional Establishments for the Cure of Stammering and for Elocutionary Instruction are conducted (in Edinburgh) by Mr MELVILLE J. BELL; and (in Dublin) by Mr D. C. BELL.

Edinburgh: No. 13 South Charlotte Street.
Dublin: No. 1 Kildare Place.

B

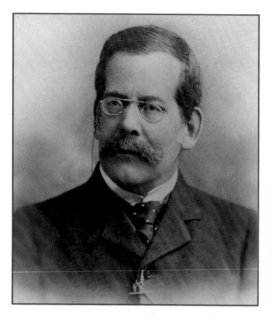

FIGURE 2–7. Henry Sweet, an expert in phonetics (aka Henry Higgins).

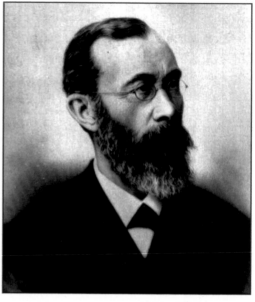

FIGURE 2–8. Wilhelm Wundt, known as the "Father of Experimental Psychology."

research center in Germany that was responsible for training the first generation of psychologists. Sigmund Freud was influenced by the Leipzig School. The school also dabbled in techniques for quantitatively measuring aspects of hearing and speech. Upon graduation, Wundt remained at the Leipzig School and developed a psychology laboratory. He is widely regarded as the "Father of Experimental Psychology." In particular, he is credited with developing the science of psychophysics, which forms the basis for the testing of hearing. Some of Wundt's students were influential in the field of communication disorders.

Edward Wheeler Scripture (1864–1945) graduated from Leipzig in 1888 under the supervision of Wundt. He was an American who developed skills in hearing measurement such as threshold testing and magnitude estimation. Scripture eventually developed a psychology laboratory at Yale University

and wrote a book comparing stuttering with lisping or "super-energetic versus sub-energetic" speech production.

Carl Seashore (1866–1949), who was born in Sweden, traveled to America and studied under Scripture at Yale University (Figure 2–9). Seashore had interests in music, voice, and hearing. He built the first audiometer with the help of Scripture. He is also the individual who developed the concept of the decibel by separating loudness magnitude into units of 40 steps each. He later became the head of the psychology department at the University of Iowa.

In 1920, Seashore was approached by **Samuel Orton** (1879–1948) who was a physician interested in learning disabilities. Orton's daughter had difficulty in speaking and reading. He suggested to Seashore that someone should be specifically educated to work with individuals having these types of difficulties. Seashore selected the most promising

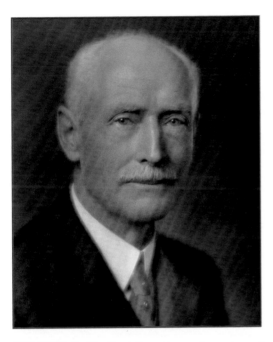

FIGURE 2–9. Carl Seashore, inventor of the audiometer.

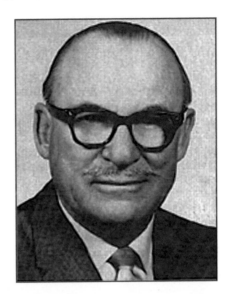

FIGURE 2–10. Lee Edward Travis, known as the "Father of Speech-Language Pathology." (Reprinted with permission from Van Riper, C. [1981]. An early history of ASHA. *ASHA Magazine, 23*(11), 855–858.)

student from the undergraduate psychology class at the University of Iowa and offered this specialized PhD to **Lee Edward Travis** (1896–1987; Figure 2–10). Travis received his PhD in 1924 and is recognized as the founding father of the speech-language pathology profession in the United States. Travis established himself as a particular expert in the area of stuttering and had many well-known students who went on to establish educational programs across the United States, including Charles Van Riper, who established the program at Western Michigan University, and Max Steer, who established the program at Purdue University.

Around the same time that Travis was completing his studies, **Sara Stinchfield Hawk** (1885–1977) was awarded a masters degree in 1920 from the department of psychology at the University of Iowa (Figure 2–11). Her thesis topic pertained to the area of stuttering. In 1922, Hawk became the first person in the United States to receive a PhD degree specifically designated in the area of speech pathology, awarded from the University of Wisconsin. Both Hawk and Travis were among the 25 founding members of the American Speech and Hearing Association established in 1925.

Raymond Carhart (1912–1975) is referred by many to be the "Father of Audiology" in the United States (Figure 2–12). He is credited with coining the word *audiology* to designate the science of hearing. Carhart was a professor of speech at Northwestern University. When World War II broke out, he was commissioned as an officer in the U.S. Army where he developed an aural rehabilitation program for individuals who were deafened as a result of war exposure. His wartime efforts working with thousands of hearing-impaired

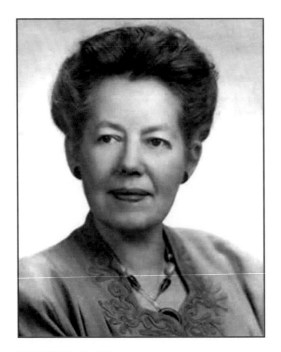

FIGURE 2–11. Sara Stinchfield Hawk. The first person to obtain a PhD in speech-language pathology.

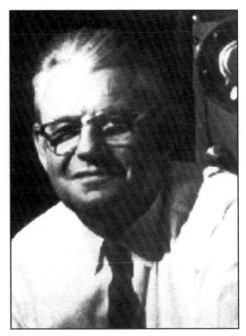

FIGURE 2–12. Raymond Carhart, known as the "Father of Audiology."

soldiers served as the basis for the development of a new discipline that is now audiology. Upon conclusion of the war, he returned to Northwestern and proceeded to develop a specific program in audiology.

Finally, the efforts of **Hallie Quinn Brown** (1849–1949) have been overlooked by many historians in regard to her contributions to speech-language pathology in the United States (Figure 2–13). She was a renowned American elocutionist and educator in the late 19th century and a significant figure in the history of speech-language pathology in the United States. She was born the daughter of two former slaves. She taught reading and provided elocution training to children and women, most notably African Americans from plantations who had been denied the opportunity of a proper education.

EDUCATIONAL PREPARATION

People who choose to become either audiologists or speech-language pathologists are entering a clearly defined field of professional practice. So what does it mean to be a *professional*? A professional can be defined as a person who is trained to do a special job in exchange for payment. This often is the case when considering people in the sports world, where it is easy to distinguish a professional athlete from an amateur athlete, through their being paid. Another form of professionalism is in regard to occupations that require education or training pertinent to a specialized field, as distinguished from general education. Training for professionals who work in communication disorders has devel-

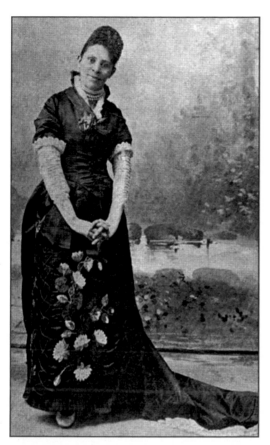

FIGURE 2–13. Hallie Q. Brown, American elocutionist and educator in the late 19th century.

oped from different starting points and within different philosophical contexts in various countries. The educational requirements to become an audiologist or speech-language pathologist share many commonalities, but they are not identical. There also are differences between countries in regard to the educational requirements for each profession. The differences between countries can be broadly categorized as reflecting an American model or British model of education. These models are presented separately.

The American Model

A primary feature of the model of education used in the United States is the emphasis on a liberal arts and sciences education at the undergraduate level followed by a period of intensive and concentrated education at the (post) graduate level. To become eligible to practice as either an audiologist or speech-language pathologist in the United States, a graduate-level education is required.

FYI

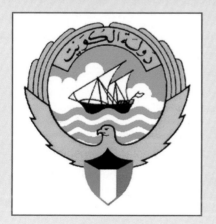

There are hundreds of university programs worldwide that educate audiologists and speech-language pathologists. Many countries offer no formal educational programs, requiring residents of these countries to travel abroad to obtain their professional qualification. One of the newest communication disorders programs is the University of Kuwait. Students receive academic coursework in English and apply this to the clinic setting speaking Arabic.

An example of the typical educational model for both degrees is provided in Table 2–2. As undergraduates, students pursue a bachelor's degree in a major usually called Communication Disorders. This major encompasses fundamental aspects of both audiology and speech-language pathology. The first two years of undergraduate education involve coursework covering a wide range of general education courses. These courses serve to satisfy the liberal arts and sciences foundation for the bachelor's degree. The final two years of undergraduate education focus more specifically on coursework in audiology and speech-language pathology, which satisfy the major requirements for the degree. The bulk of this coursework centers on normal aspects of hearing and speech and an introduction to some of the more common communication disorders such as child language disorders and phonological disorders. Upon graduation, the student holds a pre-professional bachelor's degree in communication disorders. To satisfy the educational requirements to become an audiologist or speech-language pathologist professional, the student must obtain a graduate degree. Students are allowed to choose freely whether to pursue graduate education in audiology or speech-language pathology.

For those wishing to pursue a clinical career in audiology, the requisite degree is a Doctor of Audiology (AuD) degree, which ranges from three to four years of graduate study beyond the bachelor's degree. The first two years of graduate study involve detailed coursework and on-site clinical education in audiology and hearing science. The final year involves an extensive off-campus

Table 2–2. American Model for the Education of Audiologists and Speech-Language Pathologists

Audiology	Speech-Language Pathology
Undergraduate Education	**Undergraduate Education**
Four-Year Bachelor's Degree	Four-Year Bachelor's Degree
Years 1 and 2 "Related" Areas of Study	Years 1 and 2 "Related" Areas of Study
Years 3 and 4 "Major" Areas of Study	Years 3 and 4 "Major" Areas of Study
Minimal Fieldwork	Minimal Fieldwork
Graduate Education	**Graduate Education**
Three-/Four-Year Doctor of Audiology (AuD) Degree	Two-Year Master's Degree
Years 1 to 3 Audiology Coursework	Years 1 to 2 Speech-Language Pathology Coursework
1,800 Hours of Fieldwork	400 Hours of Fieldwork
Year 4 Externship	Three One-Semester Externships
Clinical Fellowship Year	Clinical Fellowship Year
National Examination	National Examination
Obtain CCC-A	Obtain CCC-SLP

full-time clinical experience (an externship), where students acquire a considerable number of fieldwork hours. The AuD degree also requires student to complete a research project.

For those wishing to become a speech-language pathologist, the requisite degree is a master's degree, which takes two years of full-time study to complete. Across the two years of study, students complete coursework in speech, language, and swallowing disorders, and engage in a mix of on-campus and off-campus clinical experiences. Students who complete either the AuD or master's in speech-language pathology are eligible to work after graduation. The first year of professional employment is referred to as the clinical fellowship year. During the clinical fellowship year, the individual works in his or her respective profession; however, periodic oversight is provided by a work colleague who holds professional membership status in the American Speech-Language-Hearing Association (ASHA). Membership status is designated by the acronym CCC, which refers to the **Certificate of Clinical Competency.** Individuals who complete the one-year clinical fellowship make a formal application to ASHA to be awarded the CCC.

All audiologists and speech-language pathologists working in the United States generally are expected to hold the CCC in order to practice in their respective professions. There is also an expectation that these individuals will continue to up-skill throughout their professional careers. ASHA requires audiologists and speech-language pathologists to attain a minimum of 30 hours of professional development education every three years. Failure to do so can result in a loss of CCC status and limits a person's ability to practice professionally.

The British Model

The British model of audiologist and speech-language pathologist education is in widespread throughout the United Kingdom, Australia, India, Ireland, New Zealand, and South Africa. The British model places less emphasis on a liberal arts education compared with the American model. Instead, education is more concentrated on the essential coursework and clinical competencies for becoming either an audiologist or speech-language pathologist. The British model for the education of audiologists and speech-language pathologists allows for one of two paths. One path involves completion of a concentrated four-year undergraduate degree. As first-year university students, they immediately begin studying their major. By conclusion of the four-year degree, these students are likely to have taken the same number of courses in audiology or speech-language pathology as an American student. The second path involves completion of a two-year master's degree in audiology or speech-language pathology. To obtain a master's degree, it is not mandatory to hold a bachelor's degree in communication disorders, but rather a degree that is compatible with audiology or speech-language pathology such as psychology, health, linguistics, biology, engineering, or education. Similar to the United States requirement, most countries require audiology graduates to complete a clinical fellowship year as part of the first year of professional experience prior to becoming full-fledged members of their respective professional associations. This is not necessarily the case for speech-language pathology graduates. Examples of the typical British educational models for audiology and speech-language pathology degrees are provided in Table 2–3.

Qualities of an Audiologist and Speech-Language Pathologist

Individuals who work as either audiologists or speech-language pathologists interact with people of all ages and backgrounds. One of the prime attributes of becoming a successful professional is having good people skills, such as knowing how to interact effectively with others who have various disorders and a range of backgrounds. People are individuals, with as many similarities from one person to the next as there are differences. An effective audiologist or speech-language pathologist is able to relate to a wide range of clients and bring out their best performance,

Table 2–3. British Model for the Education of Audiologists and Speech-Language Pathologists

Audiology	Speech-Language Pathology
Path 1 Undergraduate Degree	**Path 1 Undergraduate Degree**
Four-Year Bachelor's Degree	Four-Year Bachelor's Degree
Year 1"Related" Areas of Study	Year 1"Related" Areas of Study
Years 2 to 4 Audiology Coursework	Years 2 to 4 Speech-Language Pathology Coursework
350 Hours of Fieldwork	350 Hours of Fieldwork
Three One-Semester Externships	Three One-Semester Externships
Path 2 Master's Degree	**Path 2 Master's Degree**
Bachelor's Degree in Related Areas (Psychology, Biology, Engineering, Health)	Bachelor's Degree in Related Areas (Psychology, Biology, Linguistics, Health, Education)
Years 1 to 2 Audiology Coursework	Years 1 to 2 Speech-Language Pathology Coursework
350 Hours of Fieldwork	350 Hours of Fieldwork
Three One-Semester Externships	Three One-Semester Externships
Clinical Fellowship Year	
National Examination	
Obtain CCC	

whether it is related to testing the hearing of an elderly individual or promoting language development in a young nonverbal child. The two professions are not physically demanding, but they can be emotionally and intellectually challenging. These professionals need to approach problems objectively and provide support to their clients and families. Many disorders are complex and not fully understood, so professionals should be able to tolerate challenge and uncertainty. Because a client's progress may be slow, audiologists and speech-language pathologists must have patience and compassion. Another quality of being a good audiologist or speech-language pathologist is to have sharp listening skills and exceptional observational skills. They also should be able to effectively communicate test results and possible treatment choices to their clients in a manner that is easily understood.

PROFESSIONAL WORK SETTINGS

Speech-language pathologists and audiologists can be found in a range of work settings. In some instances, the professionals work side by side. Alternatively, some forms of professional practice have quite unique work settings. A description of some of the more common work settings is provided below.

Education

By far, the largest employer of speech-language pathologists are public and private schools, and specialized schools such as those designated for hard of hearing and deaf children. The type of work performed by a speech-language pathologist in educational settings may involve employment at a single school or serving as an **itinerant speech-language pathologist** that entails traveling between many schools and having a caseload of clients in each school. Some audiologists are employed in deaf education centers or in public school systems, where they may be involved in performing routine audiological assessments on students. Higher education settings such as colleges and universities also employ audiologist and speech-language pathologist lecturers and professors to teach students pursuing a career in communication disorders. Approximately 50% of the speech-language pathologist workforce and 10% of the audiologist workforce can be found in educational settings.

Hospitals

Approximately 40% of speech-language pathologists and 60% of audiologists are employed in health care settings, including hospitals and residential or nonresidential health care facilities. The two primary hospital settings are: (1) acute care and (2) rehabilitation care. An **acute care hospital** is one where the patient has recently been admitted because of a planned surgery or an accident or trauma. The type of patient seen by the speech-language pathologist in an acute setting may be someone who has had their larynx removed as a result of throat cancer, or possibly an individual who recently experienced a stroke, or motor vehicle accident. In these situations, the speech-language pathologist often will first visit the patient in the hospital bed shortly after the medical condition has been treated. The speech-language pathologist will diagnose whether a communication disorder exists, as well as the severity of the disorder. A patient might eventually transfer from an acute care hospital to a **rehabilitation hospital** where she or he is now being managed on a longer term basis. The speech-language pathologist typically is employed to provide treatment to the patient to assist with their eventual discharge from the hospital and transitioning to communicating in the outside environment. Once discharged, the individual could still have a communication disorder and likely would receive services via a residential (e.g., nursing home) or nonresidential facility. The type of client seen by an audiologist in a hospital setting may be an individual who receives a hearing assessment as part of a routine physical examination. Newborn infants routinely receive a hearing assessment prior to being discharged from the hospital. Sometimes audiologists can be found in the operating room of hospitals, where they may monitor a patient's hearing during delicate operations that can affect the hearing mechanism.

Private Practice

Individuals engaged exclusively in private practice account for approximately 5% of the speech-language pathologist workforce and 20% of the audiologist workforce. The type of client seen by a speech-language pathologist private practitioner is generally one who is not in a medically acute condition. Rather, the speech-language pathologist may see children with mild communication disorders that typically do no qualify for

therapy services in a school setting. Or the speech-language pathologist may offer a unique or specialty type of service, such as working exclusively with individuals who have voice problems or individuals who may speak English as a second language and are receiving assistance with reducing the strength of their foreign accent. Audiologists may work independently or with other private practitioners such as ear, nose, and throat physicians. A major facet of this type of job setting is the prescription and fitting of hearing aids. It is not unusual for some audiologists to hold full-time employment in another setting but also engage in a minimum level of private practice.

Research

A small percentage (approximately 5%) of speech-language pathologist and audiologist professionals work exclusively in research settings. These individuals are not engaged in clinical practice or education, but rather in scientific investigations of basic and applied aspects of communication sciences and disorders. One well-known institution in the United States is the Boys Town National Research Hospital in Omaha, Nebraska that focuses on childhood deafness, visual impairment, and related communication disorders. A well-known hearing research laboratory in Melbourne, Australia is the Bionic Ear Institute.

Industry

One particular work setting that is unique to audiologists is their employment in the hearing aid industry. Around 5% of audiologists work in the

---

FYI

There is a severe shortage of audiologists and speech-language pathologists worldwide. In addition to this overall shortage, less than 25% of the workforce is made up of males. This sex imbalance is also found in other allied health professions such as nursing, physiotherapy, and occupational therapy.

---

industry and may serve as sales representatives for large hearing aid companies. These individuals are experts on current hearing aid devices on the market and provide consultation to practicing audiologists about the latest product advancements.

PROFESSIONAL CODE OF ETHICS

To be a professional involves behaving with dignity and in an ethical manner, and in such a way that people trust your judgment. **Ethical behavior** refers to doing the right thing and encompasses attributes such as: (1) honesty, (2) respect, and (3) responsibility. Being honest involves truthfulness and refraining from lying and cheating. Respect involves tolerance and openness toward others regardless of personal or cultural differences. Responsibility means taking your professional duties seriously and accepting culpability for your decisions. Many professional organizations have established a series of behavioral guidelines that govern the day-to-day activities of a professional. These guidelines are referred to as a **code of ethics**, and are a list of common sense rules and regulations that refer to doing the right thing when individuals are engaged in their chosen professional practice (see Appendix 2–A: ASHA Code of Ethics).

Most professional associations will establish an ethics board that is designed to handle any complaints raised against individual members. Individuals who are found to be in violation of any of the established codes may run the risk of being sanctioned by their professional association. The level of sanctioning can range from a reprimand that could involve payment of a fine, to the temporary suspension of professional licensure, or in extreme cases, to being handled by state or national law enforcement agencies.

The audiologist and speech-language pathologist professions adhere to a code of ethics, an example of which is established by ASHA as provided in Appendix 2–A. There are slight differences in the code of ethics developed by audiologist and speech-language pathologist associations worldwide, but some of the common tenets are that audiologists and speech-language pathologists:

1. Should safeguard the welfare of the clients they serve.
2. Should maintain high standards of professional competence.
3. Should maintain accurate and up-to-date information about the nature, management, and treatment of communication disorders.
4. Should uphold the dignity of the profession and accept the profession's self-imposed standards.

CULTURAL CONSIDERATIONS AND COMMUNICATION DISORDERS

Population centers throughout the world are becoming increasingly diverse both culturally and linguistically. To effectively meet the needs of a diverse population, audiologists and speech-language pathologists need to be sensitive to issues that can influence both the identification and management of communication disorders. Multilingual and culturally diverse clients are those who use languages and dialects other than that of the audiologist or speech-language pathologist, or do not share the same cultural background as the audiologist or speech-language pathologist. Clients may belong to a different culture and communicate in a language different from the audiologist or speech-language pathologist, or may share the same language to some degree while belonging to a different culture. If misunderstood or misinterpreted, the audiologist or speech-language pathologist may inadvertently mistake certain communication behaviors as signs of a disorder. There also are cultural differences in beliefs about health, disability, and delivery of clinical services. The differences can influence how an individual would either perceive a communication disorder or accept certain treatment for the disorder. Professionals providing services to individuals from different cultural backgrounds need to be aware of unique perspectives or communication styles common to those cultures. The complexities of communication in a multicultural environment are depicted as a series of layers in Figure 2–14. These layers apply to both the client and the professional providing services to the client. Some observations about different cultural styles that should be considered by audiologists and speech-language pathologists when communicating with individuals of differing cultural and linguistic backgrounds are listed below (Roberts, 2001).

Sharing Space

People from different cultures share physical space differently. In some cultures, it is quite acceptable for people to stand in close proximity to one another while talking, whereas in other cultures people like to keep farther apart. For example, Hispanics might view Americans as being distant because they prefer more space between speakers. On the other hand, Americans often view individuals who come too close as invading their private space.

Touching

The rules for touching others vary from culture to culture. In Hispanic and other Latin cultures, two people engaged in conversation often are observed touching and individuals usually embrace when greeting each other. In other cultures, people are more restrained in their greetings. Most Arabic cultures do not customarily shake hands with individuals of the opposite sex.

Eye Contact

The simple act of looking at another person when speaking can have different cultural connotations. Avoidance of direct eye contact is sometimes seen

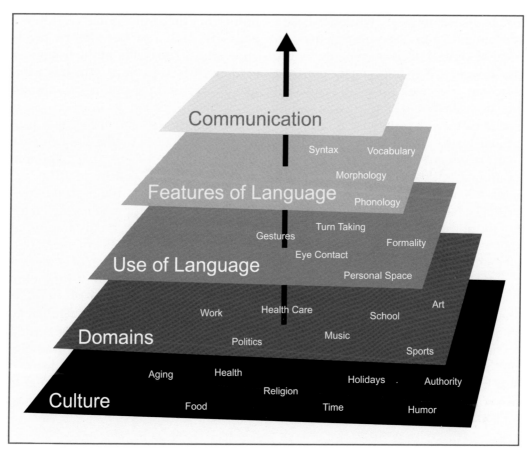

FIGURE 2–14. Depiction of the various layers of communication within a cultural context.

as a sign of attentiveness and respect, whereas sustained direct eye contact may be interpreted as a challenge to authority. Among African Americans, it is not unusual for the listener to avert their eyes, whereas European Americans prefer to make direct eye contact while listening.

Time Ordering

The statement, "business before pleasure" refers to the belief that we must take care of our responsibilities before enjoying ourselves. The notion of completing one activity at a time is called *monochronic,* and many mainstream cultures perceive time in this manner. However, some cultures are *polychronic* where several activities occur at the same time. Many Polynesian cultures are polychromic with social interactions interwoven throughout a work activity.

CURRENT ISSUES IN THE PROFESSIONS

Evidence-Based Practice

The notion of **evidence-based practice** has its origins in the field of medicine where it is known as evidence-based medicine. Evidence-based practice is a form of clinical decision-making by the practitioner to help improve the patient's outcome. The need for evidence-based practice was driven by the desire to shift health care away from basing decisions primarily on opinion and past practices, many of which had not been sufficiently examined to determine their effectiveness. A simple way of conceptualizing evidence-based practice is based on asking the questions, "Why am I practicing this way?" and "Is there evidence that can guide me to a better outcome in my practice?" The processes of evidence-based practice can be illustrated in the shape of a triangle (Figure 2–15). Two points on the triangle represent the professional's search for best practice based on their personal experience as well as that found in the academic and research arena. The third point of the triangle represents the professional's acknowledgment of his or her client's needs and values. The center of the triangle is evidence-based practice, which is a collection of the three points that should guide the professional's practice.

Two types of evidence guide professional practice. The first is evidence that demonstrates effective treatment approaches (i.e., what to do). The second type of evidence demonstrates ineffective treatment approaches (i.e., what not to do). Both are equally important in helping to improve the patient's outcome. The implementation of evidence-based practice in the field of communication disorders is only just beginning, as it is in most professions. Similar to what has been found in medicine, audiologists and speech-language pathologists cannot rely on what they learned several years ago (e.g., as students) to carry them through a lifetime of profes-

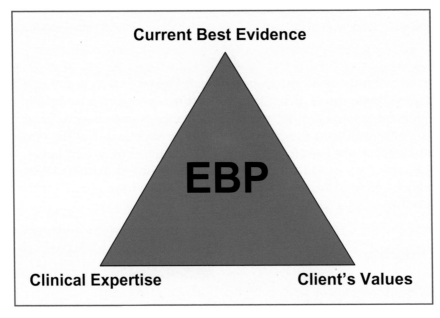

FIGURE 2–15. Evidence-based practice triangle illustrating the processes and responsibilities of professionals who adopt evidence-based practice.

sional practice. On average, research in any particular area of health can be expected to double every 10 years. Keeping this in mind, for practice to be effective, the information we base our practice on needs to be constantly updated. As expert clinicians, audiologists and speech-language pathologists should consistently seek new information to improve therapeutic effectiveness (Ratner, 2006). Many professional associations require their members to regularly attend professional development events, such as workshops and conferences, to keep abreast of current and best practices.

Professional Licensure

Whenever we try to help others, we inevitably risk harming them. Most health professions, namely in medicine, are practiced with tight regulations imposed by local and national governments. These regulations are designed to safeguard the public from potential harm, whether it is emotional, physical, or financial. They attempt to ensure that professionals work within a well-defined scope of practice in which the education and training of the professional is suited to the health problem at hand. The concepts of **beneficence** and **nonmaleficence** are used to determine whether a particular profession should require licensure. Beneficence refers to "doing good" and implies that positive steps are taken by the professional to prevent harm to the patient or to remove the patient from harm. Nonmaleficence refers to an obligation by the professional "not to harm" the patient. Beneficence and nonmaleficence can be seen as two ends of the same continuum of patient care.

Health care workers are committed to helping others and should, therefore, consider the principles of beneficence and nonmaleficence. This has prompted many countries to license (or regulate) various health care professions in a manner similar to what is found in medical practice. At present, there is surprisingly little worldwide consistency toward the regulation of the audiologist and speech-language pathologist professions by government bodies. Yet it would appear that both professions have the potential for causing patient harm. Table 2–4 provides examples of some of the harm that can occur to patients who have a communication disorder and are seen by an incompetent audiologist or speech-language pathologist. The United Kingdom and South Africa require professional licensure of all audiologists and speech-language pathologists, whereas Australia, Canada, and the United States vary

---

FYI

Audiologists and speech-language pathologists who choose to work in a private practice usually are required to purchase professional liability (or malpractice) insurance. These insurance policies are designed to protect the client from an audiologist or speech-language pathologist who fails to exercise a competent degree of skill and care in the performance of their duties.

Table 2–4. Examples of Harm That Might Be Caused by an Unqualified or Incompetent Audiologist or Speech-Language Pathologist

Audiologist Error	Potential Harm
Misdiagnosis of brainstem tumor.	Failure to treat the problem, resulting in worsening of the tumor.
Misdiagnosis of hearing loss in a newborn.	Delayed/disordered speech, cognitive, learning outcomes.
Failure to identify conditions of chronic otitis media in preschool children with speech and language difficulties.	Permanent sensorineural hearing loss, poor educational achievement.
Taking of deep ear impressions.	Serious physical and mental harm can be caused if the deep ear impression is performed incorrectly.
Failure to provide necessary environmental support for communicatively impaired patients who have demonstrated physical weakness (stroke, paralysis).	Injury due to fall.
Purchase of unnecessary hearing aids.	Financial harm.
Speech-Language Pathologist Error	**Potential Harm**
Initiation of feeding too soon or inserting objects into the mouth during dysphagia treatment.	Patient choking and/or aspirating leading to aspiration pneumonia and possible death.
Providing therapeutic services to an individual with a perceived voice problem without first referring to an otolaryngologist.	Overlooking possible cancer of the larynx, resulting in surgical removal of larynx and possible death.
Failure to identify seizure activity in speech disordered clients, such as those with traumatic brain injury or cerebral palsy.	Permanent brain damage, coma, death.
Incorrect choice of augmentative devices for nonverbal patients.	Limitation of communication competence if choice is below the patient's abilities. Frustration, withdrawal, decreased motivation to attempt communication. Inappropriate educational and vocational placement.

in regard to the total number of states or provinces that require licensure. At present, neither profession is regulated in New Zealand, although steps are being taken to mandate licensure.

Currently, a conviction for practicing as an audiologist or speech-language pathologist without a license is a minor misdemeanor in countries where no professional licensure is required.

Professional Reciprocity

Audiologist and speech-language pathologist professions are practiced throughout the world. A question that often arises is whether it is possible to work outside one's home country. The answer is yes. However, each country may have its own unique requirements, as can been seen in the different educational models presented earlier in this chapter. Generally, the first step in seeking employment in another country is to contact the professional association of the specific country. A list of the various professional associations of audiologists and speech-language pathologists found in various English-speaking countries is provided in Table 2–1. The association will determine whether the applicant's education and professional experiences are equivalent to that found within the country. The process of **reciprocity** is a situation whereby two countries accept the validity of professional credentials granted by the other country. This can be a lengthy process that involves providing evidence of language proficiency, educational background, and clinical experience. There are few, if any, countries that allow for immediate reciprocity. Although there is a common universal thread to these professions, namely, to improve communication abilities, there are some subtle and not so subtle differences across countries.

A worldwide effort is now underway to streamline the process for speech-language pathologists to work abroad. A case in point is the recent pact between a handful of countries referred to as the **Mutual Recognition of Credentials Agreement**. The Mutual Recognition of Credentials Agreement was originally established in 2004 and currently includes ASHA, the Canadian Association of Speech-Language Pathologists and Audiologists (CASLPA), the New Zealand Speech-Language Therapists Association (NZSTA), the Irish Association of Speech and Language Therapists (IASLT), the Royal College of Speech and Language Therapists (RCSLT), and Speech Pathology Australia (SPA). The premise of the Mutual Recognition of Credentials Agreement is that under certain terms and conditions an individual's credentials are deemed substantially equivalent. Each country may still require applicants from another country to achieve certain competencies prior to the start of employment; however, the steps toward working in the country of interest are *fast tracked*. No such agreement is currently available for the audiologist profession. That is not to say that an audiologist educated in one country cannot work in another, but rather the steps toward having one's credentials recognized in another country are likely to take a bit longer than for a speech-language pathologist.

An additional resource for those interested in working in another country is the International Directory of Communication Disorders (IDCD). The IDCD is a compilation of Internet resources focusing on communication disorders, including national associations, international associations and groups, educational programs, and employment opportunities (Bleile, Ireland, & Kiel, 2006). The IDCD also contains personal accounts of international experiences of persons in the profession, sample Code of Ethics, and examples of volunteering and employment opportunities. The purpose of the IDCD is to facilitate international connections between professionals in audiology and speech-language pathology. The IDCD is a free resource for persons in the professions (http://www.comdisinternational.com/purpose.html).

THE PROFESSIONS OF AUDIOLOGY AND SPEECH-LANGUAGE PATHOLOGY ON THE WORLD WIDE WEB

Listed below are websites that provide further information on the professions of audiology and speech-language pathology. At the time of publication, each website was freely accessible.

A Guide to Internet Resources in Audiology

http://www.worldaudiology.com

A Guide to Internet Resources in Speech Pathology

http://www.abacon.com/internetguides/spath/weblinks.html

American Speech-Language-Hearing Association

http://www.asha.org/students/

Audiology and Speech-Language Pathology Professions Videos

http://education-portal.com/degree_in_speech_therapy.html

http://youniversitytv.com/careers/audiologist

http://youniversity.com/careers/speech-pathologist

http://www.youtube.com/user/UniCanterburyCMDS/videos

Mutual Recognition of Credentials Agreement

http://www.asha.org/about/certification/MultilateralMRA.htm

STUDY QUESTIONS

1. Describe the classifications used for the various types of communication disorders.
2. Who are some of the pioneers that contributed to the creation of the audiologist and speech-language pathologist professions?
3. Compare and contrast the two models for educating audiologists and speech-language pathologists.
4. What are the qualities that make for a good audiologist or speech-language pathologist?
5. List and describe cultural styles that should be considered by audiologists and speech-language pathologists when communicating with clients.

REFERENCES

American Speech-Language-Hearing Association. (2003). *Code of ethics* [Ethics]. Available from http://www.asha.org/policy

Bleile, K. M., Ireland, L., & Kiel, T. (2006, December). The professions around the world: New Web-based directory goes global. *ASHA Leader,* 11(17), 8–9, 26–27.

Denes, P., & Pinson, E. (1973). *The speech chain: The physics and biology of spoken language.* New York, NY: Anchor Books.

Ratner, N. B. (2006) Evidence-based practice: An examination of its ramifications for the practice of speech-language pathology. *Language, Speech, and Hearing Services in Schools, 37,* 257–267.

Roberts, P. (2001). Aphasia assessment and treatment for bilingual and culturally diverse patients. In R. Chapey (Ed.), *Lan-*

guage intervention strategies in adult aphasia (3rd ed.). St. Louis, MO: Lippincott, Williams & Wilkins.

Van Riper, C. (1981). An early history of ASHA. *ASHA Magazine, 23*(11), 855–858.

APPENDIX 2–A

ASHA Code of Ethics (2003)

PREAMBLE

The preservation of the highest standards of integrity and ethical principles is vital to the responsible discharge of obligations by speech-language pathologists, audiologists, and speech, language, and hearing scientists. This Code of Ethics sets forth the fundamental principles and rules considered essential to this purpose.

Every individual who is (a) a member of the American Speech-Language-Hearing Association, whether certified or not, (b) a nonmember holding the Certificate of Clinical Competence from the Association, (c) an applicant for membership or certification, or (d) a Clinical Fellow seeking to fulfill standards for certification shall abide by this Code of Ethics.

Any violation of the spirit and purpose of this Code shall be considered unethical. Failure to specify any particular responsibility or practice in this Code of Ethics shall not be construed as denial of the existence of such responsibilities or practices.

The fundamentals of ethical conduct are described by Principles of Ethics and by Rules of Ethics as they relate to the conduct of research and scholarly activities and responsibility to persons served, the public, and speech-language pathologists, audiologists, and speech, language, and hearing scientists.

Principles of Ethics, aspirational and inspirational in nature, form the underlying moral basis for the Code of Ethics. Individuals shall observe these principles as affirmative obligations under all conditions of professional activity.

Rules of Ethics are specific statements of minimally acceptable professional conduct or of prohibitions and are applicable to all individuals.

PRINCIPLE OF ETHICS I

Individuals shall honor their responsibility to hold paramount the welfare of persons they serve professionally or participants in research and scholarly activities and shall treat animals involved in research in a humane manner.

Rules of Ethics

1. Individuals shall provide all services competently.
2. Individuals shall use every resource, including referral when appropri-

---

Reprinted with permission from American Speech-Language-Hearing Association. (2003). Code of Ethics [Ethics]. Available from http://www.asha.org/policy.

ate, to ensure that high-quality service is provided.

3. Individuals shall not discriminate in the delivery of professional services or the conduct of research and scholarly activities on the basis of race or ethnicity, gender, age, religion, national origin, sexual orientation, or disability.

4. Individuals shall not misrepresent the credentials of assistants, technicians, or support personnel and shall inform those they serve professionally of the name and professional credentials of persons providing services.

5. Individuals who hold the Certificates of Clinical Competence shall not delegate tasks that require the unique skills, knowledge, and judgment that are within the scope of their profession to assistants, technicians, support personnel, students, or any nonprofessionals over whom they have supervisory responsibility. An individual may delegate support services to assistants, technicians, support personnel, students, or any other persons only if those services are adequately supervised by an individual who holds the appropriate Certificate of Clinical Competence.

6. Individuals shall fully inform the persons they serve of the nature and possible effects of services rendered and products dispensed, and they shall inform participants in research about the possible effects of their participation in research conducted.

7. Individuals shall evaluate the effectiveness of services rendered and of products dispensed and shall provide services or dispense products only when benefit can reasonably be expected.

8. Individuals shall not guarantee the results of any treatment or procedure, directly or by implication; however, they may make a reasonable statement of prognosis.

9. Individuals shall not provide clinical services solely by correspondence.

10. Individuals may practice by telecommunication (for example, telehealth/e-health), where not prohibited by law.

11. Individuals shall adequately maintain and appropriately secure records of professional services rendered, research and scholarly activities conducted, and products dispensed and shall allow access to these records only when authorized or when required by law.

12. Individuals shall not reveal, without authorization, any professional or personal information about identified persons served professionally or identified participants involved in research and scholarly activities unless required by law to do so, or unless doing so is necessary to protect the welfare of the person or of the community or otherwise required by law.

13. Individuals shall not charge for services not rendered, nor shall they misrepresent services rendered, products dispensed, or research and scholarly activities conducted.

14. Individuals shall use persons in research or as subjects of teaching demonstrations only with their informed consent.

15. Individuals whose professional services are adversely affected by substance abuse or other health-related conditions shall seek professional assistance and, where appropriate, withdraw from the affected areas of practice.

PRINCIPLE OF ETHICS II

Individuals shall honor their responsibility to achieve and maintain the highest level of professional competence.

Rules of Ethics

1. Individuals shall engage in the provision of clinical services only when they hold the appropriate Certificate of Clinical Competence or when they are in the certification process and are supervised by an individual who holds the appropriate Certificate of Clinical Competence.
2. Individuals shall engage in only those aspects of the professions that are within the scope of their competence, considering their level of education, training, and experience.
3. Individuals shall continue their professional development throughout their careers.
4. Individuals shall delegate the provision of clinical services only to: (1) persons who hold the appropriate Certificate of Clinical Competence; (2) persons in the education or certification process who are appropriately supervised by an individual who holds the appropriate Certificate of Clinical Competence; or (3) assistants, technicians, or support personnel who are adequately supervised by an individual who holds the appropriate Certificate of Clinical Competence.
5. Individuals shall not require or permit their professional staff to provide services or conduct research activities that exceed the staff member's competence, level of education, training, and experience.

6. Individuals shall ensure that all equipment used in the provision of services or to conduct research and scholarly activities is in proper working order and is properly calibrated.

PRINCIPLE OF ETHICS III

Individuals shall honor their responsibility to the public by promoting public understanding of the professions, by supporting the development of services designed to fulfill the unmet needs of the public, and by providing accurate information in all communications involving any aspect of the professions, including dissemination of research findings and scholarly activities.

Rules of Ethics

1. Individuals shall not misrepresent their credentials, competence, education, training, experience, or scholarly or research contributions.
2. Individuals shall not participate in professional activities that constitute a conflict of interest.
3. Individuals shall refer those served professionally solely on the basis of the interest of those being referred and not on any personal financial interest.
4. Individuals shall not misrepresent diagnostic information, research, services rendered, or products dispensed; neither shall they engage in any scheme to defraud in connection with obtaining payment or reimbursement for such services or products.
5. Individuals' statements to the public shall provide accurate informa-

tion about the nature and management of communication disorders, about the professions, about professional services, and about research and scholarly activities.

6. Individuals' statements to the public—advertising, announcing, and marketing their professional services, reporting research results, and promoting products—shall adhere to prevailing professional standards and shall not contain misrepresentations.

PRINCIPLE OF ETHICS IV

Individuals shall honor their responsibilities to the professions and their relationships with colleagues, students, and members of allied professions. Individuals shall uphold the dignity and autonomy of the professions, maintain harmonious interprofessional and intraprofessional relationships, and accept the professions' self-imposed standards.

Rules of Ethics

1. Individuals shall prohibit anyone under their supervision from engaging in any practice that violates the Code of Ethics.

2. Individuals shall not engage in dishonesty, fraud, deceit, misrepresentation, sexual harassment, or any other form of conduct that adversely reflects on the professions or on the individual's fitness to serve persons professionally.

3. Individuals shall not engage in sexual activities with clients or students over whom they exercise professional authority.

4. Individuals shall assign credit only to those who have contributed to a publication, presentation, or product. Credit shall be assigned in proportion to the contribution and only with the contributor's consent.

5. Individuals shall reference the source when using other persons' ideas, research, presentations, or products in written, oral, or any other media presentation or summary.

6. Individuals' statements to colleagues about professional services, research results, and products shall adhere to prevailing professional standards and shall contain no misrepresentations.

7. Individuals shall not provide professional services without exercising independent professional judgment, regardless of referral source or prescription.

8. Individuals shall not discriminate in their relationships with colleagues, students, and members of allied professions on the basis of race or ethnicity, gender, age, religion, national origin, sexual orientation, or disability.

9. Individuals who have reason to believe that the Code of Ethics has been violated shall inform the Board of Ethics.

10. Individuals shall comply fully with the policies of the Board of Ethics in its consideration and adjudication of complaints of violations of the Code of Ethics.

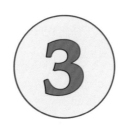

ANATOMICAL PROCESSES OF SPEECH AND HEARING

OBJECTIVES

After reading this chapter, the student should be able to:

- Label major anatomical structures and systems for speech, language, and hearing.
- State the physiological functions of these structures and systems.
- Identify individuals who have made historical contributions to understanding the anatomy of speech and hearing.
- Describe the essential physiological processes involved in the production of speech.
- Describe the essential physiological processes involved in hearing.
- Understand how impairments in one or more systems can cause communicative disabilities.
- Relate the anatomy and physiology of these structures and systems to the professional responsibilities of the audiologist and speech-language pathologist.

INTRODUCTION

Anatomy is the study of the structure of organisms and the relations of their parts. The word **anatomy** comes from the Greek *ana* meaning "up" or "through," and *tomie* meaning "a cutting." Anatomy was once a "cutting up" because the structure of the body was originally learned through **dissection** of human cadavers. However, less invasive methods are now available to examine the living body, using such devices as endoscopic cameras and body scans (e.g., CAT-scan, MRI-scan). **Physiology** is the study of the functions of living organisms and their parts. This word is also Greek in origin with *physis* meaning "nature," and *logia* meaning "to speak." So physiology involves describing the nature of things. **Gross anatomy** and physiology involves examination of the structure and function of body parts that can be seen with the naked eye. **Cellular anatomy and physiology** (or histology) entails examining those body parts best seen under the microscope. Traditionally, both gross and cellular anatomy and physiology are foundation courses that beginning medical students are required to take as part of their degree program. This is no different for students of the audiology and speech-language pathology professions. To fully appreciate the nature of normal communication and disorders of communication, knowledge about the structure and function of the speech and hearing mechanism is essential. This chapter provides some introductory exposure to speech and hearing anatomy and physiology. The material presented is referred to in later chapters concerning communication disorders resulting from anatomical and physiological abnormalities of the speech and hearing mechanism.

SPEECH ANATOMY

The human anatomy involved in the production of speech is grounded in biological structures and processes used for doing nonspeech things such as breathing, swallowing, and coughing. The structures can be divided into three subsystems: (1) respiratory, (2) laryngeal, and (3) articulatory. As human beings, we have learned to exploit these structures that were originally designed for basic survival, and to use them to communicate with other human beings. A survey and description of the structure and function of the respiratory, laryngeal, and articulatory systems is provided.

Respiratory System

The respiratory system consists of the lungs, trachea, pharynx, oral and nasal passages, diaphragm, and rib cage. The general location of each of these anatomical structures is shown in Figure 3–1. The respiratory system is divided into the **upper respiratory tract** (including the oral and nasal cavities, and pharynx) and the **lower respiratory tract** (the trachea, bronchi, and lungs). Air is inhaled primarily through the nostrils into the **nasal cavity**. The nasal cavities are lined with mucous membranes that are covered with tiny hairs known as cilia. These features within the nasal cavity serve to warm, moisten, and fil-

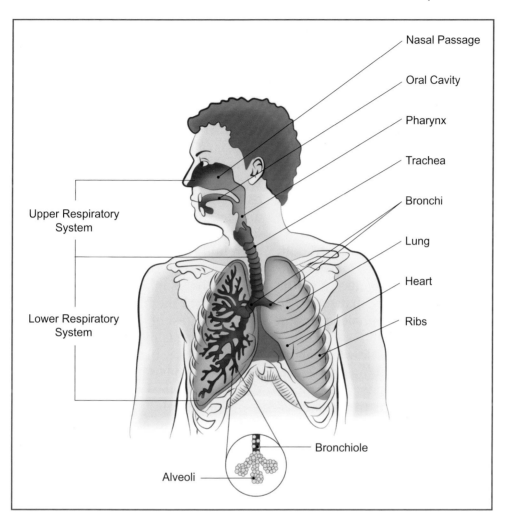

FIGURE 3–1. Anatomical features of the human respiratory system.

ter the air of possible contaminants. For most of us, breathing is breathing, and it does not matter whether it is from the mouth or nose. **Mouth breathing** may appear to be a harmless form of breathing; however, there are many negatives associated with breathing through the mouth. Excessive mouth breathing is problematic because air is not filtered and warmed as much as when inhaled through the nose, as it bypasses the nasal cavity. The dust and dirt deposited in the membranes cannot be disposed of as they are by the nasal cavity and, therefore, remain to produce irritation and inflammation. Mouth breathing is thought to contribute to a higher than average occurrence of upper respiratory infections, and may also exacerbate the occurrence of asthma. Excessive mouth breathing may also be indicative of situations in which the nasal cavity is obstructed, thereby preventing nasal breathing to occur naturally. In cases such as this, mouth breathing is done out of necessity. Situations like enlarged

---

FYI

At rest, a healthy adult breathes about 14 to 16 times per minute. After exercise it could increase to over 60 times per minute. New babies at rest breathe between 40 and 50 times per minute. By age five, it decreases to around 25 times per minute.

---

adenoids can lead to excessive mouth breathing. **Adenoids** (e.g., tonsils) consist of a paired mass of tissue in the back of the nasal cavity that serves to filter out debris that is inhaled through the nose.

The **pharynx** is a hollow tube about five inches (12.7 cm) long that starts behind the nose and ends at the top of the trachea. The tube is made of muscles that encircle the throat. At the bottom of the pharynx the tube splits with one tube running down the front of the neck, called the trachea (i.e., windpipe). The second tube running down the back of the neck is called the **esophagus** (i.e., food tube). The pharynx serves a twofold purpose. During the process of eating, food enters the oral cavity and is readied for swallowing. The food is directed down the pharynx. The muscles surrounding the pharynx contract and push the food toward the esophagus and onward to the stomach. During the process of breathing, air inhaled through the nose is directed toward the pharynx and down through the trachea toward the lungs.

The trachea is the principal tube that carries air to and from the lungs and is made up of elastic tissues and about 20 rings of cartilage. It is designed to be flexible, so that we can twist and turn our head and neck while, at the same time, being able to breathe normally. The trachea branches into two main tubes supplying air to the right and left lung, respectively. These are called **bronchial tubes**. An inflammation of these airway tubes is called bronchitis. The tubes continue to divide again and again becoming narrower and narrower, referred to as **bronchioles**. The very end of these airway tubes look like spongy sacs known as **alveoli**. Tiny blood vessels surround each of the alveoli. It is at this point in the process of breathing when oxygen that is inhaled into the lungs is delivered to the bloodstream and carried to the rest of the body. Each cell in the body needs oxygen at all times. At the same time, these tiny sacs remove carbon dioxide from the blood, which is exhaled from the body.

Collectively, the bronchial tubes, bronchioles, and alveoli serve to make up the lungs. The **lungs** are so large that they occupy most of the space in the chest. The lungs are cone shaped. Although the lungs come as a pair, they are not exactly the same size as is often found for other paired anatomical structures such as our eyes or nostrils. Instead, the lung on the left side of the body is a bit smaller than the lung on the right. This extra space on the left leaves room for the heart to occupy space within the chest. The lungs are protected by 12 sets of rib bones creating the **rib cage**. Beneath the lungs is the **diaphragm** muscle, which extends across the bottom of the rib cage. The diaphragm is the principal muscle of respiration. When we inhale to take a breath, the diaphragm is drawn downward and the rib cage is expanded and elevated. The combined actions of the rib cage and diaphragm serve to enlarge the overall chest area, and air then passes into the lungs to fill the larger space. We rely heavily on the diaphragm for our respiratory function, so that when the diaphragm is impaired, it can seriously compromise our breathing.

The primary functions of the respiratory system are to help sustain life through the exchange of gases. When a person takes a breath, the air taken in comprises several gases. The mixture is mostly composed of oxygen, nitrogen, and carbon dioxide. Oxygen is an odorless gas that makes up about 20% of air and is essential to life because it is used for chemical reactions that occur in the cells of the body. Oxygen is brought in and utilized by the body, whereas carbon dioxide and nitrogen are expelled from the body.

A **respiratory cycle** consists of two phases, an inhalation phase and an exhalation phase. During the **inhalation phase**, the muscles are used to expand the size of the lungs so that outside air naturally flows inward toward the lungs. The process of inhalation is viewed as an active muscular process. During the **exhalation phase**, the lungs recoil back to their original size and naturally expel air out toward the oral/nasal cavities. The process of exhalation is viewed as a passive muscular process. An example of **active** and **passive** mus-

cular process is seen by raising your arm to the side. The process of arm raising involves active muscular movement. Lowering of the arm simply involves releasing control of these same muscles.

During quiet, restful breathing, the amount of time dedicated to each phase of the respiratory cycle is approximately equal. During the process of speaking, the respiratory cycle is dramatically altered. The inhalation phase composes only 10% of the cycle, whereas exhalation composes 90% of the cycle (Figure 3–2). The reason for this is obvious; we need to prolong exhalation in order to produce strings of words and sentences on one breath. Two ways in which we are able to prolong the exhalation phase are to: (1) inhale a larger amount of air than would normally occur during quiet breathing and (2) prolong expiratory airflow using vocal tract resistance. The balloon analogy is useful to consider in regard to understanding vocal tract resistance (Figure 3–3). Blowing up a large balloon is analogous to inhaling a large amount of air into the lungs. Upon releasing air from the balloon, one could either let the balloon naturally deflate or pinch the end of the balloon (i.e., create resistance) to prolong the expiratory airflow. Ways in which we prolong expiratory airflow for speech include vocal fold resistance (vibration) and oral cavity resistance

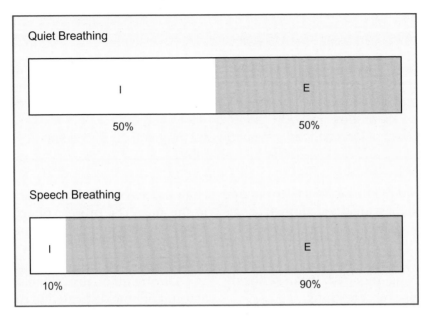

FIGURE 3–2. Comparison of the inspiratory and expiratory proportions of the respiratory cycle required for quiet breathing and speech breathing.

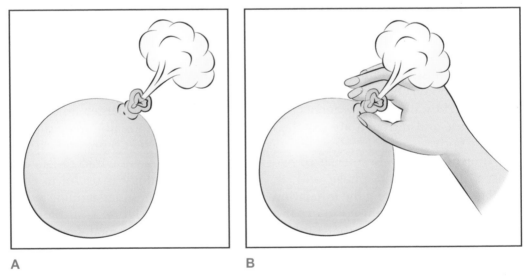

FIGURE 3–3. Balloon analogy for breathing during quiet and speech production (**A**) shows no resistance during expiratory airflow, and (**B**) shows resistance to airflow resulting in longer expiratory airflow.

(consonant articulation). These structures impede air flow and serve to alter the expiratory phase. In addition, the respiratory muscles relax gradually so that the air is not pushed out of the lungs in a short rush.

Laryngeal System

The anatomical structures that form the laryngeal system include cartilages, muscles, and bone. The **larynx** (pronounced "lare-rinks") is not a single structure but rather a framework of many structures; these major structures are shown in Figure 3–4. The largest of these is the **thyroid cartilage**, which is approximately in the middle of the larynx. The thyroid cartilage is formed by two large plates that are joined anteriorly (in the front) to create a slight bump in the neck. This bump is called the laryngeal prominence (or Adam's apple) and is most visible in adult males. The thyroid cartilage has nothing to do with the thyroid gland, which is also located in the neck. A leaf-shaped cartilage that arises from above the laryngeal prominence is the **epiglottis**. This structure does not play an important role in producing speech, although during swallowing, the tip of the epiglottis helps to direct food away from the lungs and toward the stomach. Located above the thyroid cartilage is the **hyoid bone**, which is shaped like a horseshoe and situated very high in the neck. This bone serves as a point of attachment for muscles of the tongue (from above) and for muscles of the larynx (from below). It is sometimes called a "floating bone" because it has no direct attachments to other bones. At the base of the larynx lies the **cricoid cartilage**. The cricoid cartilage is ring-shaped and rests directly on top of the trachea. Collectively, the hyoid bone, thyroid cartilage, and cricoid cartilage compose the structural framework of the larynx from top to bottom.

Inside the laryngeal framework lie the **vocal folds** (i.e., vocal cords). The technical name for the vocal folds is the thryoarytenoid muscle. The name of the muscle specifies the precise location of the vocal folds within the larynx. This is a paired muscle that makes up the right and left vocal folds. The vocal folds are attached at the front of the larynx at a point inside the thyroid cartilage (just below the Adam's apple). The vocal folds are attached at the back of the larynx to the **arytenoid cartilages**, which sit on top of the cricoid cartilage. The arytenoid cartilages swivel to allow the vocal folds to open and close, as well as shorten and lengthen. During quiet breathing, the vocal folds remain open to allow air to flow in and out of the lungs. The space between the open vocal folds is called the **glottis**. In most cases, the vocal folds remain in an open position; otherwise, we would be unable to breathe. You can purposely close the vocal folds when you wish to hold your breath. The primary reason for closing the vocal folds is to either swallow or speak. During swallowing, the vocal folds close to prevent food and liquid from entering the trachea. These materials need to be directed into the esophagus. During the production of speech, we inhale air and then close the vocal folds. The vocal folds lie stretched across the top of the trachea. As we begin to exhale, air pressure is built up under the closed vocal folds. When a sufficient amount of pressure is achieved, the vocal folds are forced open and vibrate rapidly during expiratory airflow. Think of how you can make a squealing noise by blowing through two blades of grass held between your thumbs—it is a similar action. The process of converting the air pressure from the lungs into audible vibrations is called **phonation**. The basic rate at which the vocal folds vibrate is referred to as the **fundamental frequency** (F0) of voice. It is the F0 of

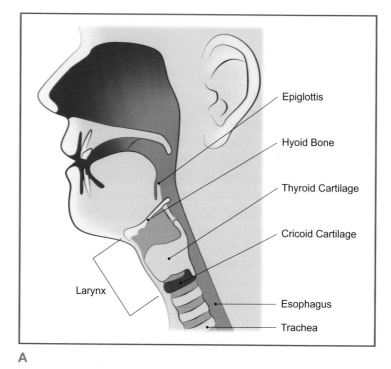

FIGURE 3–4. Anatomical features of the human laryngeal system presented as a side (lateral) view (**A**) and a view from above (superior) (**B**)..

our voice that is perceived by others as being our voice pitch. For young children, F0 is approximately 350 cycles per second (or hertz, Hz). For women and men, the average F0 is around 240 Hz and 120 Hz, respectively. The reason for the lowest F0 being found among men is due to the fact that the vocal folds are large and bulky and naturally vibrate at a slower rate compared with those that would be short and thin, as found in women and children (Figure 3–5). A visual depiction of vocal fold vibration is found in Figure 3–6.

Articulatory System

The term **articulation** refers to movement of one structure against another. Speech articulators are those structures that are in contact with another structure for the purpose of creating the sounds of speech. The major structures that form the articulatory system are shown in Figure 3–7. The system runs from the larynx to the lips and includes a combination of cavities, muscles, and boney structures. The entire articulatory system is contained within the **vocal tract**. The term tract refers to an extended area of land or space. In this case, vocal tract refers to an extended area of space within the body that is used for vocalization. The vocal tract consists of three cavities: (1) the mouth or **oral cavity**, (2) the nose or **nasal cavity**, and (3) the throat or **pharyngeal cavity**. Each of these cavities plays a role in the production of speech and also in the process of respiration, as noted earlier. The articulators within the vocal tract can be categorized as either movable or fixed.

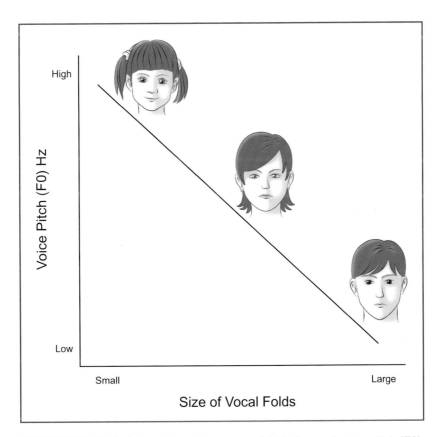

FIGURE 3–5. Relationship between vocal fold size and voice pitch (F0).

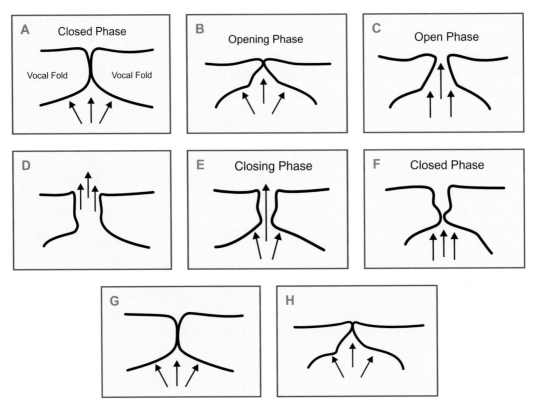

FIGURE 3–6. Frontal view of the vocal folds showing the sequential steps involved in the process of vocal fold vibration. The arrows indicate the buildup and direction of airflow from the trachea through the vocal folds.

Movable articulators are those that make contact with either another movable structure or a permanently fixed structure. The movable articulators include the lips, tongue, soft palate, pharynx, and mandible. The **lips** are two folds of tissue that surround the mouth and play a role in eating, speaking, and of course kissing. The lips are required to produce consonant sounds such as /p/, /f/, and /m/. An exception to this might be found in **ventriloquism**, which is the art of speaking without moving the lips, so that an illusion of the voice coming from another source is created.

The **tongue** probably is the most important speech articulator. This mus-cle is extremely strong, as it must move food around in our mouths as we chew. The tongue is required for the produc-tion of all vowel sounds and a major-ity of consonants such as /s/, /l/, and /th/ (e.g., the consonants in the word "sloth"). The **soft palate** (or velum) is the soft tissue located at the back of the roof of the mouth. The soft palate is dis-tinguished from the hard palate at the front of the mouth in that it does not contain bone. The very tip of the soft palate is called the **uvula**, which is a tiny "punching bag" of flesh. The soft pal-ate serves to close off the oral and nasal cavities by articulating with the back of the pharynx. This process is known as **velopharyngeal closure**. All vowels and

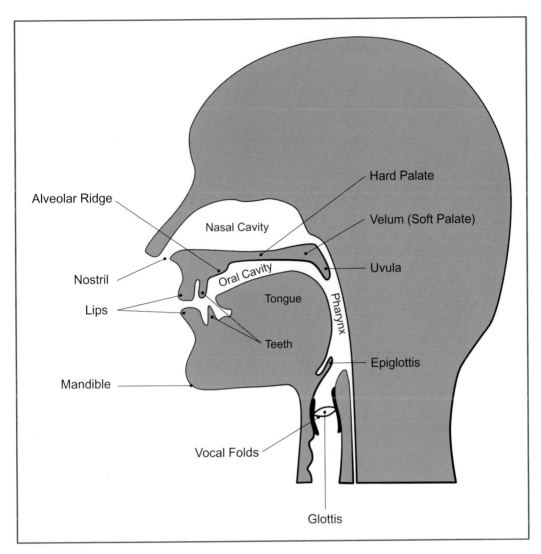

FIGURE 3–7. Anatomical features of the human speech articulatory system.

consonants, with the exception of /m/, /n/, and /ng/ (e.g., the consonants in the word "meaning") involve velopharyngeal closure. That is, most sounds are only articulated within the oral and pharyngeal cavities. If the soft palate was to remain lowered during the production of consonants and vowels, our speech would become highly nasalized because the flow of speech would be simultaneously directed through the oral and nasal cavities. The pharynx is not only a cavity within the vocal tract but a movable articulator. The muscular walls of the pharynx move and squeeze the soft palate to assist with velopharyngeal closure. The **mandible** forms the lower jaw and holds the lower teeth in place, and works as a bilateral hinge with a connection to the temporal bone on each side of the skull. It serves as a "fine tuner" of speech articulation and moves continuously during typical speech production. Although

---

FYI

The term **glossectomy** refers to surgical removal of all or part of the tongue. A glossectomy is performed to treat cancer of the tongue. Removing the tongue is indicated if the patient has a cancer that does not respond to other forms of treatment. In most cases, however, only part of the tongue is removed (partial glossectomy). Many people are still able to produce speech even when a considerable portion of the tongue is removed.

---

it is not imperative for the mandible to move to produce speech, when it does, the quality of speech markedly improves. An example of this fine tuning is demonstrated in what is known as **pipe speech**. Pipe speech (speaking with a tobacco pipe clenched between the teeth) imposes constraints on jaw movement although speech can still be articulated. Once the pipe is removed from the mouth, speech becomes noticeably clearer.

Fixed articulators are those that cannot be moved by muscles. They include the hard palate, alveolar ridge, and teeth. The **hard palate** is the front portion of the roof of the mouth that is made of bone, and also serves as the base of the skull. It is used for the articulation of sounds such as /sh/ (as in the word "shoe"). The **alveolar ridge** is located on the roof of the mouth between the upper teeth and hard palate. It contains the sockets of the teeth and can be felt with the tongue in the area right behind the upper teeth, where there is a change in the angle of the roof of the mouth. Speech sounds such as /t/, /d/, and /z/ (e.g., the consonants in the phrase "tie dyes") are articulated with the tongue at the alveolar ridge. The **teeth** are also involved in the articulation of speech sounds. The upper and lower central incisors (i.e., front teeth) are necessary for articula-

tion of consonants such as /v/, /f/, and /th/ (e.g., as in the words "vie" and "faith").

THE PROCESS OF SPEECH PRODUCTION

As noted in Chapters 1 and 2, the process of speech production involves the encoding of a message. The starting point for speech encoding is the brain. The centers of the brain responsible for generating language organize the message to be spoken and send neural commands to the anatomical structures involved in speech production. The details of brain anatomy and the nervous system are provided in Chapter 9; however, it is important to recognize that without the brain's control of the respiratory, laryngeal, and articulatory systems, speech production would be impaired, if not impossible.

The normal process of speech production entails a transformation of aerodynamic into acoustic energy. The anatomical and physiological processes involved in the generation of speech can be depicted in the formula $S * T = P$. The S symbol refers to the **source**. To produce speech, there needs to be a source of energy that provides the driving force behind the act of uttering a sound. The anatomical system that provides the source for speech production is the respiratory system. The *T* symbol refers to a **transfer function**. The concept of a transfer function is similar to that of a filter, in which the original source is altered or transformed. In the case of speech production, the original source (i.e., the air flowing upward from the respiratory system) is transformed by movements from the **laryngeal system** and the **articulatory system**. The final symbol in the formula, *P*, refers to the **product** in the generation of speech. The end-product reflects the contributions of the respiratory system, laryngeal system, and articulatory system to the acoustic generation of sound. This acoustic energy is ultimately perceived by a listener as words and sentences. An anatomical representation of S * T = P is provided in Figure 3–8.

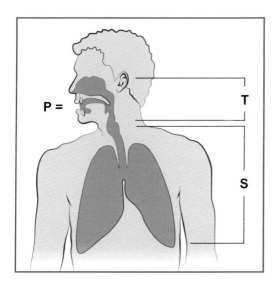

FIGURE 3–8. The process of speech production according to the S * T = P formula. *S* refers to the source of speech, namely, the respiratory system. *T* refers to the transfer function of the vocal tract involving the laryngeal and articulatory systems. *P* is the end product of the contributions from the various systems.

HEARING ANATOMY

The act of hearing is referred to as **audition**. The anatomical aspects of audition can be divided into two main components, the **peripheral auditory system** and the **central auditory system**. The peripheral auditory system consists of structures spanning from the outer ear to the auditory nerve. The central auditory system begins at a point beyond the auditory nerve and terminates at the auditory centers in the brain. A basic survey and description of the structure and function of the peripheral auditory system and central auditory system is provided.

Peripheral Auditory System

Outer Ear

A depiction of the outer ear, as well as the entire peripheral auditory system is shown in Figure 3–9. The outer ear consists of two parts: (1) auricle and (2) the ear canal, or the external auditory meatus. The **auricle**, sometimes called the **pinna**, is the most visible part of the entire auditory system and is composed of elastic cartilage (Figure 3–10). Some of the prominent landmarks of the auricle include the **helix**,

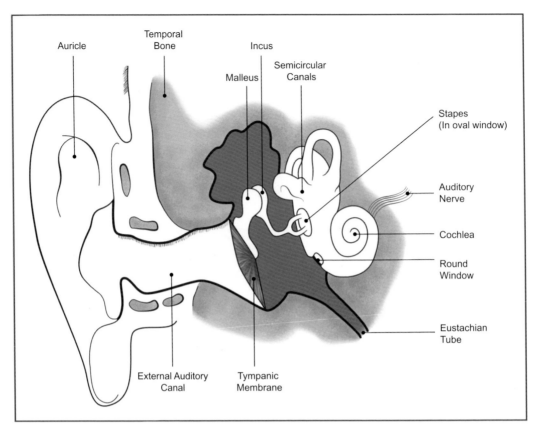

FIGURE 3–9. Cross-sectional view of the peripheral auditory system showing some anatomical detail of the outer, middle, and inner ear structures.

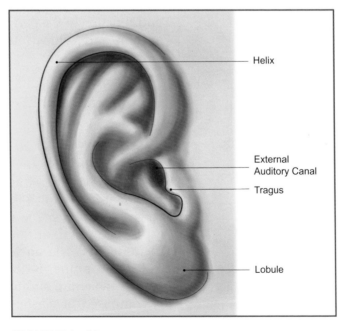

FIGURE 3–10. Landmarks of the auricle.

which is the outer rim. The **tragus** is the small cartilaginous notch that is in front of the external opening of the ear. The **lobule** is the dangling fleshy part of the auricle and is the location where ears are normally pierced. The auricle serves two purposes. The first is to protect the middle ear from damage, particularly the eardrum. The auricle also serves to help eliminate **front-back confusion** by assisting in distinguishing sounds that arise from in front of the listener from those that arise from behind the listener. Movement of the auricle is particularly advanced in several types of animals, which developed as a means of detecting predators. One need simply watch the ears of a dog or cat when presented with sounds coming from various directions. As humans, our auricles have evolved into fixed, immobile structures. However, it is not uncommon to find an individual who is hard of hearing to cup a hand behind the ear as an aid to improved localization of sound. The **external auditory meatus** is a 2.5-cm canal that runs from the auricle to the eardrum. The term meatus refers to a natural opening or canal. The outer one third of the canal, that is nearest to the auricle, is made of elastic cartilage. The inner two thirds of the canal are carved into the **temporal bone** of the skull. The entire canal is lined with skin and very fine hair. The ear canal also contains glands known as ceruminous glands. These glands secrete a substance called **cerumen**, commonly referred to as earwax. Cerumen plays an important role in preventing the ear canal from drying out. Cerumen also has been found to be useful in preventing intruders, such as insects, from entering the ear because they find this waxy substance to be noxious. The function of the external auditory meatus is to funnel sound toward the eardrum. In addition, the general shape of the external auditory meatus serves to provide a slight "boost" in loudness for high-frequency sounds, which are found to resonate in the canal.

Middle Ear

The middle ear is an air-filled space located entirely within the temporal bone. The major structures of the middle ear include the tympanic membrane, three miniature bones, two muscles, and the eustachian tube. The **tympanic membrane** (or eardrum) is a thin, tough, fibrous membrane that spreads out across the ear canal. The tympanic membrane is a very durable and tightly stretched membrane that vibrates as incoming sound pressure waves reach it. Suspended within the middle ear space is a series of three small bones that form a bridge between the tympanic membrane and the inner ear. These three bones are the **malleus** (or hammer), **incus** (or anvil), and **stapes** (or stirrup). They are the smallest bones in the human body and make up what is known as the **ossicular chain**, and each bone is an ossicle (from the Latin word *ossiculum* for diminutive bone). The malleus is in contact with the tympanic membrane. At the other end of the chain, the stapes is inserted into the oval window of the cochlea (inner ear). Collectively, these bones provide a mechanical link between the outer ear and the inner ear.

Two tiny muscles are located within the middle ear and make contact with the ossicular chain. The **tensor tympani** muscle runs from the front wall of the middle ear cavity and attaches to the malleus bone. The **stapedius** muscle runs from the back wall of the middle ear cavity and attaches to the stapes

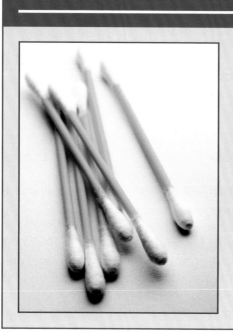
bone. These muscles provide a form of protection to the inner ear by stiffening the ossicular chain in the presence of very loud sounds, typically in excess of 90 decibels. In essence, the ossicular chain is immobilized from functioning normally and causes a decrease in the loudness of sounds entering the inner ear. The contraction of these middle ear muscles is involuntary and known as the **acoustic reflex** (see also Chapter 13). The **eustachian tube** runs from the middle ear space down toward the upper region of the pharynx (Figure 3–11). The function of the eustachian tube is to protect, aerate, and drain the middle ear. It also serves to equalize middle ear air pressure with environmental air pressure. The eustachian tube is normally closed and opens only under changes in pressure. When your ears "pop" on an airplane, the reason is that the eustachian tube has briefly opened and equalized air pressure. In adults,

the eustachian tube is approximately 35 mm long and runs from the middle ear to the pharynx along a 45° angle. In young children, the tube measures only 17 mm and is nearly horizontal in angle. This nearly flat angle in young children makes for poor drainage of fluid from the middle ear, and predisposes young children to middle ear infections.

Inner Ear

Similar to the middle ear, the inner ear is housed entirely within the temporal bone of the skull. Whereas the middle ear is an air-filled space, the inner ear is a fluid-filled space. The inner ear consists of two main organs. The **vestibular apparatus** serves as the body's balance organ and the **cochlea** serves as the body's hearing organ. A key structure in the vestibular apparatus is the **semicircular canals**, which work with the brain to sense, maintain, and regain

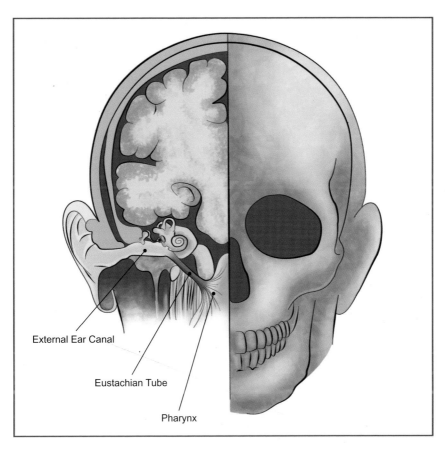

FIGURE 3–11. Depiction of the anatomical location of the eustachian tube.

balance and a sense of where the body and its parts are positioned in space. Most causes of dizziness are inner-ear problems associated with the vestibular apparatus. Specialty occupations such as astronauts or fighter pilots require an unusually intact vestibular apparatus that allows them to function during potentially dizzying environmental situations.

The cochlea has an appearance that is somewhat like that of a small snail. Indeed the term cochlea is Greek for the word snail shell. The cochlea has approximately 2.75 turns in humans. The largest turn (that nearest the stapes) is the **basal** end of the cochlea and the smallest turn is called the **apical** end.

A helpful way to visualize the cochlea is to examine the structure from the inside. A cross-sectional view (Figure 3–12) reveals that the cochlea consists of three compartments. The upper compartment is called the **scala vestibuli**, the lower compartment is the **scala tympani**, and the middle compartment is the **scala media** (or cochlear duct). At the apex of the cochlea is a small hole called the **helicotrema**, which connects the scala vestibuli and scala tympani compartments. Both compartments are filled with a fluid called **perilymph**. Perilymph is a fluid that is comparable in density with plasma or cerebrospinal fluid. The scala media is filled with a thick fluid

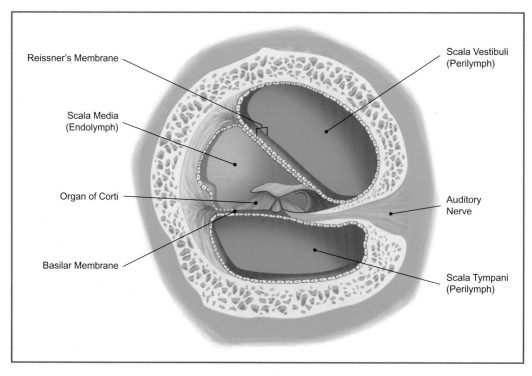

FIGURE 3–12. Cross-sectional view of the cochlea and associated landmarks.

In the figure, the following labels appear:

Reissner's Membrane

Scala Media (Endolymph)

Organ of Corti

Basilar Membrane

Scala Vestibuli (Perilymph)

Auditory Nerve

Scala Tympani (Perilymph)

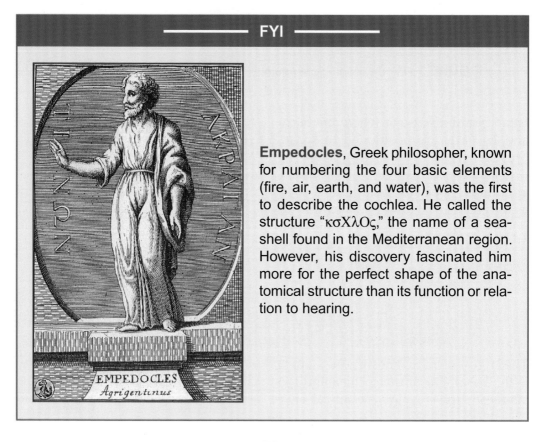

Empedocles, Greek philosopher, known for numbering the four basic elements (fire, air, earth, and water), was the first to describe the cochlea. He called the structure "κσΧλΟς," the name of a seashell found in the Mediterranean region. However, his discovery fascinated him more for the perfect shape of the anatomical structure than its function or relation to hearing.

EMPEDOCLES
Agrigentinus

substance called **endolymph**, which is a unique fluid unlike that found anywhere else in the body.

The **organ of Corti** lies within the scala media of the cochlea. This organ is responsible for converting the mechanical sound energy of the middle ear into electrical impulses. The organ of Corti sits on the **basilar membrane**, which is the wall that separates the scala tympani from the scala media. The organ of Corti consists of four rows of **hair cells** that run the entire length of the cochlea from basal to apical ends. In total, there are approximately 20,000 hair cells. At the top of each cell, a minute fiber from the auditory nerve is attached. These hair cells sense the sounds received from the middle ear and transmit the signals to the auditory nerve that, in turn, forwards the signal to the brain. A fascinating feature of the organ of Corti is its

tonotopic organization (Figure 3–13). When sounds of varying pitch (Hz) enter the cochlea, the hair cells in the cochlea do not all respond in the same way as different regions of the cochlea are selectively responsive to different frequencies of sound. The basal end of the cochlea vibrates most at high-frequency tones, and the apical end vibrates most at low-frequency tones. Assuming that each hair cell reflects a specific frequency, the normal range of hearing extends from 20 Hz up to 20,000 Hz. Research has shown that humans are unable to perceive sounds lower than 20 Hz. The **auditory nerve** is a bundle of over 30,000 nerve fibers that carries hearing and balance information from the inner ear to the brain. The nerve consists of the cochlear branch, carrying information about hearing to the brain, and the vestibular branch, carrying

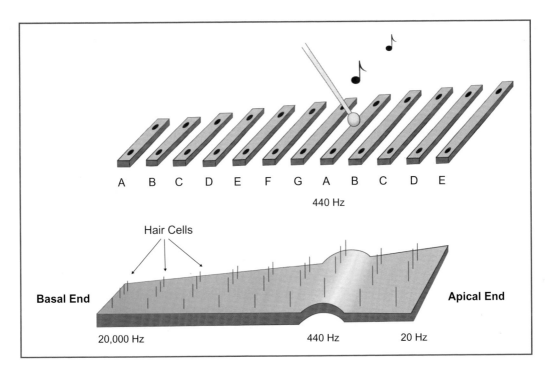

FIGURE 3–13. Schematic representation of tonotopic organization found within the cochlea (basilar membrane).

FYI

Echolocation, also called biosonar, is the process of determining the distance and direction of objects by using sound. Animals such as bats, shrews, dolphins, and whales emit pulses of high-frequency sound that bounce off things in their surroundings like insects, branches, or fish. The reflected sounds, or echoes, are picked up by their sensitive ears to locate food or obstacles in darkness, such as in caves and in the ocean.

---

information about balance. The fibers from the auditory nerve extend into the brainstem, where its fibers make contact with the cochlear nucleus, the next stage of the auditory system.

Central Auditory System

Once the electrical impulses generated in the cochlea are transmitted through the auditory nerve, the nerve fibers carry information about the sound to the brainstem. Figure 3–14 shows a simplified diagram of the central auditory system. All of the nerve fibers from the auditory nerve terminate at the **cochlear nucleus**, which is located in the medulla region of the brainstem. The cochlear nucleus is one of the most studied structures of the central auditory system in humans and animals and reflects a high concentration of neurons. Beyond the cochlear nucleus, the auditory system is characterized by a neural pathway in which a majority of the nerve fibers cross the midline of the brainstem. Prior to this crossing over, sound that entered one ear involved anatomical structures on the same side of the head. The auditory pathway courses upward through higher regions of the brainstem, including the pons and midbrain. At various locations along the way, the pathway terminates at clusters of **brainstem**

nuclei. Eventually, the auditory pathway exits the brainstem and enters the temporal lobe of the brain. The precise location in the temporal lobe where the final process of hearing takes place is the **auditory cortex** (or Heschl's gyrus). Sound entering the left ear is ultimately processed in the auditory cortex of the right hemisphere and vice versa.

THE PROCESS OF HEARING

Each part of the ear serves a specific purpose in the act of detecting and interpreting sound. The usual manner by which humans hear is via an airborne signal. Once sound is generated, it travels through the air in a disturbance called a sound wave. The outer ear serves to collect and channel the sound wave toward the middle ear. Thus, its function is to act as a transmission line in carrying the signal from one point to another. The sound is then transformed into mechanical energy by the tympanic membrane of the middle ear and the ossicular chain. The mechanical vibrations in the middle ear are an exact copy of the original airborne sound wave vibrations. As the vibrations reach the last bone in the ossicular chain (stapes),

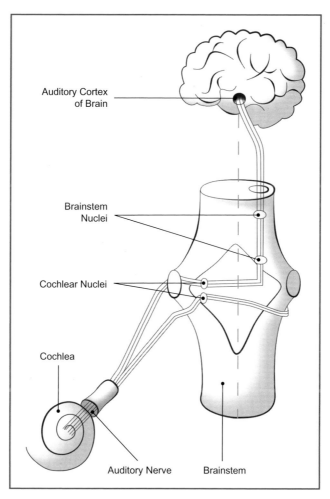

FIGURE 3–14. Simplified depiction of the anatomical structures composing the central auditory system.

they enter the fluid-filled inner ear via the oval window of the cochlea. The mechanical vibrations of the stapes at the oval window are then **transduced** into a hydraulic wave, called a traveling wave. This wave enters the cochlea and displaces (stimulates) hair cells within the cochlea. The stimulation of specific hair cells is converted to nerve impulses that are an exact match to the frequencies composing the original airborne sound wave. The transduction of mechanical energy to nerve impulses continues all the way to the brain. The physical characteristics of the original sound are preserved at every energy change along the way until the sound becomes one the brain can recognize and process. Figure 3–15 provides a simplified breakdown of the process of hearing. Although this process is viewed as a linear (left to right) one, it is worth noting that there are various points in the hearing process where the original sound is channeled backward. However, this is beyond the scope of this introductory chapter.

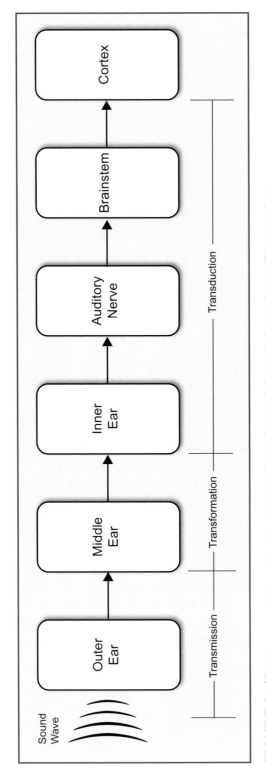

FIGURE 3–15. Process of hearing showing the flow of sound through the entire auditory system.

HISTORIC ASPECTS OF ANATOMY AND PHYSIOLOGY

Henry Gray (1827–1861) was an English anatomist and surgeon (Figure 3–16). His most famous accomplishment occurred in 1858, when he published *Gray's Anatomy: Descriptive and Surgical.* Intended for medical students, physicians, and surgeons, the first edition of the book contained 750 pages and 363 figures. **Henry Vandyke Carter** (1831–1897) assisted Gray by providing the illustrations for the book. In 1861, at the age of 34, Gray contracted smallpox from his nephew and died. *Gray's Anatomy* has lived on as the authoritative anatomy text and an indispensable teaching tool. The book has more than double the number of pages from its first appearance in 1858. Details about

speech and hearing anatomy can be found in the book. Gray accomplished much as a young man; imagine what he could have accomplished had he lived a full life.

Gray's contribution to the fields of anatomy and physiology were immense and covered the entire range of the human body. A number of individuals made contributions that more directly impacted the fields of audiology and speech-language pathology. For example, **Bartolomeo Eustachi** (1510–1574) was a 16th-century Italian physician (Figure 3–17). In 1562 and 1563, he produced a remarkable series of reports (treatises) on various parts of the body including the kidneys, teeth, and the ear. In his report concerning the ear, he provided an accurate description of the tensor tympani and stapedius muscles, as well as the *tuba auditiva*, which has since been referred to as the eustachian

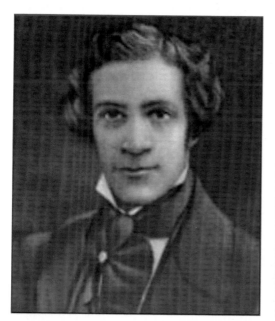

FIGURE 3–16. Henry Gray, an accomplished anatomist and surgeon in the early 1800s.

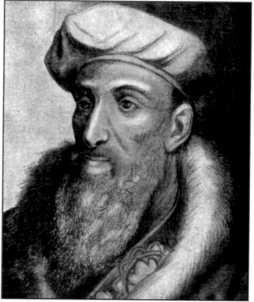

FIGURE 3–17. Bartolomeo Eustachi, the 16th-century Italian physician who studied anatomical features of the ear.

tube. The discovery by Eustachi of the connection between the middle ear and the pharynx is thought to have later inspired Shakespeare to write his play *Hamlet*, a story in which Hamlet's father is killed by poison poured into his ear.

Antoine Ferrein (1693–1769) was a French anatomist who was the first person to coin the term vocal cords. In 1741, while dissecting corpses, he discovered in the center of the larynx two muscular shelves that ran horizontally (front to back). He concluded that speech and song were produced entirely by the vibration of these bands of muscles caused by air being blown outward from the lungs. He compared the structures with that of a violin, in which the strings or "cords" work to produce sound. Vocal fold is the modern term for vocal cord; the change in terminology came about because of a better understanding of the anatomy and function of the larynx. Rather than looking and functioning like a stringed instrument, the vocal folds more closely resemble a lip of tissue.

Alfonso Corti (1822–1876) was born in Italy (Figure 3–18). As a medical student, he enrolled first at the University of Pavia, and later at the University of Vienna where he became interested in the field of anatomy. Corti began his scientific career studying the cardiovascular systems of reptiles. Later he turned his attention to the mammalian auditory system. In the years 1850–1851, he worked in the laboratory of Albert von Kölliker at the University of Würzburg (Germany) and examined more than 200 cochleas from cats, dogs, pigs, sheep, rabbits, and rats. It was there that he developed new coloring techniques in microscopic anatomy, which enabled him to describe individual components inside the cochlea. Prior to

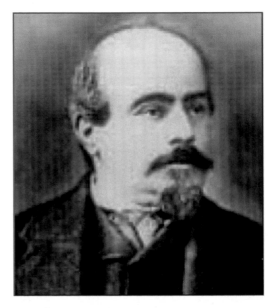

FIGURE 3–18. Alfonso Corti provided detailed anatomical descriptions of the inner ear.

this time, it was notoriously difficult to preserve inner ear structures because they quickly deteriorated once removed from their fluid-filled compartments. In 1851, he published a paper describing a structure located on the basilar membrane of the cochlea containing hair cells that convert sound vibrations into nerve impulses. This structure came to be known as the organ of Corti. His work was the starting point of our knowledge of the cochlea.

Sir Victor Negus (1887–1974) was born in London and received his medical education in laryngology at King's College Hospital in 1912 (Figure 3–19). He had a long and meritorious career in laryngology. He was a pioneer in detailing the anatomy of the human and animal larynx. In 1929, he published a monumental work entitled *The Mechanism of the Larynx* that had a profound influence on laryngologists, anatomists, and many other scientists throughout the world. In this publication, he was able to demonstrate which structures of the human larynx serve to differentiate man from other species.

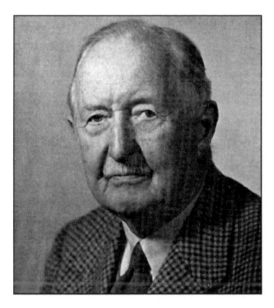

FIGURE 3–19. Sir Victor Negus, a pioneer in detailing the anatomy of the human and animal larynx.

The work of Negus on the structure of the larynx eventually contributed to the development of theories regarding the evolution of man and speech. In particular, Phillip Lieberman and Edmund Crelin (1971) argued that man's need to produce a wide range of sounds for communication led to the development of a unique two-tube (oral and pharyngeal) vocal tract. The two tubes are reflected in a clear separation between the oral cavity and the larynx, which rests low in the neck. All other animal species have a single-tube vocal tract, reflected by the close approximation between the oral cavity and larynx (Figure 3–20). This single-tube anatomy allows for easy ingestion of food and drink with no danger of food entering the lungs. This anatomical configuration also permits breathing to occur simultaneously. Anthropologists believe a single-tube vocal tract is a form of "survival" anatomy that allows animals to smell danger while eating. The two-tube vocal tract of adult humans is less efficient for eating,

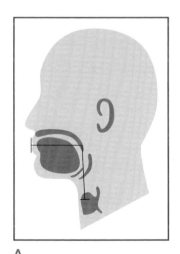
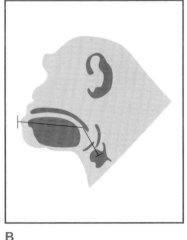
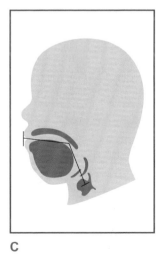

A   B   C

FIGURE 3–20. Comparison of the vocal tract anatomy of an adult human, nonhuman primate, and human infant. Only adult humans have a distinct two-tube vocal tract, whereas nonprimates and human infants have a sloping one-tube vocal tract.

and actually makes humans more susceptible to choking because of the large gap between the oral cavity and the esophagus. Additionally, adult humans cannot breathe and drink simultaneously. Most interesting, human infants do not show a two-tube vocal tract at birth but rather a single-tube vocal tract. With the larynx located high in the neck, it is not possible for liquids to enter the airway, which is what makes it possible for an infant child to suckle the nipple while still being able to breathe. As the child grows, the larynx slowly descends to form a two-tube vocal tract. Among animals, the single-tube vocal tract does not permit the production of a wide range of sounds, although the two-tube vocal tract allows for a wide range of speech sounds, prompting theorists that the lowering of the larynx in man is an anatomical specialization for human speech.

Willard R. Zemlin (1929–1998; Figure 3–21), born in Minnesota, made an enormous contribution to the field of speech and hearing science through his work in basic anatomy and physiology. Zemlin was a faculty member in the department of speech and hearing science at the University of Illinois. He was the first speech-language pathologist in the world to develop a textbook on the anatomy and physiology of the speech and hearing mechanism that was designed for students in communication disorders. Based on his own dissection work, Zemlin set about detailing essential anatomy, using line drawings and photographs. The result was the publication of the classic textbook, *Speech and Hearing Science, Anatomy and Physiology*, first published in 1964. The book continues to be in widespread use.

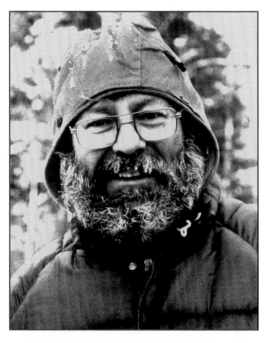

FIGURE 3–21. Willard Zemlin, who was interested in the anatomy and physiology of the hearing and speech mechanisms. From the Willard R. Zemlin Memorial website. Permission granted by Eileen Zemlin.

CULTURAL CONSIDERATIONS AND ANATOMY AND PHYSIOLOGY

It is no surprise that people come in all shapes and sizes. This observation led to the development of **anthropometry**, which is the scientific study of the measurements of the human body. The field was established to assist in understanding human physical variations and aid in anthropological classification. The term is derived from the Greek terms *anthropos*, meaning "man," and *metron*, meaning "measure." Anthropometry was first introduced in the late 19th century to the field of criminology, as a supposedly useful means of identifying criminals based on their physical characteristics. Paris police clerk Alphonse Bertillon (1853–1914) devised a system that was used to identify people held in police custody, based on classification of facial and bodily characteristics, and the description of scars and tattoos. Eventually, it was discovered that use of physical characteristics as a form of criminal profiling was not effective and served to perpetuate social racism. Probably the most infamous abuse of anthropometrical research occurred in the years leading up to, and surrounding, World War II. Anthropometric studies performed by German Nazis were used in the classification of Aryan and non-Aryan races, and led to the decimation of countless individuals who did not fit into established categories.

Putting these extreme examples of anthropometric misuse aside, contemporary anthropometry studies continue to be conducted for various purposes (Figure 3–22). One particular body measurement that is currently used in criminology is fingerprinting. Academic anthropologists often investigate the evolutionary changes in human body shape and size, stemming from ancestors from different environmental settings. For example, there is undisputable evidence that human populations exhibit similar climatic variation to other large-bodied mammals, such as the finding that indigenous individuals who reside in colder climates tend to be larger than individuals residing in warmer climates and that individuals in cold climates will tend to have shorter, thicker limbs than those in warm climates. Health practitioners use body measurements as an index of physiological development

and nutritional status. Determining a child's weight at a given age provides information about the child's overall nutritional status. Measuring a child's weight and height can be used to detect acute malnutrition. Measuring mid-upper arm circumference provides an index of muscle wastage. Measurement of skin fold thickness is related to the amount of subcutaneous fat as an index of over- or undernutrition.

Differences in body shape and size are also a consideration in the field of disabilities, including communication disorders. Anthropometry of people with disabilities, such as those confined to a wheelchair, is important in the design of home facilities, as well as work spaces. Anthropometry has been used with increasing frequency to characterize syndromes and to establish ranges of variation within syndromes. There is research revealing that approximately one third of children with autism have macrocephaly (i.e., large skull) and indicating that autism is sometimes associated with abnormal physical development (Woodhouse et al., 1996). Noting anatomical differences in the structure and function of a person's oral-peripheral speech mechanism is a routine consideration in the speech-language pathologist's assessment of communication disorders. Finally, audiologists are routinely confronted with anatomical differences in ear anatomy that are a major consideration in the appropriate fitting of hearing aids. Clearly, anatomical and physical differences between people across all walks of life are the norm rather than exception. Anthropometry has evolved to serve a useful role in the clinical evaluation and management of individuals with known and suspected disabilities.

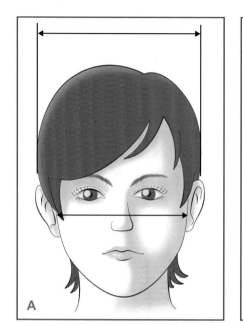

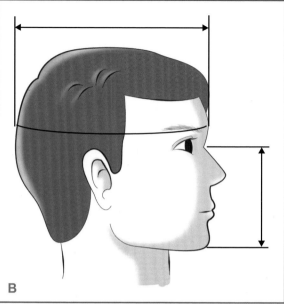

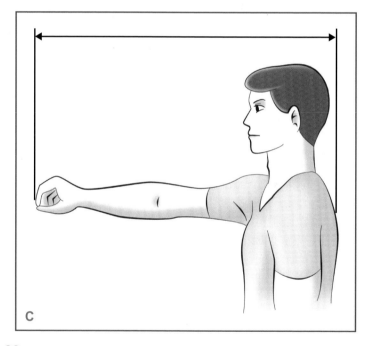

FIGURE 3–22. Examples of anthropometry for various parts of the body. *continues*

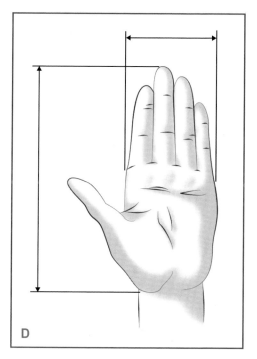

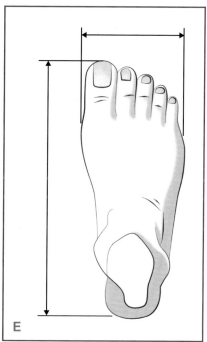

FIGURE 3–22. *continued*

Brain Imaging

The process of neuroimaging allows scientists with a noninvasive view of the brain's anatomy and physiology. There are a variety of techniques available to researchers such as **computerized tomography** (CT), **electroencehpalography** (EEG), **positron emission tomography** (PET), and **magnetic resonance imaging** (MRI). Each technique provides a specialized view of the brain. The use of MRI has become perhaps the most important tool for evaluating regions of the brain affected by injury. A variation of MRI is known as diffu-

sion MRI. A diffusion MRI looks at how water molecules move around within the brain. The way these molecules move around is dependent upon the structure of the brain. So diffusion MRI is a very sensitive measure of brain activity occurring at a cellular level. Research is currently underway using diffusion MRI to examine the unique brain pathways that help support speech and language. Such information may serve to help clinicians better understand the full extent of brain injuries that affect speech and language, and could lead to better treatment programs (Turken & Dronkers, 2011).

Ossicular Chain Replacement

One of the continuing goals of scientists and engineers is to develop technologies that reduce the severity of physical disabilities. An example of this technology can be found in regard to hearing loss resulting from middle ear defects. In severe cases, the treatment of middle ear defects can now be treated with either a partial or total ossicular replacement prostheses (PORPs and TORPs, respectively). The ability to replace existing middle ear bones with artificial bones was made possible through the development of the surgical microscope and the development of ear-microsurgery. The various design aspects of ossicular prostheses have presented their own unique challenges to the engineers involved in the development of these products. Currently, the primary consideration that goes into the PORP or TORP is that they be of approximately the same weight as the original ear bones, as this is of vital importance for a prosthesis to function properly. Such implants typically result in substantial improvement in the hearing of those who receive them, although current technology does not allow for the complete restoration of a person's hearing. Through continued development, it is possible that use of ossicular implants might someday completely correct one's hearing.

Hair Cell Regeneration in the Cochlea

A key anatomical feature of the cochlea is the thousands of hair cells that run along the entire length of the basilar membrane. These hair cells serve to transmit electrical impulses to the brain that represent frequencies as high as 20,000 Hz. At present, once cochlear hair cells are damaged, their function cannot be restored, so the death of a hair cell ultimately results in an irreversible hearing loss. The greater the number

of hair cells destroyed, the greater the hearing loss. The loss of hair cells can result from prolonged exposure to loud noise, drugs, or disease. However, it has been known for 20 years that hair cells can be regenerated in cold-blooded vertebrates. Researchers discovered that, after being exposed to loud sounds, birds have the remarkable ability to regenerate and replace dead hair cells and return their hearing to near normal, leading to the question, "Why can't humans also regenerate damaged hair cells?" Unfortunately, hair cell regeneration is not as simple as it might seem. Human ears are very complex organs, so it is no surprise that hair cell regeneration is also a complex process. The most promising area of research is the controversial method of using **stem cells** to replace the destroyed hair cells. Human stem cells would be most effective for this process by coaxing new hair cells to grow. Hair cell regeneration as a treatment for hearing loss is still years away, but researchers are making important gains in demonstrating the likelihood of using this technology to improve hearing (Stone & Rubel, 2013).

ANATOMY AND PHYSIOLOGY ON THE WORLD WIDE WEB

Listed below are websites that provide further information on the topic of anatomy and physiology of speech and hearing. At the time of publication, each website was freely accessible.

Bartleby.com Edition of *Gray's Anatomy of the Human Body*
http://www.bartleby.com/107/

W. R. Zemlin Memorial Website
http://zemlin.shs.uiuc.edu/

How the Ear Functions Video
http://archive.org/details/
HowtheEa1940

The Larynx and Voice Video
http://archive.org/details/
larynx_and_the_voice

STUDY QUESTIONS

1. List and describe the three subsystems of speech anatomy.
2. Who are some of the pioneers that contributed to our understanding of hearing and speech anatomy and physiology?
3. List and describe the two main components of hearing anatomy.
4. Explain the processes of speech production.
5. Explain the process of hearing.

REFERENCES

Lieberman, P., & Crelin, E. S. (1971). On the speech of Neanderthal man. *Linguistic Inquiry, 2*, 203–222.

Stone, J., & Rubel, E. (2013, January). A hair cell away from hearing repair? *ASHA Leader*, 38.

Turken, A., & Dronkers, N. (2011, February). The neural architecture of the language comprehension network: Converging evidence from lesion and connectivity analyses. *Frontiers in Systems Neuroscience*.

Woodhouse, W., Bailey, A., Rutter, M., Bolton, P., Baird, G., & LeCouteur, A. (1996). Head circumference in autism and other pervasive developmental disorders. *Journal of Child Psychology and Psychiatry, 37*, 665–671.

SECTION 2

Developmental Communication Disorders

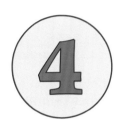

CHILD LANGUAGE DISORDERS

OBJECTIVES

After reading this chapter, the student should be able to:

■ Distinguish between speech, language, and communication.

■ Differentiate elements of language (phonology, morphology, syntax, semantics, and pragmatics).

■ Understand basic concepts of each element of language, such as *morpheme* or *phoneme*.

■ Explain the course of normal spoken language development.

■ Understand the distinctions between different disabilities that are characterized by a language disorder, including specific language impairment, intellectual disabilities, and autism spectrum disorders.

■ Know the difference between language disabilities and cultural language differences.

■ Understand the definition and implications of a language disorder.

■ Understand basic principles of formal, standardized language assessment.

■ Understand basic principles of informal language assessment.

INTRODUCTION

Language is the expression of human communication through which information can be experienced, explained, and shared. This sharing is based on a system of signs, sounds, and gestures that convey meaning. Language provides the foundation upon which communication, problem solving, and synthesizing knowledge take place. A disorder of language, therefore, can have a profound impact on a person's ability to learn and function competently in the world. A language disorder is impairment in the ability to understand and/or use words in a communicative context. Some characteristics of language disorders include improper use of words and their meanings, inability to express ideas, inappropriate grammatical patterns, reduced vocabulary, and an inability to follow directions. Children may hear or see a word but not be able to understand its meaning. They may have trouble getting others to understand what they are trying to communicate. Concern regarding a child's language development is one of the most common reasons for parents of preschool children to seek the advice of their family doctor. Although some children initially may take longer than normal to acquire language, they may show rapid improvements. For other children, their language difficulties may be more persistent, requiring intervention by a speech-language pathologist. A long-term deficit in language can adversely affect an individual's academic progress, as well as social relationships. The focus of this chapter is to provide background on normal aspects of language development and then to use this information as a basis for describing child language disorders.

TERMINOLOGY AND DEFINITIONS

Language is complex and involves multiple domains, such as nonverbal language, oral language (i.e., listening and speaking), and written language (i.e., reading and writing). A classic framework for describing the various strands of language was proposed by **Lois Bloom** and **Margaret Lahey** in 1978 (Figure 4–1). They divided language domains into three areas of skill that contribute to overall communicative competence. These skills consist of: (1) **language form**, (2) **language content**, and (3) **language use**. The form of language is created through the features of phonology, morphology, and syntax. **Phonology** refers to the knowledge a person has of the consonant and vowels sounds in the language. Although the number of sounds that exist in a language is limited, a nearly endless num-

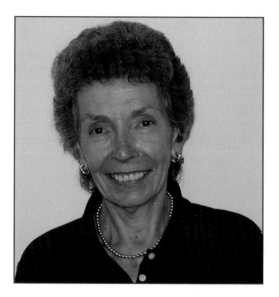

FIGURE 4–1. Lois Bloom developed a framework for describing the various strands of language. Permission granted by L. Bloom.

ber of words can be constructed from these sounds.

Morphology refers to the smallest meaningful unit of language. Morphology involves the stringing together of sounds (phonemes) and includes such structures as prefixes and suffixes. Morphemes are of two types, free morphemes and bound morphemes. A **free morpheme** is a stand-alone word. Examples of free morphemes are *play*, *safe*, and *elephant*. Each of these words contains only one morpheme because they cannot be divided into smaller units and still retain their meaning. Examples of **bound morphemes** include prefixes and suffixes, such as those attached to the words: *playing*, *unsafe*, and *elephants*. Each of these words contains two morphemes, and each morpheme within the word contributes uniquely to the word's overall meaning. However, the morphemes "ing," "un," and "s" have no meaning in and of themselves unless they are attached, or bound, to a free morpheme. **Syntax** refers to the rules used in combining words to make a sentence. As with the sounds of language, the rules for combining words to structure a sentence in a particular language are finite. For example, the rules of English require that a noun occurs before a verb in a sentence, such as, *"He is running,"* as opposed to *"Running is he."*

The content of language includes the meanings of individual words and words in combination. Another name for language content is **semantics**. The words we use symbolize concepts. If there was no meaning to what was being said, there would be no point in using language. The meaning of words constrains how words may or may not be used together. For example, the sentence, "I saw the tree swimming in the lake" would make little sense, although it is syntactically correct. Con-

tent involves knowledge of vocabulary and the relationships between words. Words can have denotative or connotative meaning. **Denotative** is the literal (dictionary) meaning of a word. **Connotative** involves use of words for a meaning other than their literal meaning. For example, the denotative meaning of the word *mother* is female parent. The connotative meaning of mother could evoke alternative meanings such as *love* and *security*. Other nonliteral aspects of language content can be found in **idioms**, such as, "If the shoe fits, wear it" or "It's raining cats and dogs."

The final component in the Bloom and Lahey model is language use. Another term for language use is **pragmatics**. The pragmatic functions of language involve the use of language in context for a particular purpose or reason. Pragmatics entails three major communication skills:

1. *Using* language for different purposes, such as greeting (e.g., hello, goodbye), informing (e.g., I'm going to get a cookie), demanding (e.g., Give me a cookie), and requesting (e.g., Could I please have a cookie?);
2. *Changing* language according to the needs of a listener or situation, such as talking differently to a baby than to an adult, or speaking differently in a classroom than on a playground; and
3. *Following* rules for conversations, such as taking turns in a conversation, introducing topics of conversation, staying on topic, the physical proximity to/from a speaker, and the use of facial expressions and eye contact.

Collectively, the skills of language form, content, and use compose our language competence.

LANGUAGE DEVELOPMENT

Knowledge of the normal, developmental features of language is important for determining the existence of a language disorder. The area of expressive language development, particularly the form of language, has been studied extensively over the past 50 years. Some of the most well-established features of normal language are described next as they occur across the period of infancy to school-age development.

Infant/Toddler Language Development

The term **infant** has its origins in Latin and means "without speech." So when referring to the period of infant development, we are considering a period during which the child has yet to utter a single word. That is not to say children remain silent during infancy. The wide array of sounds made by the infant is well documented, and these sounds are thought to contribute to the child's eventual abilities to learn language. So it seems that development of language begins before a child says her first word. Indeed, some may argue that language begins in the mother's womb.

Before children begin talking, they communicate using a combination of vocal and gestural behaviors known as **prelinguistic** communication. One form of prelinguistic communication is that which occurs between mother and child. We know that as early as three months of age, infants take part in a conversational turn-taking with their mothers, called **gaze coupling**. Gaze coupling occurs when an infant turns toward the speaker and gains eye contact; it establishes a bond between mother and infant. The infant also produces a rich array of **vocalizations**. The production of vocalizations is not unique to human infants. To vocalize simply means to produce voice, and many nonhuman species also vocalize (e.g., birds, cats, chimpanzees). Among human infants, a distinct developmental pattern of vocalizations has been charted covering the first 12 months of life. The stages of vocal development are illustrated in Figure 4–2. A similar pattern of vocal development is found in infants throughout the world. This has led experts to theorize that these vocal behaviors represent necessary milestones that need to be achieved in order to acquire language.

The earliest vocalization produced by infants is **crying**. A baby's crying at birth is used as an indicator of health status. Within the first two months following birth, the infant learns to produce cries for varying reasons such as when hungry, fussy, or experiencing discomfort. Between two and four months of age,

---

FYI

It is often reported that a child's first words are either *mom* or *dad*. The reason for this is twofold. First, these are important people in a young child's daily life. Second, the /m/ and /d/ sounds are the earliest and easiest sounds for young children to articulate, which helps pave the way for saying these two words.

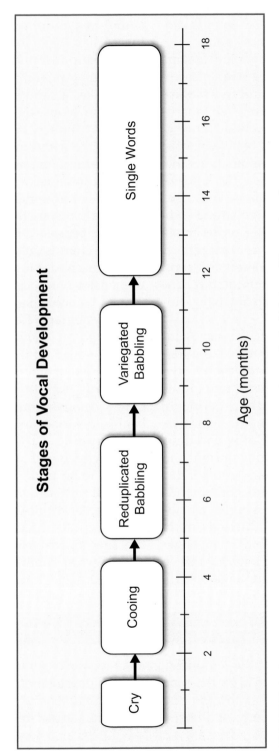

FIGURE 4–2. The stages of early vocal development from the period of birth to 18 months of age.

the infant begins to use vowel-like sounds and consonant-like sounds similar to /k/ and /g/. These sounds are referred to as **cooing** (or gooing) and are produced when the infant is in a pleasurable comfort state. Around five months of age and continuing to eleven months of age, infants produce a wide range of **babbling** sounds. These babbles consist of strings of syllable combinations that are either reduplicated (e.g., *ba-ba-ba-ba*) or nonreduplicated (*ma-ba-da-ba*; i.e., variegated) that also have strong intonation patterns. Babbling represents a rich form of vocal behavior that reflects improvements in maturation and coordination of the speech musculature. The infant is truly on the cusp of talking during the babbling period.

By the time an infant reaches his first birthday, he is referred to as a toddler. The period of toddlerhood covers the approximate ages of one to two years of life and reflects a period of rapid development in motor, cognitive, and linguistic abilities. During this time, the toddler is now standing upright and learning to walk. This is a period of discovery for the child and corresponds with the uttering of **single words**. These single word productions mark the moment when the child is no longer just producing vocalizations, but rather, **verbalizations** (i.e., language-based).

These verbalizations represent a distinct **sound-to-symbol relationship**. One of the earliest types of sound-to-symbol relationship is found in the production of **onomatopoeia**, whereby the toddler makes a sound to suggest a thing or action (cow says "moo," car goes "beep"). Children's vocabularies tend to include the names of important people in their environments and referents that they can interact with, manipulate, or change. For example, children are more likely to say something like *ball* rather than *tree* because a ball has movement, and the child is able to manipulate the object. A child's understanding (comprehension) of vocabulary normally is more advanced than his or her expressive vocabulary. Research has shown that children comprehend their first 50 words at about 13 months of age, but they cannot actually produce 50 different words until they reach 20 months of age. Another language behavior that begins to surface by 18 to 24 months is **fast mapping**. Fast mapping refers to the process by which children connect a word to an underlying concept after minimal physical exposure (i.e., seeing the object and quickly linking a word to the object). By the time a child reaches the age of two years, the production of **two-word combinations** should be apparent (e.g., "more juice" or "daddy

---

FYI

Professor Ray Kent (1984) theorized that the reason children produce repetitive strings of babbling is part of a larger human developmental process. During the first year of life, children demonstrate a number of rhythmic motoric behaviors such leg, arm, and finger movements. These rhythmic behaviors are thought to reflect a necessary activity in the development of motor control (skilled performance). Thus, babbling is just one of many rhythmic behaviors related to the development of physical coordination.

go"). Two-word combinations occur once a child achieves a single-word vocabulary in excess of 50 different words. Many of these early two-word combinations are simply a combination of two single words that are in the child's existing vocabulary. Examples of the first 50 words produced by children are shown in Table 4–1.

Preschool Language Development

The most well-charted areas of language development during the period from two to five years are morphology and semantics. During this time frame, the length of the child's expressive utterances begins to increase by leaps and bounds. This increase is accompanied by the acquisition and use of grammatical morphemes (see later discussion). By three years of age, a child is producing short phrases of three or more words.

As children gain mastery over language skills, they also become more sophisticated in their conversational abilities. Between the ages of four and five years, they can follow complex directions and enthusiastically talk about things they do. They can make up stories, listen attentively to stories, and retell stories. At this age, children usually are able to understand that letters and numbers are symbols of real things and ideas. By the age of five years, a child's expressive vocabulary is between 1,000 and 2,000 words, and a child is able to understand twice as many words spoken. They know gender and names of family members. They often play with words and make up silly words and stories. Toward the end of the preschool period, a child should have intelligible speech, although there may be some mild speech misarticulations. A summary of the language milestones covering the first six years of life is provided in Table 4–2.

FYI

A popular myth is that twin children, when learning to talk, develop their own form of communication known only to them. This has been termed **idioglossia**. However, the phenomenon is actually a case of one twin copying the immature or disordered speech pattern of their co-twin in their attempts to use language.

FYI

For years, scientists have argued that language is what sets humans apart from all nonhuman species. Although other animals can communicate, it seems that only humans are capable of using symbols (i.e., words) that have meaning. However, some researchers have suggested that apes are capable of learning sign language that provides evidence of their ability to use symbols that have meaning. The most famous of these apes was a gorilla called Koko who learned over 200 signs.

Table 4–1. Example of First 50 Single Words Produced by Three American Children

Daniel Age = 12–16 months		Will Age = 11–16 months		Sarah Age = 12–19 months	
1 light	26 nose	1 baby	26 apple	1 uh-oh	26 ticktock
2 uh-oh	27 fire	2 mommy	27 nose	2 alldone	27 ball
3 wha that	28 hot	3 doggie	28 bird	3 light	28 go
4 wow	29 yogurt	4 juice	29 alldone	4 down	29 bump
5 banana	30 pee-pee	5 bye-bye	30 orange	5 shoes	30 pop-pop = fire
6 kitty	31 juice	6 daddy	31 bottle	6 baby	31 out
7 baby	32 ball	7 milk	32 coat	7 don't throw	32 hee-haw
8 moo	33 wack-wack	8 cracker	33 hot	8 moo	33 eat
9 quack	34 frog	9 done	34 bib	9 bite	34 neigh
10 cookie	35 hello	10 ball	35 hat	10 three	35 meow
11 nice	36 yuk	11 shoe	36 more	11 hi	36 sit
12 rock	37 aoole	12 teddy	37 ear	12 cheese	37 woof-woof
13 clock	38 Big Bird	13 book	38 nite-nite	13 up	38 bah
14 sock	39 walk	14 kitty	39 paper	14 quack-quack	39 hoo-hoo = owl
15 woof-woof	40 Ernie	15 hi	40 toast	15 oink-oink	40 bee
16 daddy	41 horse	16 Alex	41 O'Toole	16 coat	41 tree
17 bubble	42 more	17 no (no)	42 bath	17 beep-beep	42 mi-mi = ferry
18 hi	43 mommy	18 door	43 down	18 keys	43 ss = snake
19 shoe	44 bunny	19 dolly	44 duck	19 cycle	44 ooh-ooh = monkey
20 up	45 my	20 wha tha	45 leaf	20 mama	45 yack-yack = talk
21 bye-bye	46 nut	21 cheese	46 cookie	21 daddy	46 hohoho = Santa
22 bottle	47 orange	22 oh wow	47 lake	22 siren sound	47 bye bye
23 no	48 block	23 oh	48 car	23 grr	48 doll
24 rocky	49 nite-nite	24 button	49 rock	24 more	49 kite
25 eye	50 milk	25 eye	50 box	25 off	50 Muriel

From Stoel-Gammon, C., & Cooper, J. (1984). Patterns of early lexical and phonological development. *Journal of Child Language, 11*, 247–271. Reprinted by permission of Cambridge University Press.

Table 4–2. Normal Language Development Across the First Six Years of Life

Age	Language Level
Birth	Cries
2–3 months	Cries differently in different circumstances; cooing/gooing
3–4 months	Babbles randomly
5–6 months	Babbles rhythmically
6–11 months	Babbles in imitation of real speech, with expression
12 months	Produces jargon-like utterances and a small number of single words; recognizes names; imitates familiar sounds
18 months	Single-word vocabulary of 5 to 20 words; understands simple instructions
2 years	Expressive utterances of two-word combinations; vocabulary is growing; waves goodbye; makes sounds of familiar animals; makes wants known; understands "no"
2–3 years	Identifies body parts; combines nouns and verbs; has a 450-word vocabulary; uses short sentences; matches three to four colors; likes to hear the same story repeated; forms some plurals
3–4 years	Can tell a story; expressive utterances of four to five words in length; vocabulary of about 1,000 words; knows last name, name of street, and several nursery rhymes
4–5 years	Expressive utterances of four to five words in length; uses past tense; vocabulary of about 1,500 words; identifies colors and shapes; asks many questions like "why?" and "who?"
5–6 years	Utterances of five to six words in length; vocabulary in excess of 2,000 words; knows spatial relations (like "on top" and "far"); knows address; understands same-different; identifies simple currency; knows right and left hand; uses all types of sentences

School-Age Language Development

As children progress through the elementary school years, their language skills continue to develop. Growth in all aspects of language occurs with obvious changes seen in the areas of semantics (vocabulary) and pragmatics (language use). It is estimated that a six-year-old child has a vocabulary of anywhere from 8,000 to 14,000 words. Beginning with the production of single words at 12 months of age, this means the child must (on average) acquire four to eight new words every day. By school age, a child should be able to speak in complete sentences with minor grammatical errors. The school-age period also marks the development of **metalinguistic**

awareness. Metalinguistic awareness is the ability to reflect consciously on the nature and properties of language. Understanding that words and sentences can have more than one meaning is a form of metalinguistic awareness. Children begin to appreciate language in terms of humor, puns, poetry, and use in different situations. The knock-knock joke told by a six-year-old captures metalinguistic awareness in the form of word play:

Knock knock.

Who's there?

Cargo.

Cargo who?

Cargo BEEP BEEP!

Written Language Development

Most of what is currently known about child language development is based on examining comprehension and production of spoken (oral) language. Less attention has been given to the relationship between oral language competency and **written language**. Yet a child's written language skills begin to surface as early as two years of age, and these abilities provide insight as to a child's overall knowledge of language (Table 4–3). Children acquire an understanding of the relationship between oral language and written language before they enter elementary school. Learning to write involves the ability to translate the sounds of a word to discrete letters (i.e., spelling). So a child's mastery in writing represents an achievement in generalizing language across modalities of communication (MacDonald, 1997). As covered in Chapter 13, the analysis of a written language sample among individuals with deafness is thought to provide an indication of a person's oral language abilities, as well.

HISTORIC ASPECTS OF CHILD LANGUAGE DISORDERS

To speak about language is to speak about the development of the human race (Butler, 1986). There is evidence to suggest that language originated during the Ice Age, approximately 30,000 years ago. When language was created, it is likely that language disorders were soon to follow, frequently as a result of a physical accident or intellectual disability. One of the earliest detailed reports of a language disorder was by the French physician **Jean-Marc Gaspard Itard** (1774–1838; Figure 4–3). The report was based on the case of the **wild boy of Aveyron**. Discovered in 1799, the boy (named Victor) had been lost or aban-

---

FYI

Children with low levels of education and who also exhibit behavioral problems are known to be at-risk for communication difficulties. These same features also place an individual at risk for criminal activity. Perhaps it is not surprising to find an unusually high number of inmates in the prison population who have some form of speech, language, or hearing disorder.

Table 4–3. Stages of Written Language Development

Stage	Age	Ability
I. Random Scribbling	2–3 years	Children make marks on paper randomly with little muscular control.
II. Controlled Scribbling	3 years	Children *write* across the paper in linear fashion, repeating patterns over again and showing increased muscular control.
III. Letter-like Forms	3–4 years	Children make mock letters. These are written lines of letters that have letter characteristics but are misshapen and written randomly. They like to pretend they are writing and are able to separate writing from drawing. They have purpose to their letter-like forms.
IV. Letter/Symbol Relationship	4 years	Children write letters to create words. They can write their name. They know the word that represents their name. They can copy words. Letter reversals are frequent.
V. Invented Spelling	4–5 years	Children make the transition from letter forms to invented spelling. They use a group of letters to form a word. Many of the letters will be consonants. They understand that letters relate to sounds. Some punctuation appears. They can copy words from their environment.
VI. Standard Spelling	5–7 years	Most of the words the children use are written correctly. They organize their words in lines with spaces between the words, and they move from left to right and from the top of the page to the bottom.

doned in childhood, apparently surviving on his own in the wild up to the age of approximately 11 years. The boy spoke no language, and Itard undertook to educate Victor. Itard believed that two things separated humans from animals: empathy and language. He wanted to be the first person to fully civilize a wild child and attempted to teach Victor to speak and show human emotion. Although initially successful in understanding language and reading simple words, Victor's abilities eventually plateaued to the point where Itard abandoned the experiment. The only words that Victor ever actually learned to speak were *lait* (milk) and *oh Dieu* (oh God). Victor died at the age of 40. This early study supported the theory that an enriching environment was vital to the acquisition of normal language.

In the early 1960s, **Roger Brown** (1925–1997) from Harvard University performed some pioneering research in the area of normal language development in a longitudinal study of three

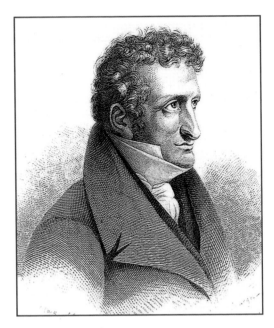

FIGURE 4–3. Jean-Marc Gaspard Itard provided one of the earliest detailed reports of a language disorder based on the wild boy of Aveyron.

as a child's speech becomes more complex, the child begins to modify words by the addition of bound morphemes, such as plural "s" or present progressive "ing," resulting in utterances such as, "Daddy going" (3 morphemes).

A great deal of what is currently known about the development of expressive language during the preschool period is based on the classic research of Brown. He was able to show that MLU reflected a child's increasing ability to combine words and produce complex utterances. He identified five stages in language development that were organized according to the child's MLU. There was an orderly development in 14 grammatical morphemes across the first five years of life that corresponded to the child's MLU (Table 4–4). The order of acquisition was similar for the three children. Brown suggested that the order in which all children acquired various grammatical morphemes was identical with the progression from simple morphemes to more complex ones. However, more recent studies have shown that by the end of the preschool period, most children have acquired a full range of grammatical morphemes in their expressive language, although the precise order in which they are acquired may not be identical.

children: Adam, Eve, and Sarah (Brown, 1973). Brown recorded the conversations of these children with their parents at home every two weeks for the first five years of life as a way of estimating the type and amount of language produced by each child. Brown calculated a measure called **mean length of utterance** (MLU). A child's MLU is calculated by taking 100 utterances produced by a child (excluding all cases where the utterance is a repetition of a statement made by an adult) and then working out the average length in morphemes. The number of morphemes in an utterance often is the same as the number of words because, in children's early multiword speech, their words usually consist only of a single morpheme. For example, the utterance, "Daddy go" consists of two morphemes. However,

TYPES OF CHILD LANGUAGE DISORDERS

Language disorders in children are characterized by deficiencies in the comprehension and/or production of spoken and written language (Figure 4–4). Deficiencies in language can have a profound impact on a child's academic, social, and

Table 4–4. Brown's (1973) Stages of Grammatical Morpheme Development and the Approximate Age at which Each Stage Should Be Attained

Stage	MLU	MLU Range	Age in Months	14 Grammatical Morphemes	Examples
I	1.75	1.5–2.0	15–30	combine basic words	more juice daddy go
II	2.25	2.0–2.5	28–36	(1) present progressive	daddy go*ing* fall*ing* down
				(2) preposition "in"	*in* house
				(3) preposition "on"	*on* top
				(4) -s plurals (regular)	my toy*s*
III	2.75	2.5–3.0	36–40	(5) irregular past tense	I *fell* down She *sat* on
				(6) -s possessives	Mommy*'s* house
				(7) uncontractible copula	*Are* they here?
IV	3.5	3.0–3.7	40–46	(8) articles	*a* ball *the* cat
				(9) regular past tense "ed"	He walk*ed* She danc*ed*
				(10) third-person regular present tense	He push*es* She *walks*
V	4.0	3.7–4.5	46–52+	(11) third-person irregular	Kathy *has* He *does*
				(12) uncontractible auxiliary	*Is* he going? What *are* you doing?
				(13) contractible copula	*Matt's* tall *I'm* short
				(14) contractible auxiliary	*They're* walking *He's* running

emotional development. Roughly 7% of preschool and school-age children exhibit significant limitations in language ability. Some language disorders in children can result from organic factors, such as intellectual impairment, hearing loss, and head injury. Often, child language disorders are functional in nature, where a specific etiology for the disorder cannot be determined.

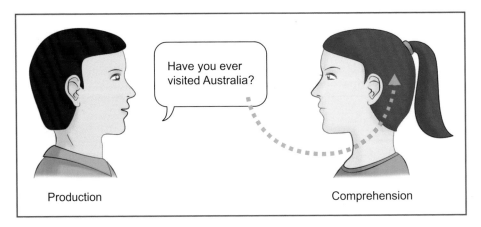

FIGURE 4–4. Conceptualization of the processes of language production and comprehension.

Later chapters in this book address language disorders resulting from specific conditions such as genetic abnormalities (Chapter 11) and hearing impairment (Chapter 12). Some common conditions indicative of language impairment are provided below.

Specific Language Impairment

Specific language impairment (SLI) is characterized by difficulty with language that is not caused by known neurological, sensory, intellectual, or emotional deficit. SLI can affect the development of vocabulary, grammar, and conversation (discourse) skills. Children with SLI may be intelligent and healthy in all regards, with the exception of an isolated difficulty with language. They may in fact be extraordinarily bright. Children with SLI usually learn to talk late. It is not unusual to first encounter a child with SLI at the age of three or four years, with limited vocabulary and short utterances. A child with SLI may do things such as omitting the plural "s" at the end

of words or omit various verbs. An example would be to say, "He drive the car" rather than "He drives the car." As children with SLI mature and the problem goes undetected, they may be described by teachers as being smart but unmotivated. SLI affects approximately 8% of five-year-old children. Although SLI is not a reading disability, 50% to 75% of children with SLI also experience problems in learning to read. If gone untreated, the impact of SLI can continue into adulthood. Studies of young adults with SLI in their thirties show that these individuals tend to have fewer educational qualifications and may have difficulty finding stable employment.

Intellectual Impairment

The acquisition of language is a remarkable human achievement. Within a few short years, children make the transition from cooing and babbling to becoming fully communicative individuals. Generally, children acquire the essential components of language by the age of three or four years. However, this may not be true for children with an intellectual disability (i.e., mental retardation). Intellectual impairment is characterized by significantly subaverage intellectual functioning, which is determined on the basis of a mathematical ratio known as an **intelligence quotient** (IQ). A standard way of determining IQ is to note the discrepancy between an individual's true, chronological age (CA) and their mental age (MA), as derived from a test of intelligence. The formula for calculating IQ is 100 * MA/CA. So two possible IQ examples would be:

- MA = 6 years / CA = 5 years (IQ = 120 which means gifted)
- MA = 6 years / CA = 9 years (IQ = 66 which means impaired)

In the late 1800s, intellectual disability was classified using descriptive terms such as idiot (IQ = 0–19), imbecile (IQ = 20–24), moron (IQ = 25–49), simpleton (IQ = 50–69), and dullard (IQ = 70–99) until these terms began to be abused by the rest of society. The terms have become obsolete, and intellectual impairment is now defined by an IQ of approximately 70 or below. Four degrees of impairment severity can be specified: mild (IQ = 50–70), moderate (IQ = 35–49), severe (IQ = 20–34), and profound (IQ = 0–19). The prevalence of intellectual impairment in the noninstitutionalized population of the United States is 7.8 people per 1,000. If institutionalized individuals are included in the prevalence rates, the number increases to 8.7 per 1,000.

Intellectual impairment is associated with limitations in learning and can have a profound effect on a child's ability to talk. At one time, it was believed that the language acquisition of all persons with an intellectual impairment represented a slow-motion version of normal language development. That is, children with an intellectual impairment demonstrated normal language behavior; however, it was behavior expected in younger, nonimpaired children. We now know there is no consistent pattern of language behavior shown in children with an intellectual impairment due to differences in the type and severity of impairment. The overall picture of early language development in children with intellectual impairment is one of differences and similarities in comparison with normal children. Impaired children appear to follow the same set of universal principles in the acquisition of word meaning, although this is not always the case for profoundly impaired children. Intellectually impaired children are found to acquire syntactic and morphological knowledge in the same order as normally developing children. Children with intellectual impairments also are able to acquire basic pragmatic skills; yet more subtle aspects of conversational competence are less commonly displayed. Intellectual impairments are associated with some of the genetic-based communication disorders covered in Chapter 11.

Autism

The brain disorder known as autism was first identified in 1943 by **Leo Kanner** (1896–1981) who described 11 self-absorbed children who had "autistic disturbances of affect contact" (Figure 4–5). Autism originally was thought to reflect an attachment disorder resulting from poor parenting. The cause of autism is still unknown, but most specialists believe it is a brain disorder that

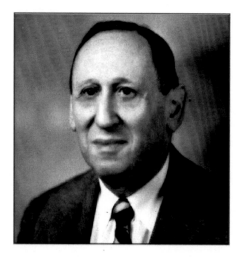

FIGURE 4–5. Leo Kanner was the first person to identify distinct features of autism.

drome, and Savant syndrome, to name a few. Details of Fragile X syndrome are covered in Chapter 11. Autism spectrum disorder is also known as a type of **pervasive developmental disorder**, because it can cause a severe impairment in thinking, feeling, language, and the ability to relate to others.

Parents are usually the first to notice autistic-like behaviors in their child. In some cases, the baby seemed different from birth, unresponsive to people, or focusing intently on one item for long periods of time. The first signs of an autism spectrum disorder also can appear in children who had been developing normally. When an affectionate, verbal toddler suddenly becomes silent and withdrawn from social activities, something is wrong. Autism is one of the most common developmental disabilities of childhood. Individuals of all races, ethnicity, and socioeconomic backgrounds can show autism. The conservative estimate of the occurrence of autism spectrum disorder is about 2 per 1,000 people, with about four times as many boys as girls affected. The number of people known to have autism

makes it difficult for the person to process and respond to the world. The term **autism spectrum disorders** is now used to capture the wide range of symptoms and behaviors that a child may exhibit. These symptoms range from mild to severe. Research has shown that many people who engage in autistic behaviors have related but distinct disorders. These include, Asperger syndrome, Fragile X syndrome, Williams syn-

---

FYI

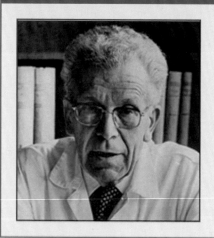

Asperger syndrome is considered a mild form of autism that is characterized by concrete thinking, obsession with certain topics, social isolation, excellent memory, and being eccentric. Individuals have an average to above average IQ, are capable of holding a job, and living independently. The cause of the condition is unknown. The condition is named after **Hans Asperger** (1906–1980), an Austrian physician who first described the syndrome in 1944.

has increased dramatically since the 1980s, partly due to changes in diagnostic practice. Some research suggests that autism spectrum disorder can be as high as 10 per 1,000 people. Current estimates suggest that approximately 500,000 individuals in England and the United States have autism spectrum disorder and over 12,000 in Australia. Autism occurs in individuals of all levels of intelligence. Approximately 75% are of low intelligence, whereas around 10% show **savant** skills such as extraordinary abilities in specific areas like music and mathematics.

Three crucial areas of development are affected by autism spectrum disorder: (1) verbal and nonverbal communication, (2) social interaction, and (3) creative or imaginative play. The communication problems of autism spectrum disorder vary, depending on the intellectual and social development of the individual. For many, speech and language develops to some degree, but not to a normal ability level. This development usually is uneven. For example, vocabulary development in areas of interest may be accelerated. Many have good memories for information just heard or seen. Some may be able to read words well before the age of five but cannot demonstrate understanding of what is read. Some may be unable to speak, whereas others might have rich vocabularies and are able to talk about topics of interest in great depth. Despite this variation, the majority of autistic individuals have little or no problem with speech articulation. Most have difficulty effectively using language. Their expressive language is likely to contain no content or information. For example, an autistic individual may repeatedly count from one to five. Others use **echolalia**, a repetition of something previously heard. One form, *immediate echolalia*, may occur when the individual repeats the question, "Do you want something to drink?" instead of replying with a "yes" or "no." In another form called *delayed echolalia*, an individual may say, "Do you want something to drink?" whenever he or she is asking

---

FYI

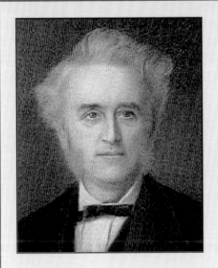

Savant syndrome is a *juxtaposition* of severe intellectual disability and prodigious (narrow) mental ability. Individuals have an IQ generally below 70. The syndrome occurs more often in males. The most common savant skills are music (playing piano by ear), art (painting or drawing), lightning-quick mathematical calculating, calendar calculating, and mechanical/spatial skills. Savant skills were highlighted in the 1988 film, *Rain Man*. The condition was first identified in 1887 by **John Langdon Down** (1828–1896), who used the term "idiot savant." The condition known as Down syndrome was also first identified by Down.

for a drink. Other distinct features of autism are a lack of eye contact and poor attention duration. Individuals with autism spectrum disorder often are unresponsive to the speech of others and may not respond to their own names. As a result, some are mistakenly thought to have a hearing problem. Children with autism spectrum disorder fail to interact with others, which adversely effects communication. The simple act of communication involves two individuals, a speaker and a listener. The child with autism fails to engage in communication, resulting in a potentially severe communication disorder.

Late Talkers

The term **late talker** is used to describe a group of children who have an impoverished expressive vocabulary, usually within the age range of 18 to 30 months of life. These children are late bloomers and are slow to acquire their first 50 words. They also take longer to begin uttering two-word combinations. By 24 months of life, most children have an expressive vocabulary of approximately 200 words, whereas late talkers may have a vocabulary of approximately 20 words. These children are developing typically in the areas of language comprehension, play, motor, and cognitive/learning skills, with the sole exception being language expression. Children who are late talkers are thought to be at risk for subsequent language problems. The challenge presented to the speech-language pathologist is determining which of these children will simply outgrow the delay and which will not. As a general rule, it is advisable for these children to be involved in language enrichment activities. Research has indicated that children who are diagnosed early show more positive outcomes in their language development.

CURRENT THEORIES REGARDING CHILD LANGUAGE DEVELOPMENT AND DISORDERS

Theories regarding the cause of a child language disorder usually attribute the disorder to biological (nature) or environmental (nurture) factors. For example, a biological cause would be seen in a child born with a profound hearing loss that interfered with his ability to hear and subsequently learn language. Alternatively, an environmental cause would be seen in a child deprived of human contact (e.g., wild boy of Aveyron), thus preventing the child from experiencing the language of others. Either of these situations would have an effect on a child's subsequent language development. However, it is equally possible for the combined effects of nature and nurture to contribute to a language disorder. One possible scenario would be a situation where a child born with an intellectual disability (a biological condition) receives inadequate language stimulation in the home environment. Needless to say, there are a wide range of situations that can contribute to a language disorder. Four major theories concerning normal language acquisition are presented. These are the: (1) behavioral, (2) nativist, (3) interaction, and (4) statistical learning theories. Regardless of the theory one may ascribe to, a

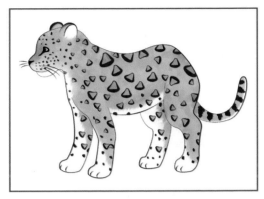
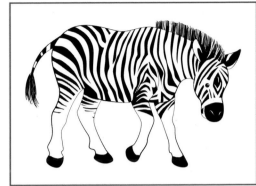
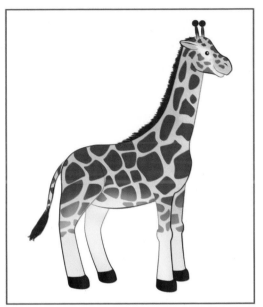
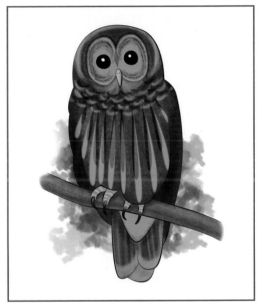

FIGURE 4–9. Example of test pictures used for standardized testing of vocabulary comprehension. The clinician would prompt the child by stating, "Point to giraffe."

sample. The child's utterances are transcribed verbatim. This is also referred to as **orthographic transcription**. The third step in this process entails analyzing the language sample in a number of ways, including calculation of the child's size of vocabulary and MLU, and noting the use of various syntactic structures and sentence types. The fourth step in the language sampling process requires interpretation of the analyses. The child's language abilities noted in the sample can be compared with reference databases of typical children to provide an indication of the child's expressive language and whether he or she may exhibit a language disorder. Computer software known as **SALT** (systematic analysis of language transcripts) is in regular use for transcribing and analyzing language samples, as well as comparing them with reference databases of typical children. The SALT program was developed by Dr. Jon Miller and

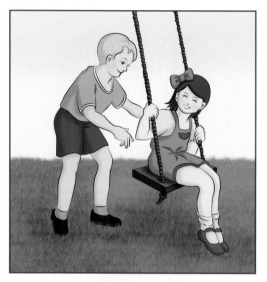
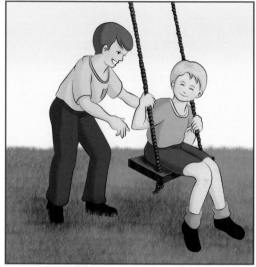
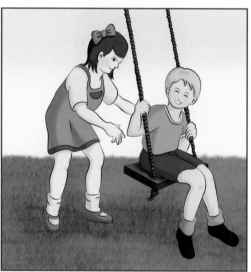
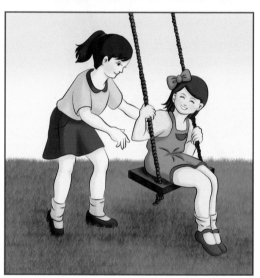

FIGURE 4–10. Example of test pictures used for standardized testing of language comprehension of sentences. The clinician would prompt the child by stating, "Point to, 'The girl pushes the boy.'"

Dr. Robin Chapman at the University of Wisconsin-Madison. An example of MLU calculation is shown in Table 4–7.

What Is the Nature and Severity of the Disorder?

On the basis of the information collected from the child and parents, the speech-language pathologist will make a number of decisions regarding the child's language abilities. The most immediate decision is a determination as to whether the child exhibits a language disorder. The disorder could be in any area of language form, content, or use. If the child's language abilities are not equivalent to those found for same-aged normally developing peers, then the initial diagnosis of a language disorder is made. If a disorder is present, the speech-language pathologist will next determine the nature of the disorder, by indicating whether the impairment is indicative of a **language delay** or **language deviance** (Figure 4–11). A language delay means that the child's language system is similar to younger, nondisordered children. The various components of the child's language system are not unusual. Rather, the child's language is trailing behind in development compared with the child's peers. Some children with a language delay may catch up without the need for treatment, such as the case with late talkers. A child demonstrating a language deviance is exhibiting a linguistic system that is unlike that of younger nondisordered children. A language deviance often is found in situations where a child may exhibit a variety of physical and or cognitive impairments. Children exhibiting a language deviance are less common than those showing a language delay. The speech-language pathologist also will make a decision concerning the severity of the language disorder that is based on determining the extent to which the child's language abilities are impaired. As a general rule, a language deviance is considered more severe than a language delay. However, a language delay also can be severe if a number of language abilities are impaired, such as vocabulary size, utterance length, and language syntax.

Table 4–7. Example of MLU Calculation: A Typical MLU Calculation Is Based on a Sample of 100 Utterances

Utterance Transcription	Number of Grammatical Morphemes
I see daddy.	3
More juice.	2
What man doing.	4
Mommy driving.	3
Ball in cup.	3
Baby pulled the wagon.	5
The girl likes eating.	6
He's falling down.	5
The bus is yellow.	4
Where mommy go?	3

Number of utterances = 10

Number of grammatical morphemes = 38

MLU = 38/10 utterances = 3.8

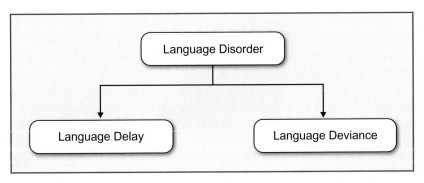

FIGURE 4–11. Classification of language disorders.

TREATMENT OF CHILD LANGUAGE DISORDERS

Treatment of child language disorders involves determining the best course of action to assist the child. There is no standard agreed-upon approach to treating child language disorders. Some approaches work better for some children than others. The particular approach and success of an approach is dependent on factors such as the child's age, attention span, and type and cause of language disorder. The set of goals and treatment strategies are unique to the child and his or her particular difficulties with language. An overarching theme in the treatment of child language disorders is to help the child improve communication. Parents and teachers can contribute a great deal to the child's success in therapy. The child may only spend a few short hours each week receiving formal therapy from a speech-language pathologist. The remainder of the time is spent outside the clinic in the home and school environment. So the speech-language pathologist is likely to provide parents and teachers with activities that can be used in these settings to help facilitate the child's language abilities. Goals developed for helping children improve their language comprehension abilities might be to help the child increase receptive (listening) vocabulary, comprehension of directions, understanding of grammar, and recognition of the role of a listener in a conversation. Examples of expressive language goals would be to expand vocabulary development and the child's use of language (pragmatics) in various speaking contexts.

Once specific goals of treatment are identified, the speech-language pathologist can opt to use either an adult-centered approach or child-centered approach in helping the child achieve these goals. Language therapy is characterized as **adult-centered therapy** if the therapist takes a direct approach to teaching specific language skills to the child. This approach has been in widespread use for many years and involves giving the child frequent prompts to produce the desired utterances. The speech-language pathologist may also use instructional materials such as charts that focus on the particular language skill being taught. The treatment goal of a session might be, for example, to get the child to correctly use verb forms such as, "is walking," "is playing," and "is eating," or learning to follow directions. Adult-centered therapy is found to be most effective with school-age children.

In contrast, **child-centered therapy** uses a less directive path to improving the child's language abilities. This approach has been referred to as "speech on the run," whereby the speech-language pathologist provides therapy by following the child's lead and using a more conversational give-and-take, rather than an instructional format. In these therapy sessions, a speech-language pathologist will interact with a child by playing and talking. The therapist may use pictures, books, objects, or ongoing events to stimulate language learning. Four therapy techniques used in child-centered therapy are: (1) self-talk, (2) parallel talk, (3) description, and (4) expansion. **Self-talk** involves the speech-language pathologist (or parent) talking out loud about what they are doing as they engage with the child. As part of self talk, the therapist provides a rich array of language models for the child in a noninvasive, natural fashion.

For example, while playing with a doll, the speech-language pathologist may say, "Oh there's my doll; she is sitting on the chair," as a natural language model for the child to overhear. **Parallel talk** involves the speech-language pathologist describing out loud what the child is seeing, hearing, or thinking during the play activity. For example, if the child is playing with a train set, the speech-language pathologist may comment, "You put the train in the tunnel" as a language model for the child to overhear. **Description** involves use of labeling or explanations by the speech-language pathologist that call attention to the child about objects or happenings in the play setting. The speech-language pathologist may say "Here comes the train." The use of **language expansions** by the speech-language pathologist requires a restatement of the child's utterance, however with a fuller and grammatically correct language model. For example, the child may say, "train go," and the speech-language pathologist responds with, "Yes. The train is going." The speech-language pathologist adds the missing parts to the utterance and elaborates on the utterance, without overtly correcting the child or interfering with the flow of communication. All four techniques are based on communicating to the child by using statements rather than questions. By avoiding posing questions to the child, there is less communicative demand placed on the child. This, in turn, results in a more natural give and take in language use between the speech-language pathologist and child. The use of these child-centered techniques is particularly effective in providing language remediation to preschool-age children.

These two therapy approaches are not mutually exclusive. It is quite pos-sible the speech-language pathologist may develop some sort of hybrid therapy approach involving both adult- and child-centered techniques. One likely situation when a hybrid approach may be used is when the speech-language pathologist wishes to implement a therapy program that involves both the home and school setting. The parents could be using *speech on the run* techniques to model general language skills for the child at home, and the speech-language pathologist could use direct therapy techniques when the child is attending school.

CULTURAL CONSIDERATIONS AND CHILD LANGUAGE DISORDERS

Assessment

As the world becomes more globally connected, the diversity of cultural and language backgrounds represented among today's children is expanding. Most speech-language pathologists working in schools are likely to be confronted with children who differ in culture, dialect, as well as primary language compared with their own. Culturally and linguistically diverse children exhibit differences in behaviors, expectations, and belief systems. They use languages other than English and/or dialectical variations different from those used in the school setting. Special considerations must be taken to address the complex issues of these populations. The percentage of children living in the United States who are Hispanic doubled between 1980 and 2004 (from 9%

to 19%) and is projected to increase to nearly 25% of the child population by 2020. Recent census statistics in England indicated that close to 4 million residents were of Asian/Indian and Black African/Caribbean background. Over 2 million Australians, or about 14% of those aged five years and over, speak a language other than English at home. Languages such as Italian and Greek, and to a lesser extent Chinese, German, and Arabic, are spoken in Australia as community languages.

Bilingualism is defined as the ability to communicate in two languages (Figure 4–12), but not necessarily at the same level of proficiency. Varying levels of proficiency can be found across the domains of reading, writing, speaking, and listening. There are two forms of bilingualism: (1) simultaneous and (2) consecutive. **Simultaneous bilingualism** also is referred to as spontaneous bilingualism. In this form of bilingualism, an individual has presumably spoken (or has been spoken to) two or more languages in the home since birth. In **consecutive bilingualism**, an individual learns one language after already knowing another. This is the situation for individuals who become bilingual as older children and adults. Consecutive bilingualism is by far the most common form of bilingualism. Most linguistically diverse children speak a form of English that varies from Standard English. These variations should not automatically be considered a language disorder.

The challenge for the speech-language pathologist when confronted with a bilingual child is to distinguish between aspects of linguistic variation that represent regular patterns in the speaker's language or dialect and those that represent true disorders in language. This is known as the difference versus disorder paradox. A **language difference** is a situation in which the language features of a community differ from the majority language. The rules are normal for the smaller community. Consider the case of a child who is speaking Spanish-accented English. The child's first or dominant language (**L1**) is Spanish, and the second language (**L2**) is English. The speech-language pathologist must determine if the child's differences with the English language are due to variation that is caused by normal linguistic processes, resulting from the competition between two languages, or a more basic problem, reflecting a language disorder. If the language of the child's L2 is found to be disordered, it is highly likely the L1 also is disordered. It is inappropriate to label a child as language disordered if the second language is in transition. It is also inappropriate to overlook a child who is speaking L2 when the L1 may be disordered.

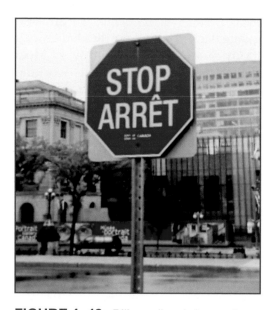

FIGURE 4–12. Bilingualism is becoming a part of our everyday world.

Great care must be taken to ensure that language assessment of bilingual children is culture-free and dialect-sensitive. Problems may arise when the language tester (the speech-language pathologist) and the child being assessed come from different linguistic or cultural backgrounds. In addition, there are few language tests that have been adapted to the bilingual population. Most tests are developed using speakers of Standard English. So, in addition to the mismatch between the speech-language pathologist and the child in regard to cultural and linguistic differences, there is also a mismatch in the tools available to evaluate the child's language abilities. According to ASHA, fewer than 2% of speech-language pathologists identify themselves as being bilingual. If the speech-language pathologist is monolingual and is not fully aware of the possible factors influencing a child's L1 on the L2, the therapist should recruit the services of an interpreter or family member as part of the assessment protocols. It is crucial that speech-language pathologists exercise diligence in distinguishing between a language difference and a language disorder.

Intervention

The traditional role of the speech-language pathologist has been to provide therapy services to individuals with diagnosed communication disorders. It is also within the scope of practice for speech-language pathologists to provide what is termed **elective therapy**. Given that a standard form of English is often required to be successful in business, economic, and educational sectors, speakers of nonstandard English may be at a disadvantage. In these cases, the role of the speech-language pathologist is to help the client acquire the desired competency in speaking a standard form of English and reducing the affects of the accent resulting from the individual's L1 or primary dialect. Normally, the services of the speech-language pathologist would not be required because the language demonstrated by the client technically is not disordered. In these cases, the client chooses to receive therapy on an elective basis.

CURRENT RESEARCH IN CHILD LANGUAGE DISORDERS

The Role of Genetics

Children with unexplained difficulties with learning and using language have puzzled researchers for many decades. The term SLI is used as the umbrella term for language disorders that cannot be attributed to retardation, autism, deafness, or other general causes. Today, research is actively taking place to identify the genetic underpinnings of language disorders. Evidence is available to show that language impairment can run in families, transferring down from one generation to the next. The gene, called **FOXP2**, was identified in a detailed study of a severe speech and language disorder that affected almost one half the members of a large family, identified only as "KE" (Lai et al., 2000). Based on examination of the genetic makeup of each member of the KE family, researchers narrowed the location of the FOXP2 gene to a region of chromosome 7 that contained about 70 genes. The discovery of this gene was the first to be linked to the normal development of communication and, therefore, allowed for the identification of some of the biological mechanisms important for speech and language acquisition. At present, it seems that disruption in this gene accounts for severe language disorders. There is now evidence that children with language impairment fall into different subtypes, including one with syntactic deficits and one with pragmatic deficits. This has led to the proposal that there are likely other genes under the regulatory control of FOXP2 that might influence language functions (Newbury & Monaco, 2010)

The Social Context of Communication

Successful communication involves social interaction. A person needs to have the necessary language abilities and social skills to engage in day-to-day communication. This interaction occurs most often among one's peers. Challenges in social communication are a defining characteristic among children with SLIs or autism spectrum disorders. The requirements for successful social communication are complex. Children must be aware of their own intentions and perspectives, as well as those of their peers. Ultimately, social communication is successful when children have both the motivation and desire to interact with others, as well as an understanding of the explicit and subtle social rules for communicating in a particular environment. Increasing emphasis is now being placed on identifying the skills necessary for children to be successful in social communication, and how these skills can be addressed in treatment of children with language disorders (Timler, 2008).

CHILD LANGUAGE DISORDERS ON THE WORLD WIDE WEB

Listed below are websites that provide further information on the topic of child language disorders. At the time of publication, each website was freely accessible.

Language Development Videos
http://www.learner.org/series/discoveringpsychology/06/e06expand.html
http://languagedevelopmentin children.net/?p=15

Autism Speaks Videos
http://www.cbsnews.com/video/watch/?id=2645143n
http://www.autismspeaks.org/video/index.php

Specific Language Impairment
http://www.ldonline.org/spears werling/Specific_Language_Impairment

Late Talkers
http://latetalkers.org/index .php?p=about

Bilingualism Video
http://arts.ucalgary.ca/lrc/home/parent-counselling-service/video-benefits-bilingualism

STUDY QUESTIONS

1. List and describe the stages of infant vocal development.
2. Who are some of the pioneers that contributed to our knowledge related to child language development?

3. List and describe three common conditions indicative of language impairment.
4. How do standardized and nonstandardized approaches to language assessment differ?
5. What is the difference between adult-centered and child-centered language therapy?

REFERENCES

Bates, E., & Carnevale, G. F. (1993). New directions in research on language development. *Developmental Review, 13,* 436–470.

Brown, R. (1973). *A first language.* Cambridge, MA: Harvard University Press.

Butler, K. (1986). *Language disorders in children.* Austin, TX: Pro-Ed.

Dunn, L. M., & Dunn, D. M. (2006). *Peabody Picture Vocabulary Test* (4th ed.). Upper Saddle River, NJ: Pearson Education.

Kent, R. D. (1984). Psychobiology of speech development: Coemergence of language and a movement system. *American Journal of Regulatory Integrative and Comparative Physiology, 246,* R888–R894.

Lai, C., Fisher, S., Hurst, J., Levy, E., Hodgson, S., Fox, M., & Monaco, A. (2000). The SPCH1 region on human 7q31: Genomic characterization of the critical interval and localization of translocations associated with speech and language disorder. *American Journal of Human Genetics, 67,* 357–368.

MacDonald, S. (1997). *The portfolio and its use: A road map for assessment.* Little Rock, AR: Southern Early Childhood Association.

Newbury, D., & Monaco, A. (2010). Genetic advances in the study of speech and language disorders. *Neuron, 68,* 309–320.

Saffran, J., Aslin, R., & Newport, E. (1996). Statistical learning by 8-month-old infants. *Science, 274,* 1926–1928.

Semel, E., Wiig, E., & Secord, W. (2003). *Clinical evaluation of language fundamentals* (4th ed.). Upper Saddle River, NJ: Pearson Education.

Stoel-Gammon, C., & Cooper, J. (1984). Patterns of early lexical and phonological development. *Journal of Child Language, 11,* 247–272.

Timler, G. (2008). Social communication: A framework for assessment and intervention. *ASHA Leader, 13*(15), 10–13.

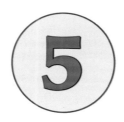

CHILD PHONOLOGICAL DISORDERS

INTRODUCTION

As children learn to speak, they begin producing single words. The words typically are only one or two syllables in length and are created using a small number of consonants and vowels. Advances in a child's age are accompanied by advances in the length of spoken utterances, as well as increases in the number and variety of consonants and vowels. Children progress through phases of speech sound acquisition so that, by no later than six to seven years of age, they should be overheard producing the entire repertoire of speech sounds. For a variety of reasons, children may be unable to accurately produce certain consonants and vowels by the age at which they are expected. Such children are described as having a **phonological disorder**. The severity of a phonological disorder can range from speech that is completely incomprehensible, even to a child's immediate family members, to speech that can be understood by everyone but with a few slightly mispronounced sounds. A phonological disorder has long been recognized as the most common type of communication disorder. In the following chapter, the nature of phonological disorders is described.

TERMINOLOGY AND DEFINITIONS

The consonant and vowel sounds composing a language are known as **phonemes**. The term **phonology** refers to the study of how sounds are organized and used in a language. Diagonal marks (/) known as **virgules** are used to signify the individual phonemes of a language (e.g., /m/, /b/, /z/, etc.). The symbols of the English alphabetic system serve as a poor example of depicting the sound-symbol relationship of the English language. The English alphabet consists of 26 letters (5 vowels and 21 consonants), yet these individual letters or combinations of these letters can represent the same or different sounds. For example, the /s/ sound is depicted differently in the words _bass_, _base_, and _face_. In the word _scissors_, the /s/ sound is written as "sc," whereas the remaining /s/ symbols in this same word are produced more like a /z/ sound. This rather fuzzy sound-symbol relationship is not unique to English. This situation prompted a group of French and English linguists to gather in 1886 and develop a symbol system called the **International Phonetic Alphabet** (IPA), which has become the standard notation system used worldwide to describe the sound patterns of various languages. The basic idea behind developing the IPA was to create an alphabet in which each sound would have its own distinctive symbol. According to the IPA system, the English language consists of 42 distinct sounds (or symbols; 18 vowels and 24 consonants). A portion of the IPA symbol system is shown in Figures 5–1 and 5–2. The figures depict the various ways in which consonant and vowels sounds can be classified. This classification relates to the pattern of articulation within the vocal tract.

Consonant Classification

When a consonant is articulated, there is almost always some form of obstruction or at least a narrowing of the vocal tract

Place of Articulation

Manner of Articulation		Bilabial	Labiodental	Lingua-Dental	Lingua-Alveolar	Lingua-Palatal	Lingua-Velar	Glottal	Examples
Stops	Voiceless	/p/			/t/		/k/		pin tin kin
	Voiced	/b/			/d/		/g/		bust dust gust
Fricatives	Voiceless		/f/	/θ/	/s/	/ʃ/		/h/	fin thin sin shin hit
	Voiced		/v/	/ð/	/z/	/ʒ/			van the zoo treasure
Affricates	Voiceless					/tʃ/			cheap
	Voiced					/dʒ/			jeep
Nasals	Voiced	/m/			/n/		/ŋ/		seem scene sing
Liquids	Voiced				/l/	/r/			late rate
Glides	Voiced	/w/				/y/			well yell

FIGURE 5–1. Categorization of consonants according to place, manner, and voicing features of articulation. Where there are voiced and voiceless consonants within the same manner of articulation, the voiceless consonant is listed in the top of the box.

Tongue Elevation	Front	Central	Back
High	i (heed) ɪ (hid)		u (hude) ʊ (hood)
Mid	e (hayed) ɛ (head)	ʌ ə (hud)	o (hoed)
Low	æ (hat)		ɔ (hawed) ɑ (hod)

Tongue Advancement

FIGURE 5–2. Categorization of vowels according to tongue elevation and tongue advancement categories.

that causes a disruption in the air flowing upward from the lungs. The three major ways of classifying the pattern of consonant articulation are according to: (1) place of articulation, (2) manner of articulation, and (3) consonant voicing.

Place of Articulation

Place of articulation refers to the location where the constriction or obstruction of the vocal tract occurs. An illustration of the various places of consonant articulation is shown in Figure 5–3. Beginning at the front of the mouth and working toward the back of the throat, the places of consonant articulation include:

Bilabial. As the name implies, a **bilabial** articulation is carried out by using both lips for consonant articulation. The bilabial consonants are /p/, /b/, and /m/.

Labiodental. In **labiodental** articulation, the lower lip and the upper teeth act together to produce the consonant sound. The labiodental consonants are /f/ and /v/.

Linguadental. Articulation of the **linguadental** consonants involves placement of the tongue between (or just behind) the teeth. The sounds /θ/ and /ð/ are included in this category.

Lingua-Alveolar. The alveolar ridge, situated just behind the upper teeth, is a common place of **lingua-alveolar** articulation for English consonants. No less than six sounds are produced there, including /t/, /d/, /n/, /s/, /z/, and /l/.

Linguapalatal. In **linguapalatal** sounds, the tongue makes direct (or close) contact to the region of the hard plate. Similar to lingua-alveolar consonants, this is a popular place of articulation for English consonants and includes /ʃ/, /ʒ/, /tʃ/, /dʒ/, /j/, and /r/.

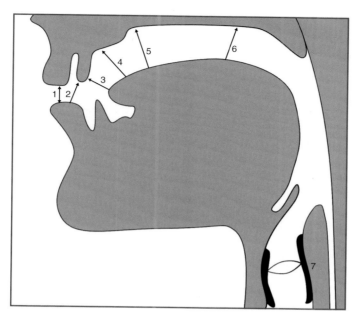

FIGURE 5–3. Cross-sectional view of the vocal tract depicting consonant places of articulation. 1 = bilabial, 2 = labiodental, 3 = linguadental, 4 = lingua-alveolar, 5 = linguapalatal, 6 = linguavelar, and 7 = glottal.

Linguavelar. The **linguavelar** place of articulation is limited to the /k/, /g/, and /ŋ/ sounds.

Glottal. The **glottal** place of articulation is located at the back of the throat at the lower end of the pharynx (i.e., near the glottis). The primary glottal consonant is /h/, although there is another, less frequently produced consonant known as a **glottal stop** /ʔ/.

Manner of Articulation

The term **manner of articulation** refers to the way in which the obstruction inside the oral cavity is made. There are six distinct manners of articulation including:

Stops. For the production of **stops**, a solid obstruction is built up somewhere within the oral cavity, initially completely blocking the airstream coming up from the lungs. This blockage is then abruptly released so the air that was compressed behind the obstruction can escape with a kind of explosive movement. The stop consonants are /p/, /b/, /t/, /d/, /k/, and /g/.

Nasals. For the production of **nasals**, the velum is lowered, allowing air to escape through the nasal cavity rather than the oral cavity. Nasal consonants in English are fairly limited in number. There are only three: /m/, /n/, and /ŋ/.

Fricatives. Where stops are produced with complete obstruction in the oral cavity, **fricatives** are produced by creating a partial obstruction of the airstream. This makes turbulence arise at or near the point of obstruction, where the airstream is forced through a greatly narrowed channel. Fricatives compose the largest class of English consonants according to manner of articulation, including /f/, /v/, /θ/, /ð/, /s/, /z/, /ʃ/, /ʒ/, and /h/.

Affricates. **Affricates** are a combination of a stop and a following fricative, where the quality of the stop remains largely the same, but the fricative part tends to be shorter than a "pure" fricative. The affricates are /tʃ/ and /dʒ/.

Liquids and Glides. The **liquids** and **glides** are consonants that differ from the other consonants by the fact that they are produced with far less obstruction in the vocal tract. Instead, there is a subtle narrowing of the vocal tract. These consonants are sometimes referred to as **approximates** because their manner of articulation seem to lie between true consonants and pure vowels. The liquid consonants are /l/ and /r/. The glide consonants are /w/ and /j/.

Consonant Voicing

The **voiced consonants** are those that require vocal fold vibration to be produced correctly. These include /b/, /d/, /g/, /v/, /ð/, /z/, /ʒ/, /dʒ/, /w/, /j/, /l/, /r/, /m/, /n/, and /ŋ/. Not all con-

sonants involve vocal fold vibration. These are referred to as **voiceless consonants** and include /p/, /t/, /k/, /f/, /θ/, /s/, /ʃ/, /tʃ/, and /h/. Collectively, all consonants can be described using the categories of voicing, place, and manner of articulation. The phoneme /b/ is an example of a voiced bilabial stop. The phoneme /ʃ/ is an example of a voiceless linguapalatal fricative (see Figure 5–1).

Vowel Classification

As noted above, consonants are characterized by an obstruction of the vocal tract, which causes a disruption in airflow. The opposite is true of vowels. Here, the characteristic feature is the absence of closure of the vocal tract, so that air can flow in a relatively unimpeded fashion. The articulation of vowels is organized according to the positioning of the tongue body within the oral cavity. The two vowel classifications are tongue elevation and tongue advancement (Figure 5–4).

Tongue Elevation

As implied, **tongue elevation** (or tongue height) refers to the distance that the tongue is moved from the base of the mouth toward the roof of the mouth for the production of vowels (see Figure 5–4).

FYI

The ability to articulate an innumerable number of speech sounds in an oral cavity that is less than three inches in length is considered the most sophisticated and coordinated activity performed by the human body.

FYI

American English uses a vowel that is found in less than 1% of the world's languages. The vowel is found in words such as *fur*, *stir*, and *her*.

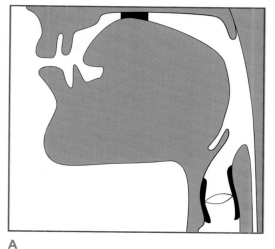

A

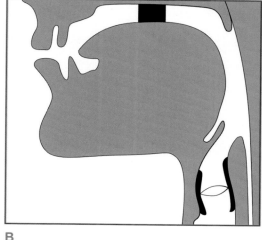

B

C

FIGURE 5–4. The articulation of vowels according to tongue elevation within the oral cavity. The three panels depict tongue articulation ranging from high (**A**), mid (**B**), and low (**C**).

There are three general locations of vowels according to tongue elevation: high /i, ɪ, u, ʊ/, mid /e, ɛ, ə, ʌ, o/, and low /æ, ɔ, ɑ/.

Tongue Advancement

The classification of vowels according to **tongue advancement** (or tongue carriage) refers to the movement of the tongue body from the back of the oral cavity toward the front (Figure 5–5). There are three locations of vowels according to tongue advancement: front /i, ɪ, ɛ, e, æ/, central /ə, ʌ/, and back /u, ʊ, o, ɔ, ɑ/. Collectively, all vowels can be described using the categories of tongue elevation and tongue advancement. The phoneme /u/ is an example of a high-back vowel. The phoneme /æ/ is an example of a low-front (see Figure 5–2).

Phonological Development

Children do not acquire all the sounds of their language at once; the process is gradual and covers the approximate age

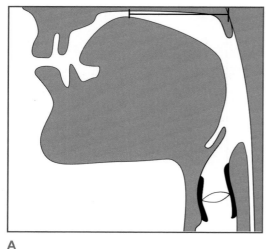

A

B

C

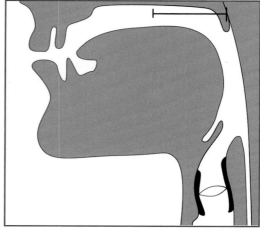

FIGURE 5–5. The articulation of vowels according to tongue advancement within the oral cavity. The panels depict tongue articulation according to front (**A**), central (**B**), and back (**C**).

range of one year to around six years of age. Although some variability is naturally expected between children, most tend to acquire the sounds of speech in an orderly fashion. As a general rule, vowels of the English language are acquired by children slightly earlier than consonants. The 24 consonants of English can be loosely organized into three phases of development (Table 5–1). The first phase contains the *early eight* consonant sounds such as the letters "m," "b," and "w." The next phase involves acquisition of the *middle eight* consonants such as the letters "t," "k," and "f." The last phase includes the *late eight* consonants such as "sh," "th," and "z." The latter sounds generally involve more precise articulatory movements compared with early developing sounds, so it is not unusual for children to require more time to master these articulations. Some children may not acquire the late eight until they reach six years of age. So it is important to emphasize that these phases are not set in stone. Children are known to show variability in the order and pace at which they acquire speech

Table 5–1. Acquisition of 24 English Consonants Organized According to the Early, Middle, and Late Periods of Acquisition (The phonetic symbol is listed on the left, and a word example in standard orthography is provided on the right.)

Early Eight (1.5 to 2 years of age)	*Word Examples*
Nasals m n	movie, north
Stops b p d	boy, pea, do
Fricatives h	hat
Glides w j	wind, yell
Middle Eight (3 to 4 years of age)	
Nasals ŋ	wing
Stops t k g	toy, cat, go
Fricatives f v	food, vine
Affricates tʃ dʒ	church, jump
Late Eight (5 to 6 years of age)	
Fricatives θ ð s z ʃ ʒ	thick, these, sew, zoo, ship, beige
Liquids l r	lamp, ramp

sounds, especially the middle eight consonants. If a child's speech does not consistently contain these various consonants by a particular age range, suspicion is raised about the possibility of a phonological disorder.

Any deviation, great or small, in the articulation of phonemes can lead to **misarticulations**, or what is simply referred to as a **speech sound disorder** (or phonological disorder). Phonological disorders affect 15% of preschool children. In a majority of cases, the type of phonological disorder demonstrated by children results from inaccurate production of consonants. This is not always the case, especially among children with severe phonological disorders who demonstrate impaired consonant and vowel production. By the time children enter school, approximately 6% continue to exhibit a phonological disorder ranging from mild to severe. For 80% of children with a phonological disorder, the condition is sufficiently severe that they will require the services of a speech-language pathologist to help them improve the quality of their speech. As noted in other chapters, many medical conditions found to occur during the childhood period seem to affect boys more often than girls. Phonological disorders are no exception. Estimates suggest that two to four times as many boys as girls exhibit the disorder. As of 2012, approximately 93% of speech-language pathologists working in the United States reported that their caseloads included individuals with a phonological disorder. There is no other speech or language disorder that receives more attention from a speech-language pathologist. Children who have a phonological disorder are more likely to have additional difficulties with their communication such as language problems and academic difficulties. A relationship can be observed between early phonological disorders and subsequent reading, writing, spelling, and mathematical abilities.

HISTORIC ASPECTS OF CHILD PHONOLOGICAL DISORDERS

A great deal of research has occurred over the past 100 years examining phonological disorders, and a large body of this historical research has centered on approaches to correcting the disorder. In the early 20th century, **E. W. Scripture** (1864–1945), who was a professor of psychology at Yale University (Figure 5–6), recommended specific treatment approaches for a speech condition he called "negligent lisping." In current times, we would refer to this phonological disorder as stopping of fricatives, where the fricative /s/ might be produced with a stop consonant /t/ ("soup" is produced as "toup"). Scripture attributed the condition to mental carelessness, and his cure for the condition consisted of teaching the individual to carefully correct his faults. To elicit correct articulation for /s/, for example, Scripture wrote:

> One cure consists [of] inserting a probe, an applicator, a toothpick, or a pencil just over the middle of the tongue and pressing it down as the person begins to speak a word beginning with "s"

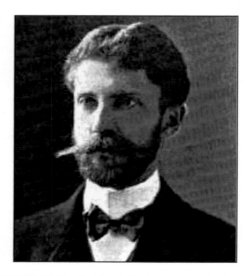

FIGURE 5–6. E. W. Scripture, early 20th-century psychologist who recommended specific treatment approaches for speech sound disorders.

> . . . He cannot close the passage completely, and instead of saying "t," he is forced to say "s." This catches his ear, and he notices the difference in sound. Constant repetition enables him to train his tongue in the new way. (Scripture, 1912, pp. 132–133)

Lee Edward Travis (1896–1987) made contributions to a number of areas in communication disorders, including phonological disorders (see also Chapter 2). He developed treatment programs that differed depending on whether the disorder was organic (anatomical) or functional (nonanatomical) in nature. Travis wrote:

> The articulatory case frequently shows inferior ability in controlling the lips, tongue, jaw and diaphragm in voluntary rhythmical movements not involved in speech. This would imply, as does the speech defect itself, that he possesses poor control of these structures in speech. (Travis, 1931, p. 223)

Grant Fairbanks (1910–1964) was a well-respected speech scientist at the University of Illinois who wrote a therapy manual known as the *Voice and Articulation Drillbook*, published in 1940 (Figure 5–7). The book was filled with a number of word- and sentence-naming activities for correcting the speech misarticulations of children and adults. Fairbanks firmly believed that good listening skills, in addition to repeated practice in producing specific misarticulated speech sounds, were essential for the correction of any phonological disorder. He wrote:

> When articulating a sound in isolation it is valuable to start with prolonged examples, since you can listen carefully, make the necessary adjustments and perceive the position of your articulators. (Fairbanks, 1940, p. xxi)

Charles Van Riper (1905–1994), a contemporary of Fairbanks, was undoubtedly one of the leading researchers in child phonological disorders and stuttering during the mid-20th century (Figure 5–8). Van Riper was a skilled speech-language pathologist who also happened to stutter. He devoted his career to developing effective treatment approaches. In his seminal publication, *Speech Correction* (Van Riper, 1947), he recommended a series of procedural steps for the treatment of phonological disorders. The steps begin with helping to establish a new sound (that is misarticulated) in a person's speech and working through increasingly complicated speaking situations, with the end goal of producing the new sound in natural conversational speech. This management program has since been referred to as the **traditional approach**, and the

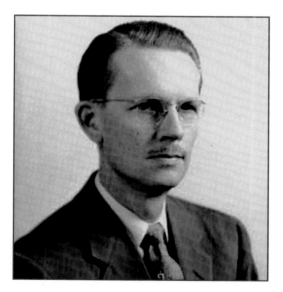

FIGURE 5–7. Grant Fairbanks, American speech scientist who wrote a manual for treating voice and speech sound disorders.

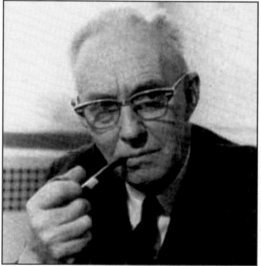

FIGURE 5–8. Charles Van Riper established what is now known as the traditional approach to treating speech sound disorders. Reprinted with permission from Van Riper, C. (1981). An early history of ASHA. *ASHA Magazine, 23*(11), 855–858.

essential components of the approach are still used today. Additional details regarding the traditional approach are provided later in this chapter.

There was a short period during the 1950s where a group of researchers attempted to link phonological disorders to a larger emotionally based disorder (Rousey, 1957). With the exception of obvious physical impairments of the speech anatomy, the assumption was that a functional phonological disorder was indicative of a **psychological disturbance**. The treatment for phonological disorders was thus focused on psychotherapy. This view was prompted by existing research at the time, which indicated that children showed considerable variability in acquiring speech sounds. This variability was attributed to developmental differences between children in their social and emotional development. A number of theories were proposed concerning the psychological underpinnings of specific consonant and vowel misarticulations. For example, substitution of the /d/ for the /ð/ ("th") sound ("the" is produced as "duh") was assumed to be related to an oral expression of aggression. That is, a pattern of speech utilized by "tough guys."

The resultant therapy focused on reducing aggression as a means of improving speech clarity. This perspective on phonological disorders was short-lived. Large-scale studies examining the acquisition of speech have since confirmed there is considerable similarity across children in achieving normal milestones. Furthermore, we now have a much clearer understanding of the patterns of speech sound misarticulations that are produced by children, which attribute the problem to either motor or language-based difficulties, as opposed to psychological difficulties.

Finally, no history of phonological disorders would be complete without mentioning the contributions of **Mildred Templin** (1913–2008; Figure 5–9). Templin earned her PhD in child development from the University of Minnesota in 1947. She conducted a series of longitudinal and cross-sectional studies of spelling, vocabulary, and cognitive behavior of children with hearing disabilities and normally developing children. Her work led to the publication of *Certain Language Skills in Children* (1957). At the time, this was a definitive work in the field. Together with her colleague Dr. Frederick Darley in 1969, she created the Templin-Darley Tests of Articulation, which are still used today to evaluate speech sound production skills in children.

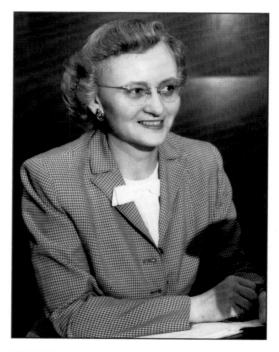

FIGURE 5–9. Mildred Templin, expert in the communication disorders of children. Printed with permission of the Trustees for the Estate of Mildred Templin.

TYPES OF PHONOLOGICAL DISORDERS

The types of phonological disorders can be organized into three categories based on the presumed cause of the disorder: (1) structural, (2) neurological, and (3) functional. Structural and neurological disorders are sometimes referred to as **articulation disorders** rather than phonological disorders, the reason being that the cause of the disorder is related to problems in the motor movements required to produce clear speech. Functional disorders are simply referred to as phonological disorders because there are no clearly identifiable motor problems. Instead, the difficulty observed in producing speech sounds appears to be related to a problem in learning to organize the sounds of the language.

Structural Cause

Structural problems involve abnormalities of the mouth that are necessary for speech sound production, such as the teeth, tongue, or palate. These abnormalities make it difficult for children or adults to produce certain sounds, and in some cases make it impossible to produce the sounds at all. The structural problem causing the speech sound disorder generally needs to be surgically or medically treated before the child receives any sort of speech therapy. Correction of the structural problem is likely to greatly assist in correction of the speech sound difficulties. One such example is a **cleft lip or palate**. Chapter 8 is specifically dedicated to this condition. A cleft lip and palate is one of the most common and obvious phonological disorders that has a structural

cause. Another structural problem contributing to a phonological disorder is **dentition**. It is not unusual for children to develop a temporary speech sound disorder during the time when primary teeth are being replaced by permanent teeth. This condition is found in nearly all first graders (see Chapter 2, Figure 2–3). Indeed, the child who loses her front two teeth experiences considerable difficulty producing consonants that require articulation between the tongue tip and central incisors (e.g., "s" and "t").

More permanent forms of dental-related articulation problems concern the alignment of the upper and lower teeth, which is referred to as **occlusion**. An uneven alignment between the upper and lower teeth is called a **malocclusion**. This situation occurs in approximately 90% of the population. There are three types of malocclusion patterns that help to create the overall appearance of our faces (Figure 5–10). A **Class I malocclusion** involves normal alignment of the upper and lower teeth with only one or two teeth slightly misaligned. A **Class II malocclusion** (or distocclusion) is an overbite. This pattern can result from one of two conditions, the first being an overly large maxilla (upper jaw) with a normal sized mandible (lower jaw). The second condition is a result of a normal-sized maxilla but a small mandible. The third type is referred to as a **Class III malocclusion** resulting in an underbite (or mesiocclusion). In this condition, the maxilla may be unusually small with a normal-sized mandible or the mandible may be unusually large with a normal-sized maxilla. In extreme instances of either a Class II or Class III malocclusion, oral surgery may be required to correct the alignment pattern. However, this

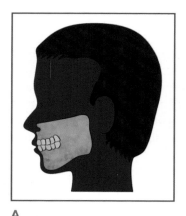 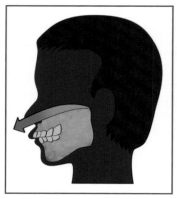 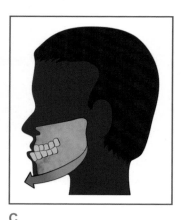

A   B   C

FIGURE 5–10. Dental and jaw alignment (occlusion) patterns. The patterns represent Class I (**A**), Class II (**B**), and Class III (**C**) malocclusions.

situation usually is prompted by other medical conditions, aside from speech problems. Most notable is a condition in which the **temporomandibular joint** works abnormally. This joint serves as the socket location where the mandible fits into the side of the skull (temporal bone). When the temporomandibular joint fails to function normally, an individual may experience severe headaches. There also are extreme instances of temporomandibular joint dysfunction when the jaw may open and stay locked (i.e., lockjaw).

Two conditions concerning *tongue mobility* contribute to a structurally based phonological disorder: **ankyloglossia** and **reverse swallow**. The first condition involves the **lingual frenulum**, which is the tendon that extends from the floor of the mouth to the underside of the tongue. A child may be born with a condition where the length of the tendon is abnormally short. The short length of the tendon restricts tongue mobility and possibly, tongue-related speech sounds. In the past, there were suggestions that clipping the tendon would help to improve speech clarity.

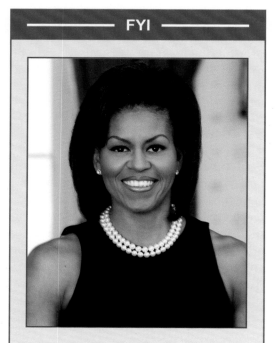

FYI

Some famous people who have a Class III malocclusion (underbite) include the U.S. First Lady Michelle Obama; television personality Jay Leno; former Prime Minister of Canada, Brian Mulroney; and film actors Casey Affleck, Keira Knightley, and Quentin Tarantino.

There is little evidence to indicate that undergoing this rather drastic surgical procedure serves to correct a phonological disorder, and it should only be considered when the tendon is so short that it impairs more basic biological functions such as swallowing. Another term for ankyloglossia is "tongue tie." An illustration of a lingual frenulum is provided in Figure 5–11.

The condition of reverse swallow also is called **tongue thrust**. The condition is reflective of an orofacial muscular imbalance. A reverse swallow normally is seen during the early infancy and toddler periods of normal development. During this time period, swallowing is achieved by pushing the tongue forward, rather than backward, to assist with the digestion of food and liquid (Figure 5–12). By the time children reach the age of six years, most have automatically changed to a normal swallowing pattern, which involves squeezing the tongue against the roof of the mouth instead of pushing it forward against the teeth. Research suggests that hereditary factors, learned behavior such as thumb sucking, and/or medical conditions may be responsible for tongue thrust. For whatever reason, a child may experience a delay or interruption in the oral maturational process and fail to progress to an adult swallowing pattern. This delay may also affect motor skills required for speech sound production.

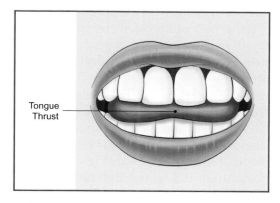

FIGURE 5–12. Illustration of tongue thrust during moments of swallowing.

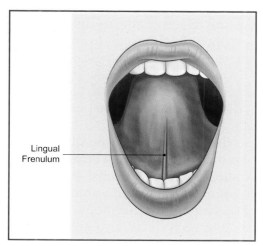

A

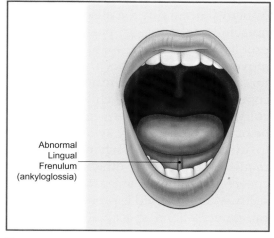

B

FIGURE 5–11. Illustration of a normal lingual frenulum (**A**) and an abnormally short frenulum (ankyloglossia) (**B**).

Neurological Cause

The second category of phonological disorders reflects **neurological** problems attributed to the nervous system. The nervous system is responsible for activating and controlling the various structures and muscles needed for producing speech sounds. Depending on the location of the nervous system impairment, an individual could show excessive speed or stiffness in the execution of speech. It is equally possible for the nervous system impairment to result in slow or labored speech production. Some neurological conditions that are known to cause a phonological disorder are **Parkinson disease** and **amyotrophic lateral sclerosis**. A portion of Chapter 9 is dedicated to speech sound disorders of this particular neurological origin. One type of neurologically based phonological disorder that has been discussed for over 25 years is **childhood apraxia of speech**. Childhood apraxia of speech is thought to be a disorder of the nervous system that affects a child's ability to organize and sequence the sounds of speech when producing words. This difficulty occurs in the absence of any muscle weakness or paralysis. The problem lies with the inability to plan movements of the speech articulators for the purpose of volitional (i.e., on command) speech. The child has difficulty making speech movements when he or she is consciously aware of trying to do so or in instances when the child is requested to do so by others. The same speech movements are produced correctly when the child is producing natural, conversational speech. A key feature of childhood apraxia of speech is that the child's misarticulations are inconsistent. Childhood apraxia of speech is a relatively rare, poorly understood phonological disorder that continues to be a topic of debate among researchers. There are varying opinions regarding the existence, cause, symptoms, and treatment of childhood apraxia of speech. There is no clearly defined set of speaking behaviors that identify the presence of childhood apraxia of speech, rather it is a spectrum of characteristics and consequently no two children with childhood apraxia of speech are alike.

Functional Cause

The third category of phonological disorder is considered **functional** because the precise cause of the disorder is unknown. In this condition, the phonological disorder results from impairments in the organization of phonemes and/or their application in speech. A child may be able to say a sound correctly but not use it appropriately in all words containing the sound. The child may also display a reduction in the total number of consonant and vowel sounds in his or her speech repertoire. In either case, the speech patterns displayed by the child are different from those of same-age peers. Phonological disorders of a functional nature make up the largest percentage of child-based phonological disorders. A functional phonological disorder can be further divided into disorders that reflect a **speech delay** or those that reflect **residual errors**. A delay is characterized by speech that is unclear (or unintelligible) and contains many consonant misarticulations. Children with a speech delay also are found to be at an increased risk for broader communication and academic difficulties. Children with a speech delay represent the most severe form of functional phonological disorder. Children with a phonological disorder who show residual errors are those who may only have one or two speech sounds that are misarticulated. The speech sound in error is usually one of the late-eight sounds such as a fricative (e.g., thumb is produced as *fumb*) or liquid consonant (e.g., radio is produced as *wadio*). This category represents a less severe form of functional phonological disorder.

CURRENT THEORIES REGARDING CHILD PHONOLOGICAL DISORDERS

A number of theories have attempted to explain the fashion in which children normally learn the sounds of their language. The same theories have been used as a backdrop for the assessment and treatment of phonological disorders. Three of these theories are the: (1) behaviorist theory, (2) natural phonology theory, and (3) optimality theory.

Behaviorist Theory

The **behaviorist theory**, developed by Mowrer (1960), suggests that a child's acquisition of consonants and vowels has its roots in early prelinguistic babbling behavior. The vocal interaction that takes place between the infant and caregiver during this early period of life sets the stage establishing the child's speech development. The child's babbling is shaped and directed toward the adult pronunciation of words through selective reinforcement of sounds that approximate the target language. According to this theory, children may not acquire speech sounds in an identical fashion. Instead, their speech development is based on the environment in which they are reared. In the case of a phonologically disordered child, a faulty environment would be viewed as contributing to the child's speech difficulties.

Distinctive Features and Natural Phonology Theory

Chomsky and Halle (1968) proposed that the unique sound systems of all the world's languages could be described according to a specific number of phonological patterns, which they termed distinctive features. By simply noting the presence or absence of these features, the phonology of a particular language could be captured. Examples of distinctive features include nasality, consonantal, vocalic, and lip rounding. This approach to describing phonology according to patterns represented a dramatic shift in the way theorists viewed a child's acquisition of speech sounds.

The early work of Chomsky and Halle was a turning point in phonological theory and led to the development of other theories examining patterns of speech sound development. Notable among these theories was the **natural theory** proposed by David Stampe (Donegan & Stampe, 1979). In this theory, a child's speech development is thought to be affected by naturally occurring phonological patterns (or "processes"), some of which remain active and others that are suppressed (or disappear) as the child learns his or her language. The child's task is to either "allow" or deliberately "suppress" various sound patterns that match those of the native language. The phonological system of a particular language is based on retaining some of these patterns while suppressing others. An example of a phonological pattern would be *final consonant deletion* (i.e., producing words that do not end with a final consonant—only vowels). A child acquiring English would learn to deliberately suppress this pattern because many of the words of English contain final consonants. On the other hand, a young child learning Mandarin would naturally accept this phonological pattern as part of the language because the words of Mandarin do not contain final consonants. The notion of phonological patterns has received widespread attention over the past 30 years as a framework to evaluate and treat the speech of children with severe phonological disorders. The theory provides an approach to treating entire classes of misarticulated speech sounds rather than individual phonemes.

Optimality Theory

Optimality theory is a general model of how grammars are structured. The theory was originally developed in the field of linguistics but has since been applied to phonological disorders. In its approach to the acquisition of phonology, optimality theory focuses on two important aspects of any phonological system: (1) the patterns that are impossible for a language and (2) the patterns that are possible. It is distinguished from other theories of phonological development in the role that is assigned to **constraints** (Geruit & Morrisette, 2005). A constraint is a limit on what constitutes a possible pronunciation of a word. The child's role in learning the sounds of the language is to learn these constraints. For example, in English some of the various phonological constraints are:

- No word may end in /tp/, although /pt/ is possible.
- No word may start with /tl/ or /dl/, but /pl/, /bl/, /tr/, and /dr/ are possible.
- No word may start with /mr/ or /nr/, although /br/ and /fr/ are possible.

ASSESSMENT OF CHILD PHONOLOGICAL DISORDERS

The goal of assessment is to obtain and establish an accurate profile of the child's speech sound production abilities. The diagnosis of a phonological disorder depends greatly on the age of the child in question. Children who are three years old may show mispronunciation of words, but these mispronunciations are expected (normal) for their age. On the other hand, an eight-year-old child who makes the same mispronunciations may have a phonological disorder. Listed below are some of the fundamental steps in performing a phonological assessment. These steps include: (1) speech sampling, (2) collection of a phonetic inventory, (3) describing speech patterns, (4) estimation of age expectancy, (5) severity estimation, and (6) performing an oral-facial examination.

Speech Sampling

The first step in determining whether a phonological disorder exists is to collect a sample of the child's speaking behavior. There are numerous ways of collecting the sample that vary according to **speech spontaneity** and **structure**. Spontaneity refers to whether the child is asked to speak freely or whether the child is required to say specific words or sounds. Structure refers to the particular environment in which the speech sample is being collected. At one end of the continuum, the sample could involve collection of spontaneous speech in a typical environment such as the child's home. The advantage of this approach is that the sample is natural and reflects normal speaking behavior. A particular disadvantage to this approach is that it is time-consuming and may not elicit a broad sample of speech from the child containing all possible consonants and vowels. On the other end of the continuum, the speech sample may be based on having the child name specific pictures that result in a one-word response. This type of activity usually occurs in a clinic setting. The advantage of this approach is that the child is required to deliberately produce specific consonants and vowels, although a disadvantage is that this is not a typical, natural setting of free speaking. In spite of this unnaturalness, picture-naming is the preferred approach to speech sampling. A number of commercially available tests exist that are designed to sample a child's phonology using a **picture-naming task**. The pictures composing the test have been chosen because they contain consonants and vowels in various locations within a word (initial, medial, and final). There is no universally accepted picture-naming

test used across English-speaking countries. A depiction of a picture-naming task and the associated scoring sheet is shown in Figure 5–13.

Phonetic Inventory

Once the speech sample is collected, the speech-language pathologist next transcribes the sample using symbols of the IPA. Based on the transcribed sample, a **phonetic inventory** is created. A phonetic inventory is a list of the consonants and vowels noted in the speech sample. The list can be organized in a number of ways, such as noting those sounds that occurred at the initial, medial, or final position of a word. The inventory provides useful information regarding a child's ability to produce the consonant and vowel sounds of the language. Sounds absent from the inventory may be indicative of a phonological disorder.

Description of Speech Patterns

On the basis of the phonetic transcription, the speech-language pathologist then compares the child's actual pronunciation of each word to the intended pronunciation of the word. Based on this comparative analysis, the speech-language pathologist is able to describe the pattern of the child's pronunciations. There are two notational systems for the description of disordered speech patterns. The first notational system is the **SODA** system. This system considers four general types of misarticulations: (1) **substitutions**, (2) **omissions**, (3) **distortions**, and (4) **additions** (SODA). Examples of these patterns are provided in Table 5–2. The speech sound misarticulations demonstrated by children with a functional phonological disorder that are of a residual nature are often described using the SODA system. The second notational system is used in

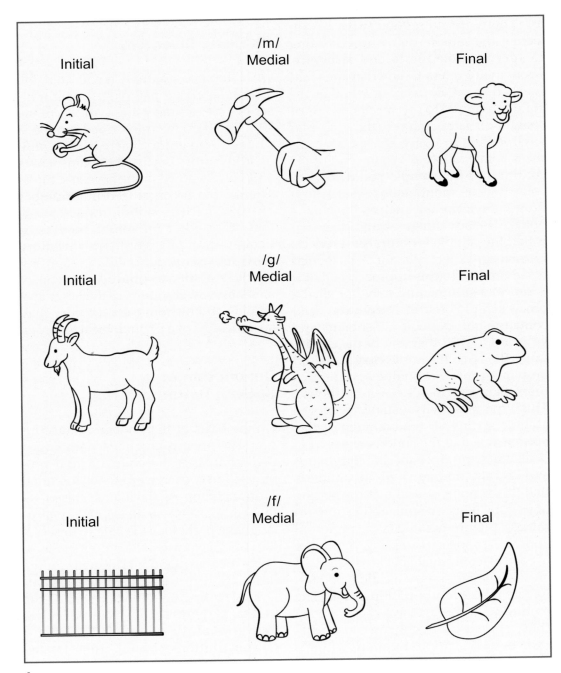

A

FIGURE 5–13. A. Example of a picture inventory test. *continues*

instances when a child exhibits a severe functional phonological disorder (i.e., speech delay). The system describes the speech pattern according to large classes of sounds that may be misarticulated; these patterns are referred to as **phonological processes** (or patterns). Examples of common phonological processes are shown in Table 5–2.

Age Expectancy Estimation

Once the speech patterns demonstrated by the child are determined, the speech-language pathologist must make a determination whether these patterns are acceptable or disordered. The child's age is an important factor when determining whether a phonological disorder

	Picture-Naming Test			
Word	**Phoneme**	**Initial**	**Medial**	**Final**
Mouse	/m/	x		
Hammer	/m/		x	
Lamb	/m/			x
Goat	/g/	x		
Dragon	/g/		x	
Frog	/g/			x
Fence	/f/	x		
Elephant	/f/		x	
Leaf	/f/			x

B

FIGURE 5–13. *continued* **B.** Corresponding test form.

Table 5–2. The SODA Patterns of Speech Misarticulations and Some of the More Commonly Occurring Phonological Processes		
Error Patterns	**Example**	
SODA Patterns		
Substitution	rabbit → wabbit	cat → tat
Omission	hat → at	blue → bue
Distortion[1]	soup → *oup	ladder → *adder
Additions	green → gareen	swim → sawim
Phonological Process		
Final Consonant Deletion	hat → ha	leaf → lea
Stopping of Fricatives	fish → pish	zoo → doo
Cluster Reduction	spoon → poon	broom → boom
Gliding of Liquids	lazy → wazy	broom → bwoom

[1]Distortions involve the substitution of a phoneme with an undecipherable sound. The * is used to denote an undecipherable sound.

exists. Normative data are available to the speech-language pathologist to guide in the decision. The normative data are presented in two ways: (1) age of mastery and (2) age of suppression. Using **age of mastery** norms involves examining each misarticulated sound produced by the child in regard to the age at which the sound should be acquired.

If a child is unable to produce a sound after the age at which it should normally be acquired, the child is assumed to be disordered in regard to the production of the sound. For example, the "g" sound is normally acquired by the age of four years (see Table 5–1). If a six-year-old child was to demonstrate misarticulations of "g," there would be cause for concern. **Age of suppression** norms refer to the age at which specific phonological processes should no longer be apparent in a child's speech. If a child still demonstrates a particular

process after the age at which it should have disappeared, the child would be exhibiting a phonological disorder. For example, the phonological pattern of final consonant deletion ("hat" is produced as "ha") should disappear by the age of 3;6 years. If a four-year-old child is observed deleting final consonants, there would be cause for concern. Some age of disappearance (suppression) norms for phonological processes are listed in Table 5–3.

Severity Estimation

For a child found to demonstrate a phonological disorder, the speech-language pathologist next determines the severity of the phonological disorder. Severity refers to the effect of the phonological disorder on the **intelligibility** of speech. Intelligibility is defined as a listener's ability to understand a speaker's words.

Table 5–3. Age of Suppression for Some of the More Commonly Occurring Phonological Processes

Phonological Process	Example	Age of Suppression
Velar fronting	gun → dun	3 years
Final consonant deletion	bat → ba	3;6 years
Unstressed syllable deletion	balloon → loon	4 years
Gliding of liquids	rabbit → wabbit	4 years
Vowelization	flower → flowa	4 years

This judgment can be based on **qualitative** and **quantitative** criteria. A qualitative criterion involves an impressionistic judgment as to the impact of the disorder on the clarity of the child's communication. This may simply involve a judgment by the speech-language pathologist using a continuum of good-fair-poor. This estimation is generally influenced by the characteristics of the phonological disorder. For example, a pattern involving a high number of consonant omissions is likely to result in a severity judgment of "poor," compared with a pattern involving a simple substitution of one sound for another such as "f" used in place of "th" (thumb is pronounced as "fumb"). Another qualitative scale of speech severity involves judgments by the child's parents or teachers in regard to how well the child communicates. For example, a teacher might be asked to rate how well they understand the child on a 10-point scale, with 1 meaning *all the time* and 10 meaning *never*.

A quantitative estimate of severity is based on more objective criteria such as: (1) the exact number of misarticulated phonemes, (2) the length of time the disorder has existed, and (3) the age of the child. A popular measure of severity is known as the **percentage of consonants correct** (Shriberg, 2003). The percentage of consonants correct is calculated from the phonetic inventory by tabulating the total number of consonants produced in a speech sample and dividing this into the total number of consonants that were only produced correctly. The formula is as follows:

$$\frac{\text{Number of correct consonants}}{\text{Total number of consonants}} \times 100 =$$

percentage of consonants correct

On the basis of percentage of consonants correct calculation, the severity of the disorder is categorized as normal to mild (85%–100%), mild to moderate (65%–84%), moderate to severe (50%–64%), or severe (below 50%).

Oral-Facial Examination

The phonological assessment continues with an examination of the child's oral-facial patterns. Assessment of the oral-facial mechanism is divided into two key areas: (1) structure and (2) function. Some individuals with a phonological disorder may show structural and/or functional peculiarities that affect speech sound production, including dental malocclusion, cleft palate, and tongue abnormalities. Structural assessment includes examination of the lips, teeth, tongue, hard palate, and soft palate. The functional assessment involves examination of the same structures in a variety of speaking and nonspeaking tasks. These tasks are designed to evaluate the **range of motion, strength, and rate of movement**. The information derived from this examination helps to guide the speech-language pathologist in determining the nature of the phonological disorder. The information also can shed light on the client's general oral-motor skills, which can be useful when developing a treatment program. A simple checklist of features considered in an oral-facial examination is provided in Table 5–4.

TREATMENT OF CHILD PHONOLOGICAL DISORDERS

Decisions about whether to treat and how often the child should be seen are based primarily on the severity of

Table 5–4. Example of a Typical Oral-Facial Examination

Oral Facial Examination

	Structure	Function
Lips	Symmetry: _____	Purse: _____
	Scarring: _____	Retract: _____
	Purse and Retract: _____	
Teeth	Alignment: _____	
	Gap or missing teeth: _____	
	Facial pattern: _____	
Tongue	Scarring: _____	Moves side to side: _____
		Moves up and down: _____
		Moves in and out: _____
Hard Palate	Vault height: _____	
	Vault width: _____	
	Scarring: _____	
Soft Palate	Symmetry: _____	Lifts on sustained "ah": _____
	Scarring: _____	Lifts on repeated "ah": _____
		Symmetry of movement: _____

the disorder. Treatment for a phono-logical disorder is important not only for the child to be able to form speech sounds, but for other reasons, as well. Children who have a speech sound dis-order may also have academic difficul-ties in subject areas such as spelling or reading. Furthermore, children whose speech articulation differs from that of their peers can find themselves frus-trated and ridiculed, and may become less willing to participate in play or classroom activities. The prognosis for children with phonological disorders generally is good. For many children, the problem resolves spontaneously. It is reported that in 75% of children with mild or moderate forms of the disor-der, and whose problems do not stem from a medical condition, the disorder is resolved by the age of six years. In many other cases, children who receive treatment eventually develop normal or close to normal speech. In some instances, there may be mild misartic-ulations that last until adulthood, but speech is completely understandable. For children with a phonological disor-der due to a structural or neurological cause, the outcome generally is depen-dent on how well the underlying cause of the problem is treated.

The types of treatment available to resolve a phonological disorder can be categorized into two primary ap-proaches: (1) the **articulation approach** and (2) the phonological approach. Within each of these approaches, there are vari-ations in management techniques.

Articulation Approach

The **articulation approach** focuses on motoric aspects of producing individ-ual consonants and vowels. Techniques

---

FYI

Children with a phonological disor-der typically receive individualized treatment from a speech-language pathologist on a twice weekly basis. The duration of each therapy ses-sion lasts between 30 minutes to 1 hour, depending on the age of the child and the severity of the disorder.

---

include the use of mirrors, tongue depressors, oral-motor exercises, and sensory motor training. Repetitive prac-tice in correctly saying the misarticulated sounds is an integral part of treatment. Two well-known techniques that use a motor-oriented framework of speech treatment are the traditional approach and maximal contrast approach.

Traditional Approach

The **traditional approach** was first developed by Charles Van Riper. This style of treatment emphasizes correct articulation of individual speech sounds. Through a series of graduated steps, the child is taught to consciously learn to produce the sound. The child has to be successful at each step before proceed-ing to the next level of speaking com-plexity. The first step involves sensori-perceptual (ear) training, whereby the child must first be able to correctly perceive the target speech sound as spoken by others before attempting to produce the sound. The ensuing steps entail teaching the child to articulate the sound in short syllables, followed by words, then sentences, and eventually, in a conversational speaking context. The sounds targeted for treatment are those that should have been mastered earliest by the child but, as yet, are not articulated correctly (see Table 5–1).

Maximal Contrast Approach

There is debate over the way children with more severe forms of a phonological disorder should be treated. A child with a severe speech sound disorder may exhibit misarticulations of early-developing, as well as later-developing speech sounds. Some speech-language pathologists believe sounds that are learned later in development should be addressed first in therapy, even if the child has not yet learned to produce some of the earlier developing sounds. Research has shown that earlier developing sounds are likely to improve on their own, so it may not be necessary to target them in therapy. The focus of the **maximal contrast approach** is to enact widespread change in children with a severe phonological disorder. Rather than targeting early developing sounds, later developing sounds are the focus of therapy. Presumably, by targeting these more difficult sounds, they assist in filling the gap for less difficult sounds.

Phonological Approach

Whereas traditional and maximal contrast approaches focus on teaching the child to articulate specific sounds correctly, the **phonological approach** focuses on having the child change his or her phonological system, using cognitive techniques such as semantic images. The phonological approach is used in cases where children have multiple misarticulations (speech delay) and highly unintelligible speech. Presumably, using

a phonological treatment approach with severely unintelligible children shortens the length of time necessary to improve their sound systems. Two phonological treatment approaches are the cycles approach and minimal pairs approach.

Cycles Approach

This **cycles approach** was developed by Hodson and Paden (1991). The general idea behind the approach is to facilitate the emergence of speech sound patterns rather than attempting to work on mastery of individual speech sounds. For example, if a child is showing the phonological patterns of final consonant deletion (e.g., "hat" is produced as "ha"), cluster reduction (e.g., "blue" is produced as "bue"), and stopping of fricatives (e.g., "see" is produced as "tee"), the treatment program would involve working on each of these patterns in a staggered fashion. A typical treatment cycle might involve working on final consonant deletion for two weeks, and then switching to cluster reduction for two weeks, followed by stopping of fricatives for two weeks. At the conclusion of this cycle, the speech-language pathologist probes to determine whether the child's overall pattern of speech sound production is improving. If not, another cycle of therapy would commence with possible changes to the particular sounds targeted during a treatment session.

Minimal Pairs Approach

A **minimal pair** refers to a situation where two words differ in pronunciation by only one sound, and the change in sound results in a change in word meaning. For instance, the words "sea"

FYI

The **electropalatograph** is a recording device that provides a form of **biofeedback** to a client with speech articulation difficulties. A specifically designed acrylic palate is created that contains touch-sensitive sensors spaced along the surface of the palate. The device is attached to the roof of a person's mouth and is capable of detecting the location and amount of contact between the tongue and palate during the articulation of speech. A visual display of the location of tongue-palate contact is provided on a computer monitor. The device is used primarily for research but is gaining popularity as an alternative approach to the treatment of some speech disorders (McLeod & Searl, 2006).

---

and "seat" differ only by the absence or presence of the last consonant [t], and this difference signals a change in meaning. For a phonologically disordered child who deletes final consonants, it is likely the child would produce "seat" as "sea." A minimal pair treatment approach might involve the speech-language pathologist presenting pictures of "sea" and "seat" simultaneously to the child. In a game format, the child would be instructed to name one of the pictures, with the speech-language pathologist guessing which picture was named. Because the child is likely to produce both words as "sea," the speech-language pathologist would deliberately point to the picture of "sea" even when the child had intended the alternate "seat." Thus, to resolve this confusion the child must learn to revise productions until the speech-language pathologist is no longer confused between the two words.

Phonological Awareness

As an adjunct to both articulation and phonological approaches to the management of phonological disorders, it is important to consider the child's understanding of the speech sound system. Treatment programs often rely on the repeated production of speech sounds and may fail to link the child's awareness with production. **Phonological awareness** refers to the ability to think about and manipulate the sound system apart from meaning. Children with impaired phonology may have incomplete (or inaccurate) awareness of their speech sound system. Training in the types of skills that deliberately involve phonological awareness has shown to help children change their disordered phonological system, as well as help children with literacy (reading) problems (Gillon, 2004). A simple phonological awareness task involves the child's recognition of words that rhyme (e.g., asking the child, "Do the words 'cat' and 'hat' sound alike?"). A more complicated phonological awareness task involves the child's ability to segment sounds and words (e.g., asking the child, "How many words do you hear in the sentence, 'I have a blue pen'?"). Examples of phonological awareness tasks, ranging in level of complexity are provided in Figure 5–14.

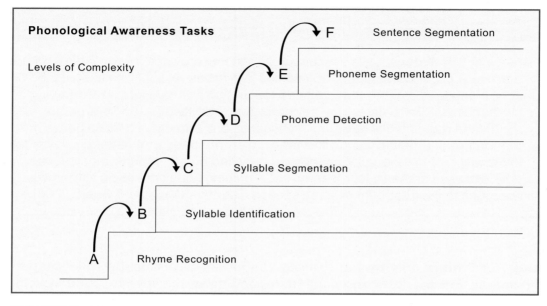

FIGURE 5–14. Examples of phonological awareness tasks according to increasing levels of complexity.

CULTURAL CONSIDERATIONS AND CHILD PHONOLOGICAL DISORDERS

English is spoken throughout the world. Although the English of England might be construed as the true mother tongue of the language, there are enormous varieties in spoken English. Each particular variety of English is often described in reference to the geographic region where the language is spoken. English is spoken around the world, resulting in geographically rich varieties of the language. We find English varieties such as British English, Irish English, Australian English, American English, New Zealand English, South African English, Indian English, and Singapore English, to name a few. Each variety is characterized by particular dialectical features, including unique vocabulary and specific phonological patterns. **Dialect** refers to a regional variety of a particular language. Dialects are distinguished by variations in vocabulary (word choice), grammar, and pronunciation. They are based on geography or socioeconomic level. **Geographic dialects** are the most common form of dialect. They are thought to be related to the immigration of certain ethnicities to specific regions of a country. The dialect reflects the vestiges (i.e., roots) of the original language. Examples of geographic dialects found in England and the United States are shown in Figure 5–15.

Socioeconomic dialects are less common, with word choice being one of the more obvious features. Individuals who vary in income level, educational level, and occupation may be found to speak differently than individuals residing within the same geographic region. For example, consider the term used in England to describe pieces of candy.

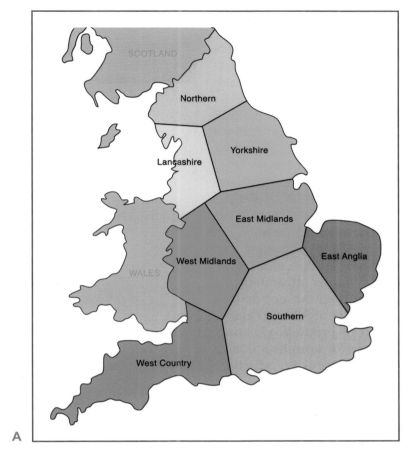

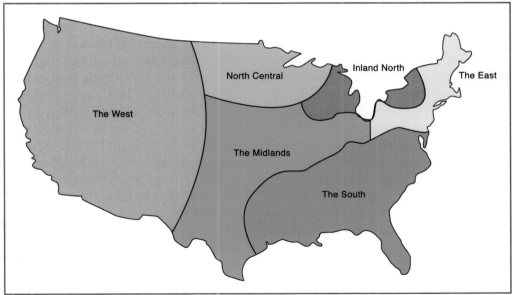

FIGURE 5–15. A. The approximate geographic boundaries for various accents of English spoken in England. **B.** The approximate geographic boundaries for various accents of English spoken in the United States.

Individuals from high economic levels often used the term "sweets," whereas someone from a lower economic class is likely to use the term "lollies."

The term **accent** refers to the manner of pronunciation of a language. Accents are found in all varieties of English. For example, a common feature of New Zealand English is the "vowelization" of postvocalic /r/ ("bear" → "bea-ah"), that is produced throughout most of the country. Yet in the most southern region of the same country, the postvocalic /r/ is clearly produced. This peculiar variation in pronunciation is attributed to a large Scottish immigrant population in the southern part of New Zealand, which is known to produce a distinct /r/. A wide range of variation is also found in American English production, including New England English, Appalachian English, and African American English. There is a popular misconception that African American English is incorrect, lazy, defective, ungrammatical, and broken English. On the contrary, evidence from many years of linguistic investigation establishes that African American English is a legitimate, rule-governed, socially constructed variety of American English (Payne, 2005). Some of the phonological patterns that are unique to African American English are shown in Table 5–5.

Bilingualism refers to the ability to communicate in two languages. This ability can found in four modalities: (1) speaking, (2) understanding, (3) reading, and (4) writing. **Multilingualism** is the ability to communicate in more than two languages. An individual who is multilingual can also be referred to as a polyglot (i.e., multiple tongues). Approximately 50% of the world's population is bilingual. Indeed, individuals who speak only one language (i.e., monolingual) are becoming the exception rather than the norm. The learning of two or more languages can occur simultaneously or consecutively. A simultaneous bilingual is one who has learned two or more languages at precisely the same time and continues to use multiple languages. Simultaneous bilinguals will not exhibit an accent when speaking various languages. A consecutive bilingual is one whose second language was learned sometime after learning a first language. In this case, the first language is referred to as L1 and the second language is L2. The majority of the world's bilinguals are consecutive and will exhibit an accent in their L2 speech. When the L2 spoken is English, the term **English as a second language (ESL)** is used.

When we encounter a foreign language, our natural tendency is to hear

Table 5–5. Some Phonological Rules of African American English

African American English Rule	Examples
Final consonant reduction	old → ole
	missed → miss
	tests → tesses
Devoicing of voiced sounds	they → dey
	feather → feavuh
	bathe → bave
	eating → eatin
Modification of voiceless sounds	nothing → nufin
	liked → lik-ted
	ask → aks
	asked → ast

it in terms of the sounds of our own language. We actually perceive it differently from the way native speakers do. Equally, when we speak a foreign language we tend to attempt to do so using the familiar sounds and sound patterns of our mother tongue. This is the well-documented phenomenon known as **phonological interference**. Our L1 (mother tongue) interferes with our attempts to produce the L2 (target language). Phonological interference can occur in many ways. Perhaps the most common interference concerns sounds in the L2 that are not found in L1. In these cases, the speaker of the L2 may either replace the foreign sound with one found in the L1 or completely delete the sound. Some aspects of accented speech are generally attributed to differences in the phonemic inventories of a speaker's native language and their second language. Some examples for French, Spanish, and Mandarin are provided below, all of which pertain to production of the phoneme /ð/ (the first sound in the English word "this"). In each of these languages, this particular phoneme is not found in the native L1.

French. In French-accented English, the French phoneme /z/ is often produced as a substitute for the English phoneme /ð/. For example, the word "thee" is likely to be produced as "zee."

Spanish. In Spanish-accented English, the Spanish phoneme /d/ is often produced as a substitute for the English phoneme /ð/. So instead of saying "this," the speaker is likely to say "dis."

Mandarin. In Mandarin-accented English, the English phoneme /ð/

> ——————— **FYI** ———————
>
> Click sounds serve as phonemes in some South African languages. Clicks are produced on ingressive (inward) airflow compared with all other phonemes, which are produced on egressive (outward) airflow. However, click sounds are sometimes found in languages when we least expect them, including English. For example, consider the ingressive sound sometimes used to express regret or disapproval, written as *tsk-tsk*.

frequently sounds like a soft "d," produced with the tongue either immediately behind the front teeth or protruding slightly from the mouth.

An issue that confronts the speech-language pathologist when evaluating the speech of an ESL speaker is determining whether the speech pattern demonstrated is indicative of a phonological difference or a phonological disorder. A **phonological difference** is a pattern where the sound productions are within the norms for the community but different from the standard. For instance, a person who produces Mandarin accented English is likely to pronounce English in the same way as other speakers of Mandarin accented English (Chen, 1999). Speech therapy is not warranted for an ESL speaker showing a phonological difference. Rather, the speech pattern is considered normal and serves a communicative function, as well as a social solidarity function. Sometimes, an accent or dialect may be a problem if it interferes with a person's goals in life. For example, an ESL speaker may choose to receive therapy to help reduce their accent, such as a Japanese executive who wishes to do business with American companies. Another situation might be where an aspiring actor from a European country wishes to "lose" his foreign accent by learning the standard form of the L2. This type of therapy would be considered "elective" as opposed to mandatory and could be provided by the speech-language pathologist.

It is possible that a bilingual speaker might show a phonological disorder. In this condition, the sound productions of the speaker fall outside the norms of the community. Referring back to a Mandarin accented English speaker, this would be a situation in which the individual's speech productions of English differ from those of other Mandarin accented English speakers. As is often the case, if the person's L2 is found to be phonologically disordered, the L1 is most likely phonologically disordered as well. In order for the speech-language pathologist to make this diagnosis, he or she would need to be aware of the phonological rules of the accent.

CURRENT RESEARCH IN CHILD PHONOLOGICAL DISORDERS

Genetic Factors

Searching for the cause of phonological disorders has typically not been of primary interest to speech-language pathologists. Rather, the research focus has been to develop effective treatment programs. This has certainly been the case for functional phonological disorders. However, recent advances in behavioral molecular genetics over the past decade have made it possible to investigate genetic factors that may contribute to phonological disorders. We typically assume that functional phonological disorders have a cause that is unknown or perhaps may even reflect learned behavior. Yet, mounting evidence suggests that at least some functional phonological disorders may actually have a genetic (i.e., organic) origin. As noted earlier in Chapter 4, researchers have now laid claim to a unique gene (*FOXP2*) located on chromosome 7 that appears to contribute to the normal acquisition of speech and language. This work has since expanded, and specific types of conditions contributing to speech sound disorders have now been found to be linked to locations on chromosomes 1, 3, 6, and 15 (Newbury & Monaco, 2010). It would seem as though some functional speech sound disorders may be more organic-based than previously thought.

Literacy Development

Most children who develop speech and language skills normally go on to develop literacy skills with no problem. We now know that a number of children who have poor oral language skills, as well as poor phonological awareness, experience difficulty learning to read and spell (Doherty & Landells, 2006). The relationship between literacy development and speech and language development is complex and is currently an active area of research. A better understanding of this relationship will lead to a more accurate and early diagnosis of difficulties in young children. In turn, this should contribute to the creation of specific intervention programs resulting in higher levels of academic achievement.

Childhood Apraxia of Speech

Although there is agreement that childhood apraxia of speech is a unique form of phonological disorder, the cause of childhood apraxia of speech remains unknown. Although there appears to be agreement that the condition is one that affects the brain's ability to send proper signals to speech articulators, results of brain imaging studies have been inconclusive. The research currently underway involves developing more sensitive protocols for diagnosing the condition (Shirberg, Lohmeier, Strand, & Jakielski, 2012), as well as searching for the underlying cause of the condition. This latter area includes a closer examination of the brain and other parts of the nervous system. Not surprising, some researchers are tying to locate possible genes that may be linked to childhood apraxia of speech.

CHILD PHONOLOGICAL DISORDERS ON THE WORLD WIDE WEB

Listed below are websites that provide further information on the topic of phonological disorders. At the time of publication, each website was freely accessible.

Phonetics Video
http://linguaspectrum.com/videos/Video_English_Lessons11.php

Information for Families
http://www.speech-language-therapy.com

Childhood Apraxia of Speech Association of North America (CASANA)
http://www.apraxia-kids.org/

Expert Information on Speech Sound Disorders
http://www.asha.org/public/speech/disorders/speechsound disorders.htm

Phonological Awareness Video
http://www.youtube.com/watch?v=tfMFeag7XJk

STUDY QUESTIONS

1. List and describe the consonant and vowel classification systems.
2. What are the three categories of phonological disorders?
3. List and describe the six steps involved in performing an assessment of child phonological disorders.
4. What are the two approaches to treating child phonological disorders?
5. What is phonological interference, and how does this influence the diagnosis of a phonological disorder?

REFERENCES

Chen, Y. (1999). *Acoustic characteristics of American English produced by native speakers of Mandarin* (Unpublished doctoral dissertation). University of Connecticut, Storrs, CT.

Chomsky, N., & Halle, M. (1968). *The sound pattern of English*. New York, NY: Harper and Row.

Doherty, I., & Landells, J. (2006). Literacy and numeracy. In J. Clegg & J. Ginsbourg (Eds.), *Language and social disadvantage*. Sussex, UK: Wiley.

Donegan, P., & Stampe, D. (1979). The study of natural phonology. In D. A. Dinnsen (Ed.), *Current approaches to phonological theory* (pp. 126–173). Bloomington, IN: University Press.

Fairbanks, G. (1940). *Voice and articulation drillbook*. New York, NY: Harper & Brothers.

Geruit, J., & Morrisette, M. (2005). The clinical significance of optimality theory for phonological disorders. *Topics in Language Disorders, 25*, 266–280.

Gillon, G. (2004). *Phonological awareness: From research to practice*. New York, NY: Guilford Press.

Hodson, B. W., & Paden, E. P. (1991). *Targeting intelligible speech*. San Diego, CA: College-Hill Press.

McLeod, S., & Searl, J. (2006). Adaptation to an electropalatograph palate: Acoustic, impressionistic and perceptual data. *American Journal of Speech-Language Pathology, 15*, 192–206.

Mowrer, O. H. (1960). *Learning theory and behavior*. New York, NY: Wiley.

Newbury, D., & Monaco, A. (2010). Genetic advances in the study of speech and language disorders. *Neuron, 68*, 309–320.

Payne, K. (2005). African American English: Nature, origin, and implications for clinicians. *ECHO, 1*(2), 95.

Rousey, C. (1957). The psychopathology of articulation and voice deviations. In L. E. Travis (Ed.), *Handbook of speech pathology and audiology*. Englewood Cliffs, NJ: Prentice-Hall.

Scripture, E. W. (1912). *Stuttering and lisping*. New York, NY: MacMillan.

Shriberg, L. (2003). Diagnostic markers for child speech-sound disorders: Introductory comments. *Clinical Linguistics and Phonetics, 17*, 501-505.

Shirberg, L., Lohmeier, H., Strand, E., & Jakielski, K. (2010). Encoding, memory, and transcoding deficits in childhood apraxia of speech. *Clinical Linguistics and Phonetics, 26*, 445–482.

Travis, L. E. (1931). *Speech pathology: A dynamic neurological treatment of normal speech and speech deviations*. New York, NY: Appleton-Century.

Van Riper, C. (1947). *Speech correction: Principles and methods*. Englewood Cliffs, NJ: Prentice-Hall.

Van Riper, C. (1981). An early history of ASHA. *ASHA Magazine, 23*(11), 855–858.

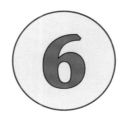

FLUENCY DISORDERS

INTRODUCTION

Most of us have met someone with a **fluency disorder** or know of someone who has a fluency disorder (Figure 6–1). The peculiarity of the disorder is undeniable and is one of the most identifiable communication disorders by both trained and untrained listeners. When a speech-language pathologist is asked to provide a general description of their occupation to a layperson, mentioning the treatment of individuals with a fluency disorder is readily recognizable. After holding a conversation with a person who has a fluency disorder one may wonder: (1) What caused the disorder? (2) Can the disorder be cured? and (3) What can I, as a listener, do to best communicate with a person who has a fluency disorder? The answers to some of these questions are still unknown, but we do know a great deal about fluency approaches that help improve a person's ability to produce speech fluently. It is interesting to note that some of the world's leading experts in the area of fluency disorders were drawn to the field because they themselves have a fluency disorder. Who would be a better expert then someone who has first-hand experience with the disorder? There is a documented history of research on fluency disorders that has led to a wealth of information on the topic. The information presented in the following chapter is an introduction to the fascinating area of fluency disorders.

TERMINOLOGY AND DEFINITIONS

The term **fluency** refers to the effortless flow of speech. Fluency encompasses

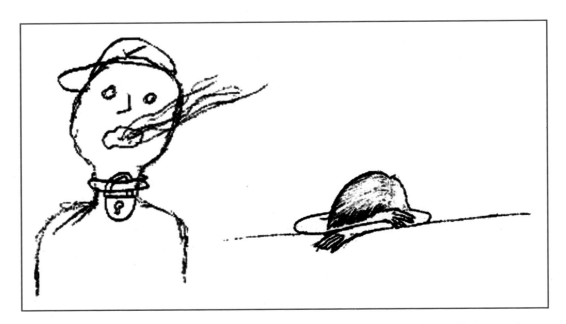

FIGURE 6–1. Pictures drawn by children in response to instructions, "Draw a picture of what it feels like to stutter." Permission granted by Andriana DiGrande, New England Fluency Program, United States.

many features that contribute to this effortless flow, such as: (1) the rate or quickness of a person's speech, (2) the silent periods or pauses that may occur within or between words, (3) the stress or emphasis placed on various syllables or words, and (4) the inflection or intonation used by the speaker during the production of an utterance. Collectively, we think of fluent speech as the pleasant sing-song pattern of talking. Fluency encompasses qualities that make speech sound natural and normal. This definition is specific to the spoken word; however, fluency can also apply to other areas of communication such as written language.

The term **disfluency** is the opposite condition, whereby a disruption or breakdown in the flow of speech occurs. A change in any single feature, or combination of features, that contribute to fluent speech, can result in disfluent speech. For example, excessively fast speaking can interfere with the correct articulation of vowels and consonants, thereby affecting the naturalness of speech. Unusually long pauses between the syllables of words can likewise affect speech naturalness. It is important to keep in mind that we all produce speech disfluencies, although this does not necessary mean we have a fluency disorder. The simple interjection of "um" between words, or changing our choice of words in mid-conversation would classify as forms of disfluency. The job of the speech-language pathologist is to distinguish between what is considered normal, natural speech disfluencies and unnatural speech disfluencies. When speech disfluencies fall outside the boundary of what is considered natural, they are deemed to represent a fluency disorder. The two fluency disorders profiled in this chapter are **stuttering** and **cluttering**.

There is a bit of confusion in the terminology surrounding fluency disorders. Students frequently ask whether the terms _disfluency_ and _dysfluency_ are interchangeable. The answer is no, although the terms have been used interchangeably as recently as the 1990s. The prefix _dis_ has its origins in Latin and is used to form words that are the opposite of the core word, such as _honor_ versus _dishonor_, and _able_ versus _disable_. Alternatively, the prefix _dys_ has its origins in Greek and refers to something bad, harsh, or wrong, such as _function_ versus _dysfunction_. We all demonstrate disruptions in fluency. To ascribe the prefix _dys_ to this condition would be too strong a description. Rather, the disruption in fluency simply reflects the opposite state. Therefore, the term disfluency is preferred for the disruptions in speech that occur normally in the majority of speakers.

HISTORIC ASPECTS OF FLUENCY DISORDERS

Observations regarding fluency disorders, specifically stuttering, can be traced back centuries. A list of notable individuals (past and present) known (or thought) to have a fluency disorder is provided in Table 6–1. Some of the earliest documented reports of individuals who stutter include Moses. There is a report in the Old Testament that Moses stuttered as depicted in the passage, "O Lord, I have never been a man of ready speech, never in my life, not even now that thou has spoken to me; I am slow and hesitant of speech" (Exodus 4:10). The Roman emperor Claudius (10 BC to 54 AD) was assumed to produce stuttered speech and showed signs of deafness. **King Louis II** of France (843–879) was also known to produce a stutter.

Table 6–1. Famous People Known to Have Displayed Stuttering

Rowan Atkinson	British actor
Lewis Carroll	Author of *Alice in Wonderland*
Winston Churchill	Former prime minister of England
Cameron Daddo	Australian actor
Charles Darwin	British naturalist
King George VI	Former king of England
Marilyn Monroe	American actor
Sam Neill	New Zealand actor
Isaac Newton	Scientist
Gareth Gates	British singer
James Earl Jones	American actor
Porky Pig	Cartoon character from Looney Tunes series
Jimmy Volmer	Cartoon character on the television series South Park
George Washington	U.S. president
Bruce Willis	American actor

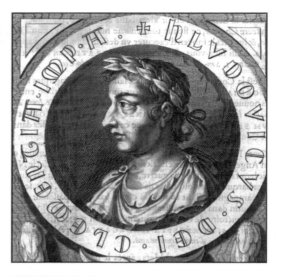

FIGURE 6–2. King Louis II of France was called "le Begue" or "the Stammerer."

He was called "le Begue" or "the Stammerer" (Figure 6–2). The 2010 film, *The King's Speech*, profiled the impact of stuttering on the life of King George VI of England (1895–1952).

Because of the unusual pattern of speaking associated with stuttering, the disorder has been of high scientific and medical curiosity. The interest has centered on determining either the cause of stuttering or how to cure stuttering. During the late 1700s and early 1800s, the root cause of stuttering was thought to be related to faulty functioning of the tongue and/or larynx. Jean-Marc Gaspard Itard (1774–1838), a physician at the Institute of Deaf Mutes in Paris (see also Chapter 4), was the first to view stuttering as a pathological condition. In his opinion, stuttering was caused by a spasm induced by a weakness of the motor organs of the larynx and tongue. The Swiss scientist **Rudolf Schulthess**

FYI

The origins of the word "stuttering" are unclear, but there are a few possibilities as to its derivation. The word *stue* is from a Greek word that means "to strike." There is a Nordic word *stytta*, which means "to stop." There is also an old German word *stutten* that means "to make a series of repeated sounds."

(1802–1833) also believed stuttering was due to spasms of the larynx and suggested using the terms *phonophobia* or *lalophobia* to describe the condition.

Toward the middle of the 19th century, there was a shift from viewing the tongue and larynx as causal factors of stuttering toward viewing stuttering as a disturbance in the breathing patterns for speech. For example, the German scholar **A. Thome** (1867) held the opinion that stuttering was a result of spasms of the respiratory organs that were linked to an individual's emotional state. The disturbance of stuttering was triggered by emotionally based disruptions in the nervous system. Two types of emotional conditions were assumed to contribute to moments of stuttering: (1) embarrassment or lack of confidence and (2) excessive rapidity of thought.

During the 1800s, approaches to the treatment of stuttering also varied widely. Believing the tongue was responsible for stuttering led Itard to develop a small forked golden plate that was placed under the tongue to provide support while speaking. More drastic treatment of the tongue was proposed by German surgeon **Johann Friedrich Dieffenbach** (1792–1847) who recommended cutting the tongue with scissors and removing a triangular wedge from the back of the tongue (Figure 6–3). **James Yearsley** (1805–1869) was a British surgeon who advocated removal of the tonsils as a form of treatment for stuttering. All of these invasive procedures were ultimately abandoned for two reasons. First, performing surgery in this region of the body carries a level of danger because the speech organs receive heavy blood supply (i.e., they are highly vascular). Therefore, surgery performed in this part of the body was risky. A surgical error could lead to con-

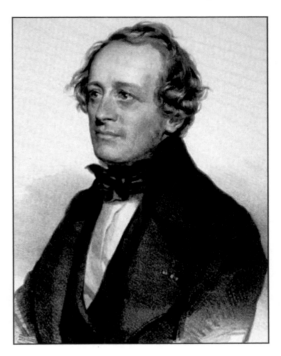

FIGURE 6–3. Johann Friedrich Dieffenbach, German surgeon who recommended cutting out portions of the tongue to treat stuttering.

siderable blood loss and subsequent death. The second reason for abandoning invasive techniques was that the various surgical procedures were not found to be successful in curing stuttering.

During the first half of the 20th century, there was continued interest in isolating the cause and cure of stuttering. Although research undertaken during this time period was less invasive than earlier years, the approaches were no less unusual. **Lee Edward Travis** (1896–1987), who is considered a founding father of the speech-language pathology profession (Figure 6–4), devoted a majority of his career to understanding the cause of stuttering. Travis held the view that people who stutter have speech centers in both cerebral hemispheres of their brain instead of just the

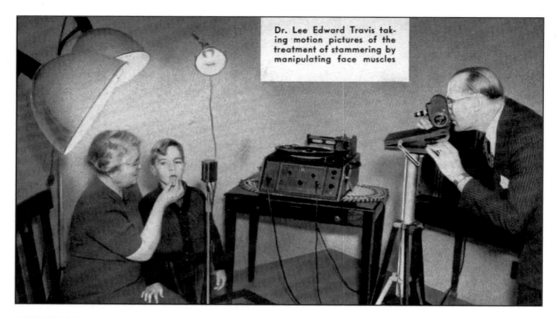

Dr. Lee Edward Travis taking motion pictures of the treatment of stammering by manipulating face muscles

FIGURE 6–4. Lee Travis (in 1940), known as the father of speech-language pathology, had a strong research interest in stuttering.

left hemisphere. According to Travis, stuttering resulted from a lack of brain dominance when it came to producing speech. As a result of this condition, when an individual began to organize the act of speech in their brain, the two sides of the brain were competing for control of the speech muscles. This competition led to a breakdown in the forward flow of speech and resulted in a stutter. This theory was based on Travis' observation that people who were left-handed or "forced" right-handers were more likely to stutter than pure right-handers. Presumably, this situation led to a lack of clear brain dominance in motor execution, which included speech execution. In the early 1930s, Travis took a group of left-handed individuals who stuttered and forced them to write with their right hand. Two of these research participants later became eminent scholars in the field of stuttering, **Charles Van Riper** (1905–1994)

and **Wendell Johnson** (1906–1965). Van Riper is quoted as saying, "Both of us [Van Riper and Johnson] wore plaster casts upon our right arms to enforce left-handedness and again I found myself doing the interminable pages of talking and writing each day." The activity did little to alleviate the production of stuttered speech.

Bryng Bryngelson (1892–1979) received his PhD from the University of Iowa and went on to have a successful career at the University of Minnesota (Figure 6–5). Bryngelson is remembered for his research on the relationship between stuttering and left-handedness. However, after spending nearly 30 years on the topic, there was little evidence to suggest that shifting handedness would alleviate the production of stuttered speech. One of Bryngelson's important contributions to the field of stuttering therapy was his concept of voluntary stuttering. By having an individual

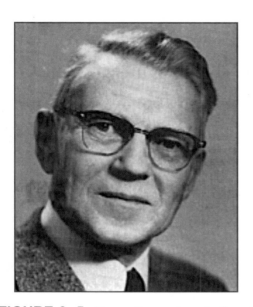

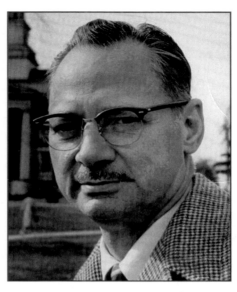

FIGURE 6–5. Bryng Bryngelson believed that a person's handedness was linked to stuttering. Reprinted with permission from Van Riper, C. (1981). An early history of ASHA. *ASHA Magazine, 23*(11), 855–858.

FIGURE 6–6. Wendell Johnson believed the development of stuttering had a strong environmental influence. Reprinted with permission from Van Riper, C. (1981). An early history of ASHA. *ASHA Magazine, 23*(11), 855–858.

who stutters do so deliberately in public settings helped to lower the anxiety associated with speaking situations. This reduction in anxiety led to a corresponding decrease in the frequency of stuttering. Gradually, deliberate stuttering was decreased with the aim of producing stutter-free speech at all times.

The area of stuttering in the early 1900s was also influenced by **Sigmund Freud's** (1856–1939) psychoanalytic theory. The cause of stuttering was felt to be a result of a deep-seeded psychological disturbance and that family relationships, especially parent-child relationships, lay at the root of the problem. An adaptation of this perspective was proposed by Wendell Johnson who felt stuttering was caused by the parents' misinterpretations of their child's speech (Figure 6–6). Parents confused

the child's normal disfluency for stuttering. According to Johnson, "Stuttering begins not in the child's mouth but in the parent's ear." In doing so, parents' required from the child a level of speaking performance that the child could not attain. The subsequent reactions of both child and parents resulted in a worsening of the child's speech, leading to stuttering. In 1939, Johnson tested this theory, in what is now known as the Iowa Stuttering Study. In this study, 12 nonstuttering children who were residents in an orphanage were induced to stutter. Of these 12 children, one half were told that they had symptoms of stuttering, and their caregivers were instructed to correct their speech disfluencies whenever they occurred. These six children eventually developed symptoms of stuttering. The other six children were part of a control group and received no instructions to correct their speech disfluencies. These children never developed stuttering. The research would nowadays be considered unethical because of the lack of protection for the participants. The University of Iowa made a public apology in 2001 and subsequently agreed to pay approximately $1,000,000 to the six children and their heirs (ASHA, 2007).

Lena Rustin (1928–2004) was an inspirational pioneer in the treatment of stuttering (Figure 6–7). Born in England, Dr. Rustin was a dedicated clinician who spent her career helping children who stutter and their families. She founded the Association for Research into Stammering in Childhood in 1991. She also was the cofounder of the Michael Palin Centre for Stammering Children in London.

TYPES OF FLUENCY DISORDERS

Stuttering

The **World Health Organization** (1977) defines stuttering as, "Disorders in the rhythm of speech in which the individual knows precisely what s/he wishes to say but at the same time is unable to say because of an involuntary repetition, prolongation, or cessation of a sound." Speech-language pathology associations worldwide such as ASHA, RCSLT, and SPA have developed their own definitions of stuttering that vary slightly from the World Health Organization definition, but the general tenets of the definition are the same. Stuttering is a disruption in the flow of speech.

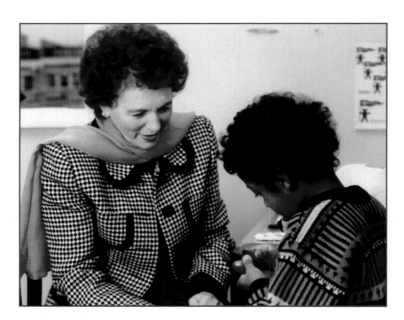

FIGURE 6–7. Lena Rustin, inspirational pioneer in the treatment of stuttering. Photo courtesy of the British Stammering Association (http://www.stammering.org).

Stuttering is also viewed as a developmental disorder. A child who eventually develops a stutter is considered to have been born with the condition; however, the condition is not perceptually apparent until the child begins using connected speech. The term **stammering** is synonymous with stuttering and is used often in the United Kingdom. Either term is appropriate and acceptable.

Stuttering is found to occur in all languages of the world, although precise estimates of its prevalence are unknown. Evidence of its occurrence around the world is provided by noting whether a word for stuttering exists in the vocabulary of the language. Table 6–2 provides some examples of various words for stuttering in languages around the world. Languages that do not have a word for stuttering does not necessarily mean the disorder is absent from the population. Rather, the condition may not be viewed as a disorder. As a general rule, stuttering is thought to occur in 1 out of every 100 individuals, or approximately 1% of the population. The percentage of stuttering in preschool children is somewhat higher with approximately 3% of children showing early signs of stuttering behavior. However, this number is reduced to 1% once children enter school. Stuttering is three times more likely to occur in boys compared with girls (3:1 ratio). There are also reports of stuttering occurring more often among twins and for the disorder to run in families across generations, suggesting a **genetic** (hereditary) predisposition for the disorder among some individuals.

The development of stuttering is not sudden. The appearance of the disorder is often equated with phases of the moon, whereby the condition waxes and wanes. There will be periods in the child's daily or weekly speaking behavior when it seems like nearly every word produced is disfluent. The same child may then show long periods of time when nearly every word is produced fluently. The **onset** of stuttering typically occurs at three years of age but may vary in children anywhere from two years to five years of age. We also know that some situations can serve to raise or lower moments of stuttering in children and adults alike. Situations that tend to require high communicative demand such as answering questions,

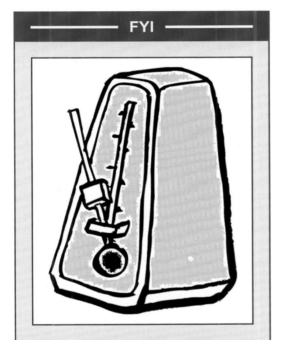

---- FYI ----

Speaking to the rhythmic beats of a metronome has been shown to help reduce stuttering. Although speaking in such a fashion sounds highly unnatural, the device has been used at the beginning of a therapy program to help gain control over severely disfluent speech.

Table 6–2. Words from Around the World Used to Refer to Stuttering

Language	Word
Afrikaans	hakkel
Arabic	rattat
Cherokee	a-da-nv-te-hi-lo-squi
Chinese (Cantonese)	hau hick
Chinese (Mandarin)	kou chi
Dutch	stotteren
Egyptian	tuhuhtuhuh
English	stuttering
Fijiian	kaka
French	begaiement
German	stottern
Hawaiian	uu uus
Hebrew	gimgum
Hindi	hakalaanaa
Hungarian	dadogo
Icelandic	stama
Italian	balbuzie
Japanese	domori; kitsuon
Korean	maldeodum
Māori	kīkiki
Nigerian	nsu
Punjabi	totalaanaa
Russian	zaikatsia; zaikanie
Spanish	tartamudez
Swedish	stamning

speaking to a stranger, or speaking on the telephone are likely to increase moments of disfluent speech. On the other hand, speaking one-on-one with a familiar individual (or even to a pet) is likely to be a situation of low communicative demand, resulting in more fluent speech.

Stuttering involves both **overt** (observable) and **covert** (nonobservable) behaviors. The combination of these behaviors has been likened to the shape of an iceberg. The tip of the iceberg that rises from the water reflects the overt behaviors, which are the audible and visible signs of stuttering (Figure 6–8). Van Riper (1982) refers to overt behaviors as the primary **characteristics of stuttering**. Yet far greater and perhaps more detrimental is the portion of the iceberg that is submerged. This portion reflects covert behaviors, which comprise feelings of fear, shame, guilt, anxiety, hopelessness, isolation, and denial. Van Riper refers to covert behaviors as the **secondary characteristics** of stuttering.

Primary Characteristics of Stuttering

A popular approach to describing overt stuttering is to differentiate and label the various types of disfluencies. The

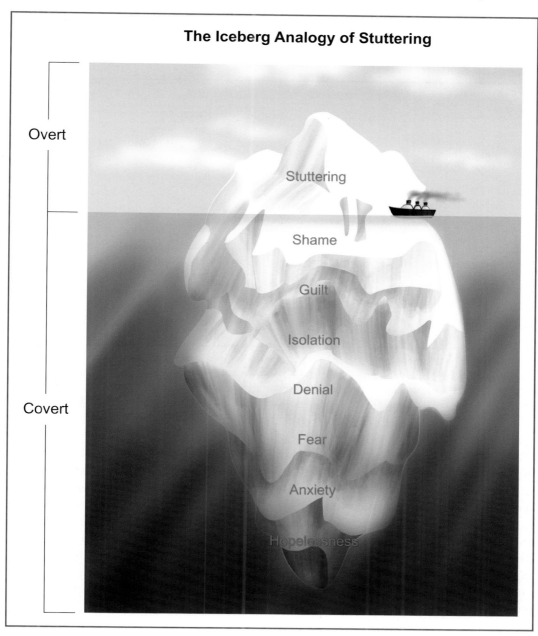

The Iceberg Analogy of Stuttering

Overt

Covert

Stuttering

Shame

Guilt

Isolation

Denial

Fear

Anxiety

Hopelessness

FIGURE 6–8. Classic depiction of the many facets of stuttering as analogous to the shape of an iceberg.

premise for identifying disfluency types is that some sorts of disfluencies are most often associated with chronic stuttering. Therefore, differentiating disfluency types should aid in the assessment and diagnosis of stuttering. Johnson (1961) identified eight disfluency types (Table 6–3). One thing to note with these various disfluency types is that some disfluencies occur within a specific

Johnson System	Yairi and Ambrose System
Table 6–3. Disfluency Notation Systems*	
(1) Part-word repetition: For example, "My t-t-t-tooth hurts."	
(2) Single-syllable word repetition: For example, "I-I-I-I want to go home."	
(3) Multisyllabic word repetition: For example, "The ba-ba-ba-baby is crying."	SLD
(4) Disrhythmic phonation (sound prolongation): For example, "MMMMMMy tooth hurts."	
(5) Tense pause (silent prolongation or "block"): For example, " . . . The baby is crying."	
(6) Phrase repetition: For example, "I want- I want- I want to go home."	
(7) Interjection: For example, "I um, well, um, want to go home."	OD
(8) Revision-incomplete phrase: For example, "My too . . . my molar hurts."	

*The Johnson (1961) system is based on the consideration of eight disfluency types. Types 1–5 are considered within-word disfluencies. Types 6–8 are considered between-word disfluencies. The Yairi and Ambrose (1992) system is based on the original Johnson system but simplified to consider two major types of disfluencies, stutter-like disfluencies (*SLD*) and other disfluencies (*OD*).

word, whereas other disfluencies occur between (or across) words. Johnson suggested that the production of **between-word disfluencies** was a common feature in the speech of people who do not stutter. The production of **within-word disfluencies** (in addition to producing between-word disfluencies) most often was associated with stuttering behavior. The typology developed by Johnson is still used in research and clinical settings; however, it has since been simplified to two broad categories of disfluencies: **stuttering-like disfluencies** and **other disfluencies** (Yairi & Ambrose, 1992). Stuttering-like disfluencies are those disfluencies indicative of chronic stuttering (i.e., part-word repetition, single-syllable word repetition, disrhythmic phonation, tense pause),

and other disfluencies are reflective of normal nonfluent speech (i.e., multisyllabic word repetition, phrase repetition, interjection, and revision-incomplete phrase). The reason for reducing the types of disfluencies to only two categories was to simplify the identification process for researchers and clinicians while still being able to capture the essence of stuttering behavior. An illustration of two common types of stuttering-like disfluencies, sound repetitions and sound prolongations, is shown in Figure 6–9.

Secondary Characteristics of Stuttering

The secondary characteristics of stuttering are more difficult to classify than

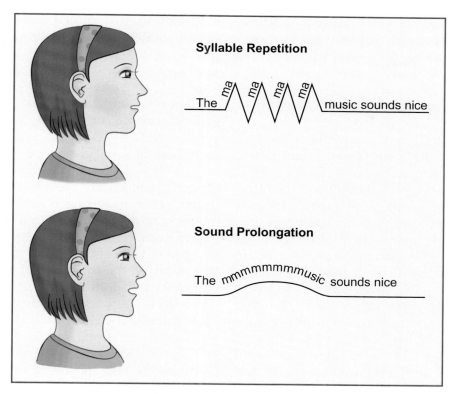

FIGURE 6–9. Illustration of a sound repetition and sound prolongation during production of the sentence, "The music sounds nice."

primary characteristics. These features of stuttering seem to develop gradually over time. Many of these behaviors may be absent among young children during the earlier years of stuttering and only begin to develop as the child grows older and stuttering becomes more fixated. These secondary characteristics can be organized into two categories: **bodily movements** and **psychosocial behaviors**. Bodily movements typically are related to facial activity that accompanies a moment of stuttering. These might include eye blinks, facial grimaces, head movements, and loss of eye contact. In more extreme cases, there also might be torso and limb movements. Some theorists believe these body movements reflect a coping strategy by the individual, whereby the behavior was used successfully at some point in time to aid the individual in speaking fluently. However, over time, these behaviors were less successful in preventing moments of stuttering. As a consequence, stuttering continued and the coping strategy (i.e., bodily movements) became uncontrollably linked to moments of stuttering. Psychosocial behaviors are the feelings experienced by the individual who stutters. A person's feelings can be as much a part of the disorder of stuttering as the speech behaviors. These feelings, which are usually negative, include fear, frustration, embarrassment, sadness, and anger, as well as overall **temperament**. As a person's stuttering worsens, these psychosocial behaviors can become more enhanced and may lead to complete withdrawal from speaking.

Nondevelopmental Stuttering

The definition of stuttering offered by the World Health Organization (1977) makes clear reference to fluency *disorders* (plural), which implies that stuttering does not occur as a single form of speech but rather in a variety of ways. Although the majority of instances of stuttering are developmental, there are forms of the disorder that arise later in life. These nondevelopmental forms of stuttering occur far less often, but this does not minimize their importance on the caseload of a speech-language pathologist. Two nondevelopmental forms of stuttering are neurogenic and psychogenic.

Neurogenic Stuttering

Conditions affecting various areas of the brain, including the cortex, cerebellum, and brainstem can cause **neurogenic stuttering**. The disfluency pattern in neurogenic stuttering is characterized by a high number of involuntary repetitions or prolongations of speech that do not seem to be a result of poor (hesitant) language formulation difficulties or as a result of psychiatric problems. Secondary behaviors may not be present, and if they do exist, they are not associated with moments of disfluency. One example of neurogenic stuttering can be found among individuals with Parkinson disease. Goberman and Blomgren (2003) suggested that stuttering in Parkinson disease is related to impairment in the amount of the neurotransmitter, dopamine, in the brain. Increases in stuttering were associated with taking medication designed to boost the amount of dopamine in the brain.

Psychogenic Stuttering

There are far fewer reports of **psychogenic stuttering** compared with neurogenic stuttering. Whereas neurogenic stuttering is associated with various known pathologies in the brain, psychogenic conditions are less obvious. Psychogenic stuttering is a condition referring to people in whom a psychological disturbance is clearly diagnosed. Because of the psychological nature of this disorder, the diagnosis of psychopathology falls outside the expertise of the speech-language pathologist. The speech disfluencies produced by the individual are strongly linked to psychological distress. The types of disfluencies are less consistent than both developmental stuttering and neurogenic stuttering. An example would be a situation where the person's speech disfluencies may change noticeably, either for better or worse. A reduction in stuttering during a person's disclosure of emotionally sensitive information is a strong indicator of a psychogenic stutter. Further evidence of a psychogenic basis for stuttering is related to response to treatment. If a person's speech fluency returns to normal or near normal, it is likely there was a psychological basis because this level of improvement is not found in developmental stuttering.

Cluttering

A third type of nondevelopmental stuttering that is considered a separate type of fluency disorder is known as cluttering. Cluttering is a disorder of speaking rate. In a person who shows cluttering, their speaking rate can be either abnormally fast, irregular, or both. Among normally fluent adult speakers, the typical rate of speaking is approximately 240 syllables per minute (spm). Individuals with cluttering will often demonstrate a speaking rate in excess of 300 spm. In cluttered speech, the rapid rate of speaking contributes to: (1) higher than normal speech disfluency, (2) types of disfluencies not like those found in stuttering, and (3) slurred speech misarticulations, such as consonant deletions and consonant substitutions during spurts of rapid speech. The general impression when listening to the speech of an individual with cluttering is that they are speaking so fast that their speech fluency deteriorates. A comparison of cluttered and stuttered speech is illustrated in Figure 6–10. Treatment for individuals with cluttering tends to focus on reducing speaking rate, which results in marked improvement in the overall fluency and clarity of their speech.

FYI

A peculiar pattern of stuttering is the production of a **disfluency cluster**, which is the production of two or more disfluencies on the same word and/or adjacent words. An example of a disfluency cluster would be the production of a sound repetition followed by a prolongation such as, "The b-b-boy wwwent." Disfluency clusters seem to only occur in the speech of people with a diagnosed stuttering disorder.

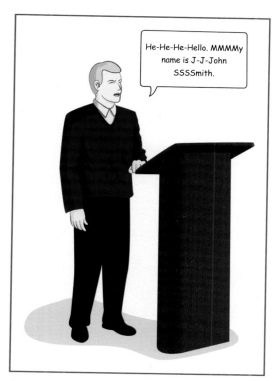

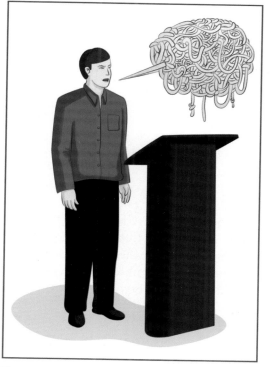

A **B**

FIGURE 6–10. The pattern of speaking found in a person who stutters (**A**) compared with the pattern of speaking found in an individual who clutters (**B**).

CURRENT THEORIES REGARDING STUTTERING

Modern theories about stuttering have been shaped over many years of research. Although stuttering is the most researched of the various communication disorders, the actual cause of stuttering remains controversial. There is no unified theory of stuttering. The general consensus is that stuttering has a multidimensional etiology. The various theories include a number of factors that may contribute to the disorder including genetics, the environment, language complexity, motor coordination, and psychological influences. In essence, modern theories suggest both nature and nurture influences on stuttering. Some of the most popular theories to date include the demands and capacities theory, covert repair theory, and the neuropsycholinguistic theory.

Demands and Capacities Theory

The **demands and capacities theory** was proposed by Starkweather (1997) and views stuttering as occurring when the intrinsic and extrinsic social demands placed on a child for producing fluent speech exceed the child's cognitive, linguistic, motor, or emotional capacities for fluent speech. Children who eventually develop stuttering have a genetic predisposition for the disorder and will encounter a mismatch between their speaking capabilities and self-imposed or environmental demands.

Covert Repair Theory

The **cover repair theory** was proposed by Postma and Kolk (1993) and links together the production of language and moments of stuttering. This theory assumes that people who stutter have an internally disordered phonological system. During the internal planning for speech, we naturally form (i.e., encode) the necessary sounds for words and sentences before physically producing speech. For people who stutter, they experience frequent planning errors in speech organization that need to be repaired before the words leave the speaker's mouth. Speech disfluencies occur when a speaker interrupts ongoing speech to repair these errors. This is why we often observe the frequent production of repetitions and pauses in people who stutter. These repairs do not occur at a conscious level.

Neuropsycholinguistic Theory

This theory was proposed by Perkins, Kent, and Curlee (1991) and is based on the assumption that producing fluent speech involves sophisticated timing between the formulation of language and the actual motor execution of speech movement. Stuttering results in a situation where there is a disruption in the timing (integration) of linguistic formulation and speech movement. People who stutter will often report experiencing a loss of control in producing speech, which is enhanced when there is time pressure to produce speech.

ASSESSMENT OF FLUENCY DISORDERS

The aim of fluency assessment is to determine whether the disfluency behavior demonstrated by an individual is typical or atypical of what we might expect of most people speaking on an everyday basis. Two questions to be addressed in

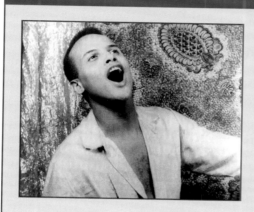
a fluency assessment include: (1) Are speech disfluencies present in the person's speaking behavior? and (2) What is the nature of the speech disfluencies? The speech-language pathologist answers these questions according to the age of the individual being assessed. The assessment will differ between children and adults because parent input is vital to the diagnosis of the condition in young children.

Are Speech Disfluencies Present?

To answer the first question, a large sample of conversational speech is collected from the person. The sample needs to be large enough so a representation of natural speaking behavior is obtained. The generally accepted minimum amount of speech is 300 words of conversation. Once this sample is collected (usually audiorecorded), the speech-language pathologist relistens to the sample and identifies and tallies moments of speech disfluency occurring across the 300-word sample. This tally is then converted to a percentage of occurrence. For example, if 21 moments of disfluency were identi-

fied across the 300-word sample, the percentage of disfluency would be 7%. Conversational speech that is 3% disfluent or higher is usually a rough indication of a fluency disorder. Alternatively, 2% disfluency or lower would be considered within normal limits for people speaking on an everyday basis.

What Is the Nature of the Speech Disfluencies?

The answer to the second question involves further analysis of the specific moments of disfluency. The stuttering typology systems developed by Johnson (1961) and Yairi and Ambrose (1992) can be used to assess the nature and severity of the fluency disorder. As a general rule, the greater the occurrence of within-word (or stuttering-like disfluencies) disfluencies, the greater the severity of the stuttering disorder. The **Iowa Scale for Rating the Severity of Stuttering** was developed by Johnson, Darley, and Spriestersbach (1963) over 50 years ago and remains quite popular. To use the scale, the speech-language pathologist must first calculate the average percentage of disfluency produced by an individual. Based on the percentage of disfluency, a corresponding severity ranking is assigned ranging from 0 (no stuttering) to 7 (very severe stuttering; Table 6–4).

A commercially available test used to determine the nature of speech disfluencies is the **Stuttering Severity Instrument** for children and adults (Riley, 1994). This test considers the frequency of disfluencies, the duration of disfluencies, and the physical concomitants of speaking to formulate a diagnosis. The use of a perceptual scale can also be used to determine the nature of speech disfluencies. Perceptual scales bypass any formal measurement of disfluent speech. The philosophy behind using a perceptual scale is that one simply needs to hear a moment of stuttering to make a judgment as to the existence and severity of the disorder. One such scale is a 9-point **severity scale** that requires a listener to assign a value ranging from 1 (not stuttering) to 9 (extremely severe stuttering) after listening to a sample of conversational speech (Figure 6–11).

Other variables that are considered when describing the nature of disfluencies are the presence or absence of secondary behaviors, including bodily movements and psychosocial behaviors. Bodily movements can be ascertained by visually examining the person during moments of disfluency. Psychosocial behaviors can be assessed by simply asking the person about their feelings and attitude toward speaking. A more thorough assessment of psychosocial behaviors can be obtained by administering the Overall Assessment of the Speaker's Experience of Stuttering instrument (Yaruss & Quesal, 2010). This is a questionnaire-based tool that is used to evaluate the perceived impact of stuttering on a person's life.

The calculation of **speaking rate** can also aid in the diagnosis of a fluency disorder, particularly in regard to cluttering. This calculation can be made using the same 300-word conversational sample that was collected for noting the frequency and type of disfluencies. It is

Severity Ranking	Descriptions
Table 6–4. Iowa Scale for Rating the Severity of Stuttering*	
0	No Stuttering
1	*Very Mild*—Stuttering on less than 1% of words
2	*Mild*—Stuttering on 1% to 2% of words
3	*Mild to Moderate*—Stuttering on 2% to 5% of words
4	*Moderate*—Stuttering on 5% to 8% of words
5	*Moderate to Severe*—Stuttering on 8% to 12% of words
6	*Severe*—Stuttering on 12% to 25% of words
7	*Very Severe*—Stuttering on more than 25% of words

*The table is a condensed version of the overall scale.

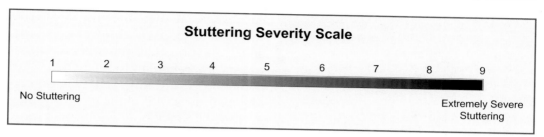

FIGURE 6–11. Example of a 9-point scale for perceptually rating the severity of stuttering.

equally important to examine a person's fluency behavior in the context of overall communication abilities. So assessment of the person's phonology and language abilities is also performed.

Once a diagnosis of a fluency disorder is made, the next step is to enroll the individual in a treatment program. There are instances when the speech-language pathologist may recommend monitoring the client rather than direct therapy. This may be the case for young children who are on the "cusp" of developing a fluency disorder or if a child appears to be at low risk for persistent stuttering.

TREATMENT OF FLUENCY DISORDERS

There is no 100% cure for stuttering. Because we still do not know what causes stuttering, it is not surprising to find that we also do not know the best way to treat stuttering. Although there is general agreement that stuttering cannot be completely remedied, a great deal can be done to help reduce the frequency of disfluent speech. Regardless of the treatment approach, there are three general goals to therapy: (1) to change the speaking behavior of the person, (2) to change the way the person feels about their speech, and (3) to change the way

the person interacts with their speaking environment. Each goal is equally important to the success of treatment. Most treatment approaches fall into one of two categories, traditional and nontraditional.

Traditional Treatment Approaches

The traditional approaches to treating fluency disorders can be broadly organized into two types: (1) fluency shaping and (2) stuttering modification (Zebrowski & Kelly, 2002). Both approaches use principles of behavior modification to change the existing pattern of speaking. Often times, the speech-language pathologist may try one or the other approach with the client to determine which seems to work best. The speech-language pathologist may also develop a hybrid approach that incorporates features of both types of therapy. Ultimately, the client's response to a particular approach serves as the best gauge to the preferred treatment approach.

The **fluency shaping** approach is designed to modify all aspects of the client's speaking behavior. That is, every syllable, word, and sentence uttered by the client is modified into an overall new pattern of speaking. This modification is made by instructing the client to: (1) speak at a reduced rate, (2) prolong the vowel portions of words, and (3) use slow and smooth speech initiation. A term associated with this pattern of speaking is **continuous phonation**, where the client attempts to maintain constant vocal fold vibration during the production of entire utterances of speaking. The aim of this treatment is for the client to become completely "stutter free." A particular criticism of this treatment approach is that the client's speech sounds somewhat unnatural as a result of the modification in overall speaking behavior.

The **stuttering modification** approach is designed to address individual moments of stuttering, as opposed to changing the entire pattern of speaking behavior. This modification is made by teaching the client to: (1) stutter with less tension, (2) use light articulatory contacts during speaking, and (3) reduce situational fears and negative attitudes of stuttering. A person applying this treatment approach will produce speech that is more natural sounding compared with speech produced with continuous phonation. A criticism of this approach is that there may still be moments of stuttering, although significantly reduced in number.

One treatment approach to working with preschool children during the earliest years of stuttering is **parent-directed therapy** (Zebrowski & Kelly, 2002). As indicated, parents are taught to play a key role in the remediation of their child's stuttering behavior. Receiving treatment in a clinical setting may typically involve only one or two (one-hour) sessions per week, which accounts for only a fraction of a child's weekly speaking activity. Therefore, by involving parents, they are taught to reinforce goals established in the clinic setting. This form of therapy places emphasis on increasing *desirable* speaking behavior instead of *undesirable* behavior. Attention is directed away from the perception of what is happening to the child, toward those things he or she is doing to both facilitate and interfere with talking. Emphasis is also placed on increasing the child's awareness of physical aspects of speaking that contribute to fluent speech, such as articulatory tension and breathing patterns.

A popular form of parent-directed therapy is the **Lidcombe Program** of early stuttering intervention (Onslow, Packman, & Harrison, 2003). The program was developed at the Australian Stuttering Research Centre and was designed primarily for preschool children who stutter. The essence of the treatment is for parents to provide direct feedback to their child about stuttered, as well as nonstuttered, speech during conversational settings.

Nontraditional Treatment Approaches

Nontraditional approaches are not used as often as traditional approaches to manage a person's stuttering. These approaches are also typically not applicable to the majority of individuals who may stutter, or show a related fluency disorder. Nontraditional approaches to treating stuttering include hypno-therapy, drug therapy, and electronic devices. **Hypnotherapy** is a psychologically based approach to the treatment of stuttering. Psychological techniques emphasizing anxiety reduction and building self-confidence are presented under hypnosis to help the individual speak confidently. By reducing anxiety and increasing self-confidence, the person's severity of stuttering presumably will lessen. Use of this technique remains controversial, but there is evidence to suggest the approach may be particularly effective for individuals with a mild stuttering disorder.

The use of **drug therapy** to manage stuttering focuses on an individual's anxiety that is often greatly heightened when anticipating moments of speaking. A number of antianxiety drugs have been shown to reduce moments of stuttering; however, only a small number of individuals tend to show a long-lasting reduction in stuttering once under the drug's influence. Those who do respond usually show only a modest reduction in stuttering (see also Current Research).

Electronic devices closely resemble hearing aids that are inserted into one ear. These fluency aids serve to alter the individual's overall speaking behavior (i.e., a form of fluency shaping). Some devices use a technology called **altered auditory feedback**. When fitted with the device, an illusion is created where the client hears his or her own voice with either a delay or slight shift in pitch. The client needs to reduce their speaking rate and prolong vowels in order to minimize the effect of the alteration, which subsequently results in fluent speech. Some devices transmit white noise, which is acoustically similar to the sound of a waterfall. By introducing noise into the speaker's ear,

they are unable to hear their own voice. This form of distraction has shown to decrease moments of stuttering in some, but not all, individuals.

The use of electronic devices is often considered at two points in the continuum of therapy. Based on consultation with an speech-language pathologist, a client may use such a device when first entering treatment to assist with gaining initial control over severe stuttering. Once control is established, the device is no longer used and the person transitions into a traditional treatment program. Alternatively, an electronic device also might be used when other forms of treatment have proved unsuccessful. The device is used on an everyday basis.

CULTURAL CONSIDERATIONS AND FLUENCY DISORDERS

Careful considerations are required in the diagnosis and management of fluency disorders among individuals from diverse cultural backgrounds. The multicultural perspectives of the client can (and should) influence clinical practice. For example, in some cultures, such as Chinese, stuttering is not considered to be a prevalent communication disorder, and thus there is less emphasis placed on correcting the disorder. In some African nations, the cause of this speech problem and its treatment are deeply rooted in folk ideas. Some of the reported causes of stuttering include tickling a baby too much or leaving a newborn child out in the rain. Corresponding treatments include praying or applying ointments to the throat. Therefore, a speech-language pathologist should not assume there is a universally agreed upon approach to the management of fluency disorders.

To illustrate this point, consider the two common traditional approaches to treating stuttering, fluency shaping, and stuttering modification. Stuttering modification therapies utilize a counseling-based methodology with a primary aim of developing positive attitudes toward communication. Although this goal may seem to hold wide universal appeal, the structuring of this form of therapy requires cultural sensitivity. Counseling has its roots in psychology, and therefore it is important to consider features such as race, language, economic class, and differing worldviews as potential barriers to the counseling process (Hickson & Christie, 1989). The stuttering modification treatment approach has the potential to become a complex and multidimensional process, especially in a context of varying multicultural perspectives and beliefs.

There are reports that fluency shaping therapies appear to have better acceptance compared with stuttering modification therapy by clients of diverse backgrounds (Cooper & Cooper, 2001). Fluency shaping approaches, at least in the earliest phases of treatment, tend to focus exclusively on gaining control of speech fluency with less emphasis on counseling. Fluency shaping has its roots in behavioral conditioning and programmed instruction, so this approach tends to bypass matters concerning cultural sensitivity. Regardless of the treatment approach selected, those that are currently available to the speech-language pathologist will likely need to be modified to make them applicable in a multicultural context.

Another multicultural consideration when dealing with fluency disorders is the influence of bilingualism.

Over 50% of the world's population is bilingual. Thus, the trend is that most people are able to speak more than one language, and people who only speak one language are becoming far less the norm. Also consider that roughly 1% of the population stutters. So in the context of bilingualism, it would seem that at some point in the career of a speech-language pathologist, they will be confronted with a bilingual speaker who stutters. There are mixed views concerning the characteristics of stuttering in bilingual speakers. Although it would seem obvious that a bilingual person who stutters in one language will show the same pattern in another language, the research to date does not support this view. Individuals are likely to stutter in both languages; however, the less dominant or least proficient language will show a higher percentage of stuttering (Howell & Van Borsel, 2011). Therefore, the bilingual person who stutters poses unique concerns in regard to diagnosis and management of the disorder. For example, can the speech-language pathologist make an accurate diagnosis of a fluency disorder when listening to a language that is foreign? Is it possible to differentiate stuttering from cluttering? Should the treatment of fluency disorders focus on only one language or both? These are important questions that still await answers.

CURRENT RESEARCH IN FLUENCY DISORDERS

Research in the area of fluency disorders has been broad and extensive over the past century. The current trends are diverse and likely to change in the years ahead. At present, there is exciting research occurring in four particular areas: (1) genetics, (2) drug therapy, (3) brain imaging, and (4) deep brain stimulation.

Genetics

Stuttering is known to run in families, which would suggest there is a **genetic** predisposition for acquiring the disorder. As with other areas of communication disorders, the search is on for identifying the possible genetic bases for stuttering. Researchers have recently discovered genetic mutations for stuttering on chromosomes 12 and 16 among families with a history of stuttering (Kang et al., 2010). The research is important because it provides additional evidence that the cause of stuttering is not due to emotional factors such as anxiety. Findings such as this could ultimately lead to a new way of treating stuttering, namely, by gene replacement therapy.

Drug Therapy

At present, there are no government-approved drugs for the medical treatment of stuttering. A wide range of drugs have been tested on individuals who stutter to determine whether symptoms of the disorder can be extinguished. Most of these drugs fall within the class of drugs known as benzodiazepines, which serve to decrease anxiety. These drugs have been found to help individuals with conditions such as epilepsy or depression, but when applied to individuals who stutter, they have been largely ineffective. The most promising research to date has come from the anti-anxiety drug known as **Pagoclone**. This drug is one of a class of medications known as nonbenzodiazepines, which have similar effects to the benzodiazepine group, but with quite different chemical structures. Unfortunately, recent results from a large multisite study occurring in the United States testing its effectiveness as a treatment for stuttering was unable to meet the prespecified criteria for success (Maguire et al., 2010). Although disappointing, this finding is unlikely to prevent further research in the area of stuttering pharmacology.

Brain Imaging

The notion of atypical cerebral functioning contributing to stuttering is not new. Dating back to the work of Lee Travis in the 1920s, there has been evidence to suggest that stuttering results from either a lack of brain dominance or competing hemispheres when it comes to producing speech. This contention has received a resurgence of interest, motivated in large part by new technologies available to directly visualize the brain, such as functional magnetic resonance imaging (fMRI) and positron emission tomography (PET) scanning. These tools are used to determine how the brain anatomy and physiology of people who stutter differs from those who do not (Beal, 2011). The use of these visualization techniques may eventually serve as a form of biofeedback for the treatment of stuttering.

Deep Brain Stimulation

The application of Deep Brain Stimulation is a surgical technique that involves the implantation of a pulse generator along with two to three electrodes within the brain (i.e., a brain pacemaker). The device sends electrical impulses to specific parts of the brain to stimulate brain activity. The device has been shown to help improve individuals with movement disorders such as Tourette syndrome or Parkinson disease. The device was recently implanted in an individual with Parkinson disease who also happened to have developmental stuttering. The researchers observed an overall reduction in involuntary movements in the patient, which included a reduction in stuttering (Thiriez et al., 2013). This has led to the suggestion that Deep Brain Stimulation may be a possible treatment for stuttering. Certainly, this would not be the first choice of treatment for individuals who stutter due to the highly invasive nature of the surgery.

FLUENCY DISORDERS ON THE WORLD WIDE WEB

Listed below are websites that provide further information on the topic of fluency disorders. At the time of publication, each website was freely accessible.

International Stuttering Association
http://www.isastutter.org/

International Fluency Association
http://www.theifa.org/

Stuttering Foundation Video
http://www.stutteringhelp.org/videos

Stigma of Stuttering Videos

http://www.cbsnews.com/video/watch/?id=4686592n

http://www.cbsnews.com/video/watch/?id=7306506n

STUDY QUESTIONS

1. What are the similarities and differences in stuttering and cluttering?
2. What are the primary and secondary characteristics of stuttering?
3. What are some of the most popular theories related to the cause of stuttering?
4. Compare and contrast the fluency shaping and stuttering modification approaches to treating stuttering.
5. Who are some of the pioneers in the area of stuttering, and what were their contributions?

REFERENCES

American Speech-Language-Hearing Association. (2007, November). Iowa stuttering study settlement. *ASHA Leader*, 8.

Beal, D. (2011). The advancement of neuroimaging research investigating developmental stuttering. *Perspectives on Fluency and Fluency Disorders*, 21, 88–95.

Cooper, E. B., & Cooper, C. S. (2001). Fluency disorders. In D. Battle (Ed.), *Communication disorders in multicultural populations* (3rd ed.). Oxford, UK: Butterworth-Heinemann Medical.

Goberman, A., & Blomgren, M. (2003). Parkinsonian speech disfluencies: Effects of L-Dopa-related fluctuations. *Journal of Fluency Disorders*, 28, 55–70.

Hickson, J., & Christie, G. M. (1989). Research on cross-cultural counseling and psychotherapy: Implications for the South African context. *South African Journal of Psychology, 19*, 162–169.

Howell, P., & Van Borsel, J. (2011). *Multilingual aspects of fluency disorders*. Bristol, UK: Multilingual Matters.

Johnson, W. (1961). *Stuttering and what you can do about it.* Minneapolis: University of Minnesota Press.

Johnson, W., Darley, F., & Spriestersbach, D. (1963). *Diagnostic methods in speech pathology.* New York, NY: Harper & Row.

Kang, C., Riazuddin, S., Mundorff, J., Krasnewich, D., Friedman, P., Mullikin, J., & Drayna, D. (2010). Mutations in the lysosomal enzyme—Targeting pathway and persistent stuttering. *New England Journal of Medicine, 362,* 677–685.

Maguire, G., Franklin, D., Vatakis, N., Morgenshtern, E., Denko, T., Yaruss, S., . . . Harrison, E. (2003). The Lidcombe Program of early stuttering intervention. In *Overview of the Lidcombe Program* (pp. 3–15). Austin, TX: Pro-Ed.

Perkins, W. H., Kent, R. D., & Curlee, R. R. (1991). A theory of neuropsycholinguistic function in stuttering. *Journal of Speech, Language, and Hearing Research, 34,* 734–752.

Postma, A., & Kolk, H. (1993). The covert repair hypothesis: Prearticulatory repair processes in normal and stuttered disfluencies. *Journal of Speech and Hearing Research, 36,* 472–487.

Riley, G. (1994). *Stuttering Severity Instrument-3.* Austin, TX: Pro-Ed.

Riley, G. (2010). Exploratory randomized clinical study of Pagoclone in persistent developmental stuttering: The EXPRESS trial. *Journal of Clinical Pharmacology, 30,* 48–56.

Starkweather, C. W. (1997). Therapy for younger children. In R. F. Curlee & G. M. Siegel (Eds.), *Nature and treatment of stuttering* (2nd ed., pp. 257–279). Boston, MA: Allyn & Bacon.

Thiriez, C., Roubeau, B., Ouerchefani, N., Gurruchaga, J., Palfi, S., & Fenelon, G. (2013). Improvement in developmental stuttering following deep brain stimulation for Parkinson's disease. *Parkinsonism and Related Disorders, 19,* 383–384.

Van Riper, C. (1981). An early history of ASHA. *ASHA Magazine, 23*(11), 855–858.

Van Riper, C. (1982). *The nature of stuttering* (2nd ed.). Englewood Cliffs, NJ: Prentice-Hall.

World Health Organization. (1977). *Manual of the international statistical classification of diseases, injuries, and causes of death, 1* Geneva, Switzerland: Author.

Yairi, E., & Ambrose, N. (1992). A longitudinal study of stuttering in children: A preliminary report. *Journal of Speech, Language, and Hearing Research, 35,* 755–760.

Yaruss, J. S., & Quesal, R. (2010). *Overall Assessment of the Speaker's Experience of Stuttering (OASES).* San Antonio, TX: Pearson.

Zebrowski, P., & Kelly, E. (2002). *Manual of stuttering intervention.* San Diego, CA: Singular.

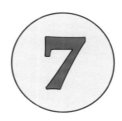

CLEFT LIP AND PALATE

After reading this chapter, the student should be able to:

- Demonstrate knowledge of the biological aspects of embryonic development that impact the process of developing a cleft.

- Understand the differences between normal lip/palate and cleft lip/palate anatomy and physiology.

- Describe the characteristics of different types of cleft lips and palates.

- Identify the impact of cleft lip and palate on speech and language development.

- Demonstrate knowledge regarding the fundamental aspects of assessing individuals with cleft lip and palate.

- Have a basic knowledge of the surgical and nonsurgical management techniques for cleft lip and palate.

- Demonstrate basic knowledge of and be able to accurately identify the articulation, voice, and resonance characteristics that are typical of clients with cleft lip and palate.

- Demonstrate basic knowledge of the team concept in the habilitation of individuals (and families) who have cleft lip and palate.

- Identify cultural issues impacting individuals with cleft lip and palate.

- Identify current research issues in the area of cleft lip and palate.

INTRODUCTION

The birth of a child is one of the most joyous experiences in a parent's life. However, it is not uncommon for expectant parents to alternate between visions of a healthy baby and worries that the baby will be born with health problems. A **birth defect** is a problem that happens while a baby is developing in the mother's body. Birth defects are defined as abnormalities of structure, function, or body metabolism that are present at birth. Most birth defects happen during the first three months of pregnancy. The majority of babies with birth defects are born to two parents with no obvious health problems or risk factors; a woman can do everything her doctor recommends to deliver a healthy child and still have a baby with a birth defect. A cleft of the lip and/or palate (CL/P) is a birth defect that affects an estimated 7,000 infants annually in the United States. According to the Centers for Disease Control and Prevention, approximately 2,700 babies are born with a cleft palate, and another 4,500 babies are born with a cleft lip with or without a cleft palate. Among the various types of communication disorders to be covered in this text, cleft lip and palate is by far the most physically obvious type of communication disorder.

TERMINOLOGY AND DEFINITIONS

A CL/P is defined as an elongated opening, resulting from failure of parts of the mouth to fuse or merge. The medical term is **schisis**, which means opening in Greek. A CL/P is an organic, developmental communication disorder. A CL/P is also a type of **craniofacial abnormality**, reflecting involvement of the bony features of the skull, as well as tissue features of the face. A CL/P is the most common congenital abnormality. Because it is present at birth, the developmental disruptions that result in a

---

FYI

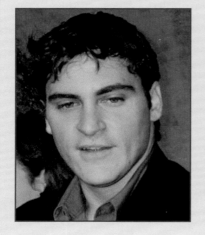

Some well-known people who were born with a CL/P include Wendy Harmer (comedian), Jesse Jackson (politician), Stacy Keach (actor), Nikki Payne (comedian), Joaquin Phoenix (actor, pictured), Peyton Manning (professional football), and Cheech Marin (comedian). According to diagnostic imaging of the Egyptian Pharaoh Tutankhamun (1341–1323 BC), he too may have had a CL/P.

CL/P occur during the prenatal period of growth.

The study of prenatal growth and the developing process of an individual is called the science of **embryology**. Human pregnancy is approximately nine months (40 weeks) in duration. This time period starts immediately after conception, when the ovum is fertilized by sperm. The prenatal period is divided into three phases of pregnancy: the first phase is **zygote**, which is the period of conception through the first two weeks of pregnancy; the second phase is **embryo**, which is the period of two weeks through the eighth week; and the third phase of pregnancy is **fetus**, which is the period of nine weeks through birth.

Physical formation of the face occurs during the period of embryonic development and early fetal development. A visual time line of facial development is provided in Figure 7–1. Late in the first month of pregnancy, the baby's developing face and mouth is effectively split into two halves with the eyes and nose spread out toward

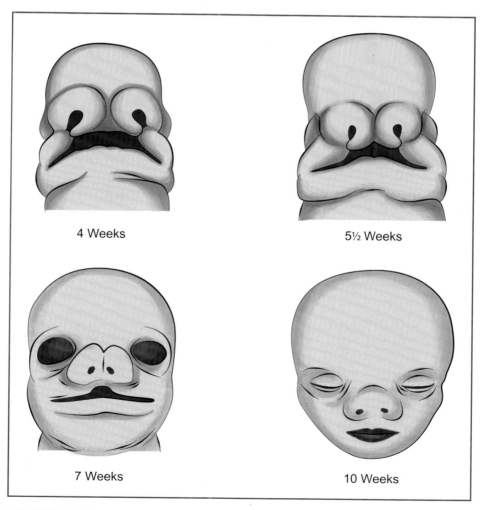

4 Weeks

5½ Weeks

7 Weeks

10 Weeks

FIGURE 7–1. Prenatal development of the face.

the sides. The two sides gradually begin growing closer together beginning around the fourth week of prenatal development. First to fuse are the lips. The face continues developing and changing shape considerably. The eyes move forward, the nose comes together, and the face appears much narrower. Following fusion of the lips, the alveolar ridge is formed, which is the boney gum ridge that serves as sockets for our teeth. Next, the fusing seam travels backward to form the hard palate and then the soft palate (i.e., velum). The tip of the soft palate is called the uvula and is recog-

nized as the teardrop-shaped tissue that hangs at the back of the throat. By the 12th week of pregnancy, the mouth is fully formed (Peterson-Falzone, Hardin-Jones, & Karnell, 2009). An illustration in the time line of palate development is provided in Figure 7–2.

Various landmarks on the face (Figure 7–3) that can be affected by a CL/P include the **columella**, which is the fleshy strip underneath the nose that separates the right and left nostrils (also called **nares**). The **philtrum** is the midline groove in the upper lip that runs from the top of the lip to the nose.

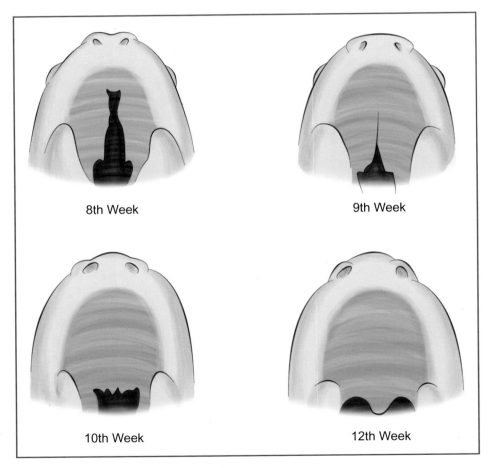

FIGURE 7–2. Major stages of hard and soft palate development during the 12 weeks of prenatal development.

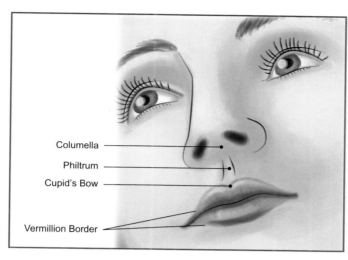

Columella

Philtrum

Cupid's Bow

Vermillion Border

FIGURE 7–3. Some anatomical landmarks of the face.

The slight curve in the upper lip directly below the philtrum is called **Cupid's bow**, said to resemble the bow of Cupid, the Roman god of love and beauty. The **vermilion border** is the edge of red pigment around the upper and lower lips of the mouth. Normally, these facial landmarks are quite prominent in children and young adults. As a consequence of normal aging, the philtrum and Cupid's bow regions of the upper lip tend to flatten and become less distinct.

a CL/P were unable to nurse, and subsequently failed to survive because of malnutrition. Others were simply left to die either because the birth defect was too hideous for society, or as a result of superstition. One of earliest reports of a CL/P was by a French surgeon **Ambroise Pare** (1510–1590) who is considered the greatest surgeon of the 16th century (Figure 7–4). When discussing a patient with a cleft, Pare first coined the phrase, *le bec-de-lièvre* with an English

HISTORIC ASPECTS OF CLEFT LIP AND PALATE

During the 1500s, research and interest in a CL/P was lacking because the deformity was thought to occur as a result of syphilis transmitted to an infant by its infected mother. An effect of syphilis was severe inflammation of the hard palate that resulted in the creation of a **fistula**, or narrow opening. At the time, surgeons viewed such openings as unrepairable. Many children born with

FYI

The occurrence of a CL/P is not unique to humans. They also are found in the animal world, including dogs and cats. Purebred dogs and cats are at the highest risk for a CL/P, and they are most common in Boston terriers, Pekingese, bulldogs, beagles, cocker spaniels, dachshunds, and Siamese cats. Heredity is considered the primary cause of a CL/P in animals.

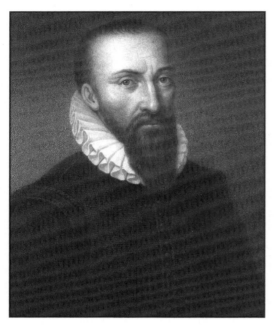

FIGURE 7–4. Ambroise Pare, considered one of the greatest surgeons of the 16th century.

transition of, "lip of the hare." He was merely observing that the lip was split, as is the lip of a rabbit (and several other animals). Among these animals, the split lip is used like forceps in picking up food (Figure 7–5).

Unfortunately, this terminology led to the development of superstition as to the cause of the disorder. For example, it was once believed that children with cleft lips were born to women who, when pregnant, were frightened by the devil, who had assumed the shape of a hare. In 1887, a passage was published in the journal of *Lancet* stating that one of the laws of heredity is that hideous physical impressions on the mind of a mother are capable of producing deformity and monstrosity in the offspring. Support of this notion was based on a report at the time of a pregnant woman attending a carnival. One of the attrac-

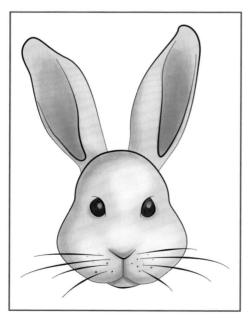

A

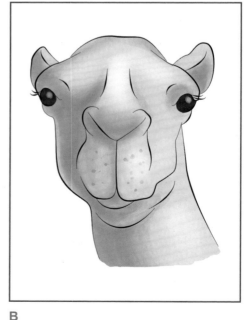

B

FIGURE 7–5. Example of two animals that have a split lip used for grasping food during eating.

tions she observed involved a trained horse pulling the trigger of a pistol, pretending to shoot a rabbit. Upon shooting, the rabbit was replaced with a stuffed (toy) rabbit that appeared to have had its head shot off. This greatly distressed the pregnant woman who later gave birth to a child resembling a rabbit. Fortunately, the term harelip is no longer in use and is considered demeaning. However, as a society, we have not yet moved beyond using names of animals to describe human conditions. For example, the phrase *pigeon-toed* is used to refer to the turning in of feet while walking, and *crow's feet* is a phrase used to refer to small wrinkles around the outer corners of the eyes.

Cosmetic surgery began in the ancient world. The Romans performed simple techniques such as repairing damaged ears. Physicians in ancient India used skin grafts for reconstructive work as early as 800 BC. The first report of surgical cleft lip repair came from China in 390 AD when an 18-year-old named Wei Yang Chi received the surgery. Chi subsequently became the Governor General of six Chinese Provinces (Rogers, 1971). The treatment consisted of cutting and stitching the edges of the cleft lip together, followed by 100 days of complete bed rest, when the patient could eat only thin gruel and was not allowed to smile or talk.

Jehan Yperman (1260–1331) was a medieval Belgian surgeon who is believed to have been the first person to provide a detailed description of cleft lip repair, although he made no mention of cleft palate repair. Yperman published a treatise on surgery that so meticulously described the details of needle-and-suture "pinning" surgery that some of his advice is still considered in modern surgical procedures (Figure 7–6).

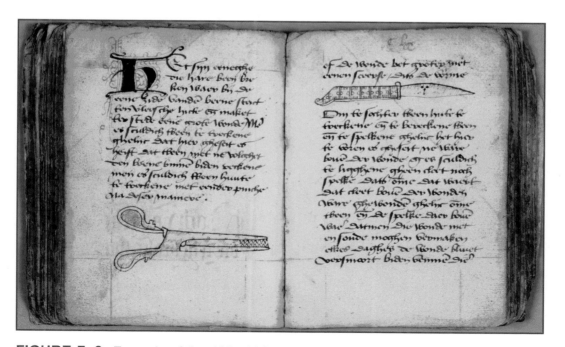

FIGURE 7–6. Example of the 13th–14th century surgical treatise written by medieval surgeon Jehan Yperman. Techniques related to cleft lip repair were included in the treatise.

The Swiss surgeon **Pierre Franco** (1506–1580) is known as the "father of cleft palate surgery." In 1556, he described in detail the principles and techniques for repairing a cleft of the palate. Because of the dangers associated with surgery in any form, especially that involving the head or face, the repair of a CL/P was almost nonexistent until the 19th century. Besides, in the absence of anesthesia, the operation was extremely painful. The first general surgery using ether was not performed until 1840, and it was not until 1860 that a cleft palate was repaired using anesthesia. It is also worth noting that the light bulb was not invented until around 1880, so many of these early surgeries were performed using lanterns. Not until the 19th and 20th centuries did CL/P surgeries become commonplace.

Some of the well-known CL/P surgeons during the 1800s included the Germans **Karl Ferdinand von Graefe** (1787–1840; Figure 7–7), **Johann Friedrich Dieffenbach** (1792–1847), **Bernard von Langenbeck** (1810–1887; Figure 7–8), and **Philip Gustav Passavant** (1815–1893). Von Graefe was a pioneer of plastic and reconstructive surgery. Dieffenbach applied his surgical talents to the correction of a CL/P, as well as other communicative disorders such as stuttering (see also Chapter 6). Von Langenbeck was a skilled surgeon who developed a procedure for the closure of the hard palate. Passavant was a dedicated surgeon who was interested in developing surgical techniques to help improve speech production. In particular, he recommended reconstruction of the velar muscles and lengthening of the soft palate as important steps to helping individuals develop normal speech.

During the time of CL/P repairs in the mid-1800s, infants and children were rarely operated on, and most patients were mature adults with speech defects that were nearly impossible to correct. However, as improvements were introduced in surgical techniques and anesthesia, the age of the patients receiving surgery gradually became younger. One of the first surgeons to recognize the

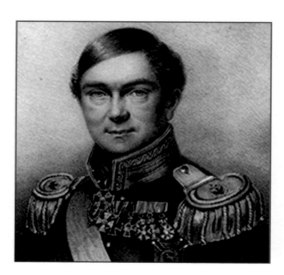

FIGURE 7–7. Karl Ferdinand von Graefe, a cleft lip and palate surgeon of the 1800s.

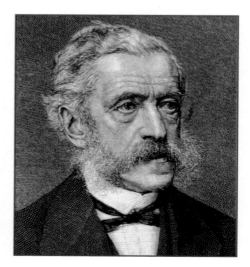

FIGURE 7–8. Bernard von Langenbeck was a skilled surgeon who developed a procedure for the closure of the hard palate.

importance of speech therapy was **Carl Casper von Siebold** (1736–1807; Figure 7–9). He conducted detailed studies of the speech difficulties of a three-year-old boy with a CL/P and noted that he had difficulty pronouncing the letters b, s, z, and r. Siebold expressed deep regret at the impossibility of correcting this defect surgically.

The effect of CL/P on speech was also studied in the United States by **Matthew Wilson** (1734–1802). Wilson served as both a minister and a surgeon during the American Revolutionary War. During this time period in the United States, it was extremely rare for surgeons to have held a medical degree. Wilson wrote a compendium of medicine called the *Therapeutic Alphabet* that contained an alphabetical listing of diseases, symptoms, and their cures. Among the various listings was a reference to CL/P and the poor speech pronunciation that accompanied the affliction. At the time, only surgery of the lip was performed. Surgery of the palate was unheard of.

Herbert K. Cooper (1897–1978) established the first CL/P clinic in the United States when his recognition of the need for multidisciplinary involvement resulted in the formation of a unique clinic in 1939. It was the first of its kind, having all the necessary dental and surgical specialists in one location. The team concept Cooper created is still the accepted standard of care for children with CL/P. The clinic remains in existence in Pennsylvania and has been renamed the Herbert Cooper-Lancaster Cleft Palate Institute.

DISORDERS OF CLEFT LIP AND PALATE

Clefts of the lip and palate can be categorized according to the affected structures and location of the cleft. The degree of clefting is related to the amount of embryonic damage to the lip and palate.

Cleft Lip

If the cleft does not affect the palate structure of the mouth, it is referred to as cleft lip. When the cleft occurs on only one side of the upper lip, it is called a **unilateral cleft lip**. The occurrence of a cleft on both sides of the upper lip is called a **bilateral cleft lip**. When the cleft results in a gap that goes all the way from the lip and mouth into the nostril, it is referred to as a **complete cleft lip**. If the gap does not extend from the mouth all the way into the nostril, it is referred to as an **incomplete cleft lip**. When the incomplete cleft lip is very minor (a groove or a notch), it is called a **microform cleft**. A microform cleft can

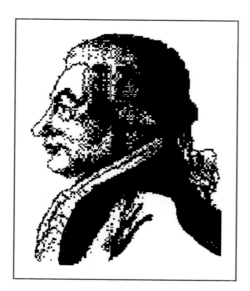

FIGURE 7–9. Carl Casper von Siebold was one of the first cleft lip and palate surgeons to recognize the importance of speech therapy for his patients.

appear as small or slight indentation in the vermilion border of the lip or look like a scar from the lip up to the nostril. Examples of the various types of cleft lip are shown in Figure 7–10.

Cleft Palate

A cleft palate can be either complete or incomplete. A **complete cleft palate** involves an opening between the hard and soft palates that extends through to the uvula. In most cases, a cleft lip is also present in conditions of a complete cleft of the hard palate. An **incomplete cleft** palate is a condition in which the hard palate may be fully developed with a cleft only found for the soft palate. In these cases, it is likely there is no cleft of the lip. Another less common and minor form of cleft palate is known as a **submucous cleft**. In this condition, there is a cleft of the muscular layer of the soft palate with an intact layer of mucosa lying over the defect. A telltale sign of a submucous cleft is a bifid (or notched) uvula. In most cases, a submucous cleft does not adversely affect swallowing and speech production. Examples of various types of clefts to the hard palate are shown in Figure 7–11.

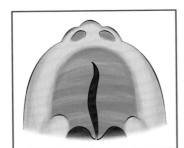 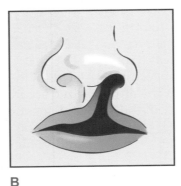 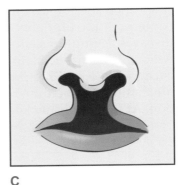

A   B   C

FIGURE 7–10. Types of cleft lip: unilateral incomplete cleft lip (**A**), unilateral complete cleft lip (**B**), and a bilateral complete cleft lip (**C**).

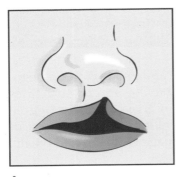 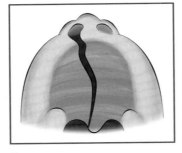 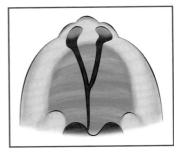

A   B   C

FIGURE 7–11. Types of cleft palate: incomplete cleft of the soft palate only (**A**), unilateral complete cleft of lip and palate (**B**), and a bilateral complete cleft of lip and palate (**C**).

FYI

Although most conditions of a CL/P are of a congenital nature, it is possible for a CL/P to be acquired. Oral cancer affecting either the hard or soft palate would necessitate removal of these structures, thereby creating a clefting condition. Cancer of either the hard or soft palate accounts for approximately 2% of all head and neck cancers.

Characteristics of Cleft Lip and Palate

Approximately 50% of all clefts involve a cleft of both the lip and palate. A cleft of the lip alone, or the palate alone, each account for 25% of all clefts, respectively. Instances when there are isolated clefts of the lip or palate alone are most often associated with birth defects affecting other parts of the body and/or brain. Ten percent of cleft lips are incomplete. Approximately 85% of cases of bilateral cleft lip and 70% of unilateral cleft lip also involve a cleft of the palate. Cleft lip and palate is more common on the left side, less common on the right, and least common bilaterally. There are sex differences in the occurrence of various types of clefts: Males are twice as likely to have a cleft lip and palate or an isolated cleft of the lip compared with females; females are twice as likely to have an isolated cleft of the palate compared with males. So across the various types of clefts, males are far more likely to be born with a cleft compared with females.

The occurrence of a CL/P varies considerably according to race. In the United States, American Indians show the highest occurrence of clefting with 7 per 10,000 live births, followed by Latinos with a prevalence of 5 per 10,000 live births. Among the Japanese population, the occurrence of CL/P is 4.5 per 10,000, and among the Chinese, the occurrence is 3.4 per 10,000 live births. Among Caucasians, the occurrence of CL/P is approximately 2 per 10,000 births. The lowest occurrence of CL/P is found among African American births with only 0.6 per 10,000 births.

The prevalence of CL/P also differs among various countries around the world. The prevalence of children born with a CL/P in the United Kingdom is around 3 per 10,000 live births, similar to what is found in Arab countries. In Australia, Canada, and New Zealand, the prevalence is approximately 7 per 10,000 births. At the extreme ends of the continuum, Cuba and South Africa show fewer than 2 children with a CL/P per 10,000 births, whereas Finland and Malta have more than 14 CL/P births per 10,000.

CURRENT THEORIES OF CLEFT LIP AND PALATE

The exact cause of a CL/P is not completely understood. Cleft lip and/or cleft palate are caused by multiple genes inherited from both parents, as well as environmental factors that scientists do not yet fully understand. About 25% of occurrences of CL/P can be attributed solely to genetic inheritance. If either parent has a cleft, the relative risks become about 5% higher for having a baby with a cleft, compared with non-clefted parents. If both parents have clefts, the risks are much greater. When a combination of genes and environmental factors cause a condition, the inheritance is called **multifactorial** (i.e., many factors contribute to the cause). By far, the majority of children born with a CL/P acquire the condition as a result of combined genetic and environmental factors. There are a number of environmental conditions that interact with one or more genes to increase the risk of CL/P. These include: (1) lack of a balanced diet, (2) maternal illness, (3) cigarette smoking, (4) alcohol consumption, and (5) chronic use of nonprescribed drugs or substance abuse. The risk of CL/P is found to be higher among pregnant women older than 35 years of age, as well as among teenaged pregnancies (Slavkin, 1992).

FYI

The cause of a CL/P most often is attributed to a combination of genetic and environmental factors. However, a group of scientists at the University of Bonn in Germany recently found that a genetic variant on chromosome 8 occurs with significantly higher frequency in people with a CL/P than those without a cleft. Although the exact gene on chromosome 8 has yet to be identified, these results point to genes playing a far more important role in the formation of a CL/P than previously thought.

ASSESSMENT OF CLEFT LIP AND PALATE

Because clefting causes very obvious physical changes, diagnosis of the condition is straightforward. As ultrasound testing becomes increasingly common in routine obstetric practice and its accuracy improves, prenatal diagnosis of a CL/P is now a reality. Developments in ultrasound technology have enabled the identification of major facial anomalies as early as 12 weeks gestation. If the cleft has not been detected in an ultrasound prior to the baby's birth, a physical examination at birth of the mouth, nose, and palate confirms the presence of a CL/P. Aside from the visible physical features that serve to confirm the diagnosis of a CL/P, there are related areas that are also assessed in regard to the child's health status, and these include: (1) feeding, (2) hearing, (3) dentition, and (4) communication.

Feeding

Normally, in order for an infant to feed (suck), the infant needs to squeeze the nipple with the lips between the tongue and alveolar ridge at the same time, maintaining suction during the act of swallowing. The muscular motions of the jaw and soft palate at the back of the mouth allow suction to draw the milk. For an infant with a CL/P, sucking is a much more difficult task. Depending on the location and severity of the cleft, it is a challenge for the infant to maintain suction of the breast or bottle. Swallowing air is likely, and babies with clefts need thorough burping. Most babies with a

CL/P are fed with a bottle, although breastfeeding is not precluded and may be attempted in some cases. It is possible the infant may need to wear a prosthetic palate called an **obturator** to help him or her eat properly. The device helps to close off the nasal cavity from the oral cavity. The infant needs to be positioned in a nearly upright position during feeding so as to prevent milk from coming through the nose (Figure 7–12). Positioning the baby upright also limits choking and helps to decrease the risk of ear infections.

Hearing

Almost all babies with a CL/P are likely to acquire **otitis media** (ear infections) at some point during the first year of life. The common occurrence of otitis media

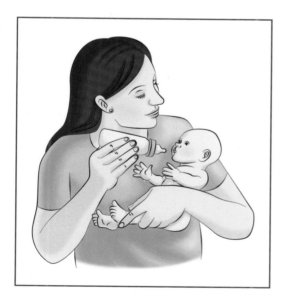

FIGURE 7–12. Feeding a baby with a cleft lip and palate. The infant is positioned in an upright position to prevent milk from entering the nasal cavity.

is due to the fact that the muscles that move the palate also open the **eustachian tube**, which runs from the back of the throat into the middle ear space (see Chapter 12). Its primary function is to ventilate the middle ear and also to drain any accumulated secretions or debris from the middle ear space. The eustachian tube is usually closed, but among children with a CL/P, these muscles are deficient or abnormal. The tube may remain open, which results in any bacteria in the child's throat traveling into the middle ear space. Although short bouts of otitis media are common in most children, persistent otitis media may cause permanent hearing loss. Treatment for this problem typically involves careful observation by the family physician and audiologist. In most instances, **pressure equalization tubes** (sometimes called "grommets") are surgically inserted through the eardrum to improve ventilation in the middle ear. These temporary tubes enable the child to hear better and serve to decrease the number of ear infections (see also Chapter 13).

Dentition

Children with a CL/P, particularly a cleft affecting the alveolar (gum) ridge, are likely to develop dental problems such as missing or malformed teeth. These dental problems may occur unilaterally or bilaterally (depending on the cleft). Because the young infant is not born with teeth, and the first set of teeth will eventually fall out, special planning is needed to solve the functional and cosmetic dental problems that a cleft can create. In about 25% of children with a unilateral CL/P, the upper jaw (maxilla) growth does not keep up with the lower jaw (mandible) growth. If this occurs, the child may need **orthognathic** surgery. This type of surgery involves manipulation of various facial bones to restore the proper anatomical and functional relationship between the teeth and jaws. Fortunately, dental experts can successfully treat most problems resulting from a CL/P.

Communication

It is common for children who are born with a CL/P to have communication problems at some time in their young lives. Children with a CL/P are likely to experience problems in two domains of communication: (1) voice and (2) speech articulation. Over one-half of them will require speech therapy during early childhood. However, many children who are born with a CL/P are able to develop normal speech by the time they enter school.

Voice

The particular voice problem associated with a CL/P concerns the ability to regulate air flowing through the nasal cavity during speech production. During normal speech production, the nasal cavity is typically closed off from the oral cavity by elevating the velum against the back of the throat (pharynx). This process is referred to as **velopharyngeal closure** (Figure 7–13). You can observe velopharyngeal closure by facing a mirror, opening your mouth, and saying "ahhh," as your doctor might have you say during a routine visit. At the precise moment of turning on your voice, you should observe the uvula elevate and press against the back of the throat. This physiological movement may be impaired in an individual with a CL/P

In cases of a CL/P, the palatal structures may be impaired resulting in a lack of closure between the oral and nasal cavities. The inability to close off the nasal cavity from the mouth is called

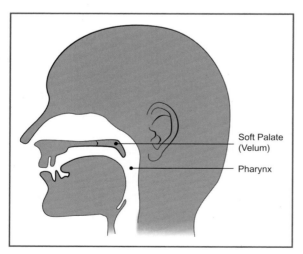
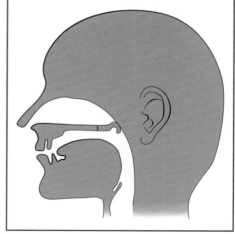

Soft Palate (Velum)

Pharynx

A   B

FIGURE 7–13. Depiction of velopharyngeal opening (**A**) and velopharyngeal closure (**B**).

velopharyngeal inadequacy. The end result is that excessive air flows through the nasal cavity, which is referred to as **hypernasal speech**. Children who have velopharyngeal inadequacy may sound like they are "talking through their noses." Prior to surgery, it is likely all children with a cleft palate will exhibit hypernasal speech. Approximately 25% of children who undergo repair of a cleft palate may still show signs of velopharyngeal inadequacy. Assessment of velopharyngeal inadequacy can be accomplished in a number of ways. By placing a mirror directly below the nose, and having the child speak, one is able to determine whether excessive nasal airflow is occurring by simply noting whether the mirror fogs up. A second approach involves either directly listening to nasal airflow or using an instrument to measure the amount of airflow exiting the nose during speech production (Figure 7–14). A commercially available instrument known as a **nasometer** has been specially created to measure nasal airflow.

Speech Articulation

Not only are the lips and palate essential for eating, but like the teeth, tongue, and other throat and mouth structures, they are also used to produce speech. When we speak, the stream of air from the lungs passes through the vocal tract and is shaped to produce the many different consonant and vowel sounds used to create strings of words. Nearly all the sounds of English involve closure of the nasal cavity, and the sounds are directed through the mouth. The only exceptions are the nasal consonants /m/ (e.g., me), /n/ (e.g., no), and /ŋ/ (e.g., sing), which all have a natural nasal quality to their production. In the case of velopharyn-

geal inadequacy, the consonants and vowels that normally are produced through the mouth are now produced through the mouth *and* nose.

Because of advances in surgical techniques, speech articulation is seldom a problem. However, if problems with speech articulation do exist, they are related to two particular classes of speech sounds. These are stop consonants (i.e., p, t, k, b, d, g) and fricative consonants (e.g., s, z, f, v, th, sh). These consonants require the buildup of a large amount of air pressure inside the oral cavity to be produced correctly. For stop consonants, air pressure is created behind a point of constriction (such as the closed lips for /p/) and then suddenly released. If the child is unable to maintain a sufficient amount of pressure at this point of constriction because of air escaping through the nose, the subsequent production of this consonant is likely to be weak. The child may acquire a **compensatory strategy** to this situation by producing a **glottal stop** (ʔ). A glottal stop is articulated deep in the vocal tract, and thus bypasses any possible nasal emission that would occur in the forward flow of speech. Acoustically, it sounds like the break separating the syllables of the interjection *uh-oh*. For the production of fricatives, high oral air pressure is required to maintain a forward flow of air friction (such as in the production of /v/). If the child is unable to maintain a sufficient amount of air pressure for fricatives, the sound will be substituted by a fricative-like sound made in the pharynx. This sound is called a **pharyngeal fricative** (ʕ) and is produced by vibrations set up between the back of the tongue and the pharyngeal wall. Acoustically, the sound resembles the /h/, but it is made with increased friction in the back of the throat.

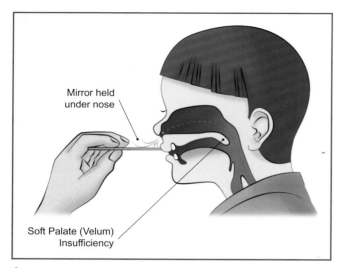

A

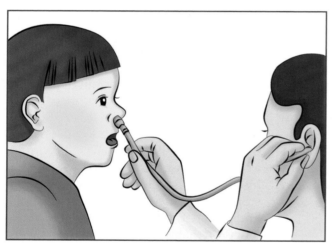

B

FIGURE 7–14. Detecting velopharyngeal insufficiency (hypernasal airflow) through the use of a mirror (**A**), listening device (**B**), and an airflow detecting instrument (**C**).

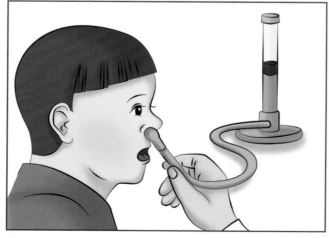

C

TREATMENT OF CLEFT LIP AND PALATE

A child with a CL/P will need to see a variety of specialists who work together as a team to treat the condition and improve the quality of life. Treatment usually begins in the first few months of an infant's life, depending on the health of the infant and the extent of the cleft. Various forms of treatment can extend until the patient reaches early adulthood (Table 7–1). The need for assembling a team of heath professionals is related to the notion of the whole child and the many facets related to human growth and cognitive development that is found across various health disciplines. The use of a team also is an ideal way of managing complex medical problems and avoids rigid compartmentalization of various specialties in medical practice. The notion that many brains are better than one prevails in working with children who have complex needs.

Table 7–1. Typical Time Line of Treatment for a Child Born with Cleft Lip and Palate

Age	Treatment
1 month	Evaluation of feeding
	Hearing evaluation
	Dental evaluation
	Emotional support for families
	Planning for upcoming surgery
3 months	Repair of cleft lip
3–12 months	Continued dental evaluations
	Hearing evaluation
	Speech evaluation
1 year	Repair of cleft palate
	Insertion of pressure equalization tubes if required
1–5 years	Annual hearing and speech evaluation
	Dental evaluation
	Evaluation of child emotional development
	Occasional lip and palate revision surgery to minimize deformity
5–9 years	Orthodontic preparation before permanent teeth erupt
	Continued speech evaluations
9–20 years	Orthodontic treatment
	Minor lip and nose surgical revisions

The concept of a **cleft palate team** was first developed by Herbert Cooper in 1939 and has continued to serve as the preferred model of health care for children with a CL/P. The principal role of the multidisciplinary team is to provide integrated case management for the child and to ensure the quality and continuity of care and long-term follow-up. A typical cleft palate team consists of:

- Audiologist, who manages ongoing hearing status.
- Geneticist, who screens child for possible syndromes and counsels parents for future pregnancies.
- Orthodontist, who straightens the teeth and aligns the jaw.
- Otolaryngologist, who monitors middle ear problems.
- Pediatrician, who monitors the child's overall health and development.
- Pediatric dentist, who makes prosthetic devices for the mouth.
- Psychologist or social worker, to support the family and assess any adjustment problems.
- Speech-language pathologist, who treats communication and feeding problems.
- Surgeon, who manages the cleft repair.

All of the specialties contributing to the cleft palate team are important and provide a valuable contribution to the well-being of a child with a CL/P. Specific forms of treatment offered by the surgeon, speech-language pathologist, and psychologist are detailed below.

Surgery

Cleft palates have to be surgically repaired before the baby is ready to speak. There is no worldwide consensus on the surgical techniques for repair of a CL/P. The decision as to when and how to repair a cleft lip or palate is based on a variety of factors such as facial growth, speech development, and psychological impact on the child and family. As a general rule, a child born with a cleft of the lip (with or without a cleft of the palate), usually has the lip repaired at approximately three months of age. Repair of the palate is usually performed between 9 to 15 months of age. The primary reason for repairing the lip earlier than the palate is to permit as near normal feeding as possible. Another reason is to improve the appearance of the child in regard to social acceptance. Repair of the palate is performed primarily for speech purposes. Without an intact hard and soft palate, it would be nearly impossible for the child to produce intelligible speech.

Other surgical treatments for cleft deformities occur during the teenage years, and may include nasal reconstruction and possible jaw alignment. However, this latter surgery is typically delayed until growth of the facial

---

FYI

Young children who have dental problems resulting from a CL/P are treated by a pedodontist. A pedodontist is a dentist specialized in handling children. Generally, treating a child may take two or three times longer than the same procedure for an adult.

skeleton is complete. In addition to the surgical procedures that are designed to repair the palatal and facial structures, there are additional procedures performed to assist with speech production. Some children may continue to demonstrate velopharyngeal inadequacy following initial palate repair. Sometimes the palate is still not able to close off the nose from the mouth. This may be because it is too short, does not stretch far enough backward and upward, or does not move quickly enough. A widely performed surgical procedure to eliminate velopharyngeal inadequacy is the creation of a **pharyngeal flap**, and is usually performed between 6 to 12 years of age (Figure 7–15). Another

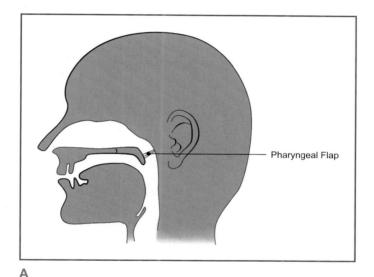

A

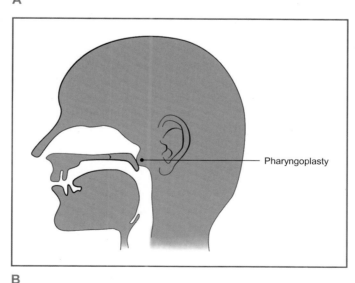

B

FIGURE 7–15. Illustration of pharyngeal flap (**A**) and pharyngoplasty (**B**).

surgical procedure is the sphincter **pharyngoplasty**. In this procedure, the surgeon moves tissue from the back of the throat closer to the back of the palate. This surgery is recommended when the surgeon decides that the palate is working as well as it can, but the back of the throat (pharynx) is not moving correctly (see Figure 7–15).

Another approach for improving velopharyngeal function is the option of a prosthetic device (i.e., obturator) for some patients. These speech aids are placed in the mouth, much like an orthodontic retainer. One common type of obturator is a speech bulb (Figure 7–16), which is designed to partially close off the space between the soft palate and the throat. An acrylic ball is attached to an acrylic (dental) retainer held by the teeth. The bulb is tailored to the vocal tract anatomy and physiology of the patient. Many professionals feel that prosthetic appliances work best in children who are at least five years of age.

Speech-Language Therapy

Since the early creation of the speech-language pathology profession, there has been high interest in the communication characteristics exhibited by individuals with a CL/P. From 1940 to 1960, many speech-language pathologists believed that children with a CL/P showed oral-motor problems that prevented them from producing clear speech. As a means of addressing this assumed problem, children with a CL/P were asked to undergo a number of activities designed to strengthen the speech musculature. Some of these strengthening exercises involved swallowing, sucking, blowing, and whistling. Tasks such as these were later discredited during the 1960s and 1970s because research failed to substantiate an improvement in speech articulation. That is, the children may have shown improvements in their abilities to blow and whistle, but these nonspeech activi-

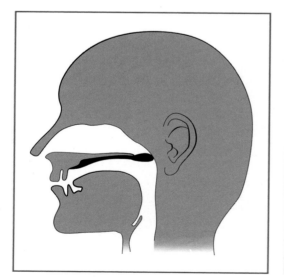

A

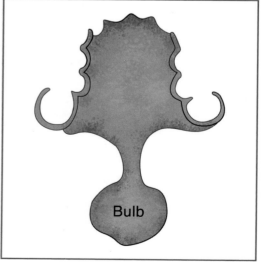

B

FIGURE 7–16. Example of a prosthetic device called a bulb obturator. The device is fit to the hard palate similar to a dental retainer. The bulb assists with maintaining velopharyngeal closure for speech production.

ties did not transfer to speaking ability. We now know that a typical child with a CL/P does not have oral motor problems.

Although current medical technology is not advanced enough to prevent the occurrence of a CL/P, most of the speech problems associated with a cleft lip or palate can be improved or even corrected. There is no doubt that a child with an unrepaired CL/P will experience severe speech difficulties. However, this is becoming the exception rather than the norm. Following surgery, only 10% of children are likely to experience a communication disorder. For those whom speech articulation difficulties may persist, the use of conventional articulation/phonology therapy approaches is preferred. A second area of concern is in regard to the child's voice, specifically the production of hypernasal speech. This condition may be corrected surgically (see previous section). However, in the event the child still demonstrates velopharyngeal inadequacy, some form of therapy may be required. The use of devices that provide the child with visual or auditory feedback regarding the amount of speech nasality has proven to be successful. The feedback guides the child in learning alternative strategies for maintaining appropriate closure between the oral and nasal cavities during speaking activities.

Psychology

Psychosocial issues are a critical part of the assessment and management of the child with a CL/P and must be addressed from the onset of care. The birth of a child is always a time of great family adjustment, and it is especially stressful when the child is born with a birth defect such as a CL/P. Parents often experience feelings of sadness, guilt, anger, and fear for their child's future social acceptance. Our society often focuses on people's appearance, which can make childhood, especially the teenage years, an emotionally challenging time for someone with a physical difference. Depending on the severity of the cleft, quality of the surgery, and the effect on speech clarity, a child with a CL/P may experience painful teasing or seclusion, which can damage self-esteem. Chan, McPherson, and Whitehill (2006) summarized the research examining the psychosocial influences on a CL/P, and found that 70% of children with a CL/P and their parents reported having to deal with teasing and ostracism because of their cleft. Teachers have been found to misjudge the intelligence of students with a CL/P with more noticeable facial disfigurement, and this may lead to reduced teacher expectations and poor school performance. Teachers also have rated school-aged children with a CL/P as more withdrawn and inhibited, compared with children without a CL/P, and this has been associated with academic underachievement of children with a CL/P. Upon entering the workforce, people with a CL/P have been viewed negatively by prospective employers. Although the majority of children and adults may not experience major psychosocial consequences as a result of a CL/P, a large systematic review of the literature suggested that behavioral problems, depression, and anxiety are associated with the disorder for some individuals (Hunt, Burden, Hepper, & Johnston, 2005). One role of the cleft palate team is to provide psychological and emotional support personnel who can help address emotional and social issues. A major goal for parents is to nurture their children so that they have a positive sense of self and ultimately make a contribution to their community.

CULTURAL CONSIDERATIONS AND CLEFT LIP AND PALATE

The management of children with a CL/P may require special multicultural considerations. The cultural variations that are likely to exist in families should be recognized so as to encourage their participation in the team approach. Traditional religious, as well as philosophical, beliefs are known to affect the attitudes of various cultural groups toward birth defects such as a CL/P. For example, Loh and Ascoli (2011) examined the cultural attitudes and perceived causes of a CL/P in Chinese, African, and Indian communities. Among the perceived causes were: (1) the will of God and (2) punishment for past wrongdoings. Bebout and Arthur (1997) surveyed a group of Cantonese-speaking Americans and found that some individuals considered the speech produced by individuals with a CL/P as indicative of an emotional disturbance and felt that persons with a CL/P could try harder to speak in a less disordered manner. Meyerson (1990) notes that Latinos from many geographic subgroups (Mexico, Central America) have attributed the cause of a CL/P to a number of folk theories including: (1) an eclipse of the moon, (2) God's punishment of sins, (3) paternal alcoholism, (4) venereal disease, and (5) emotional stress during pregnancy. Even if folk explanations or folk treatments are rejected by members of the cleft palate team, it should not be viewed as negatively influencing the goals for the patient. Unless these alternative treatments are suspected of causing physical harm or mental harm to the patient, they should be viewed as an adjunct to the treatment plan.

In many countries, there is limited medical and rehabilitation support for people with a CL/P. Individuals may go through their entire lives with an unrepaired CL/P. In 1982, an American plastic surgeon, William Magee, and his wife Kathleen, a nurse and clinical social worker, traveled to the Philippines and volunteered their time to help repair facial clefts for those who did not have access to medical care. The country's demand for repair of clefts far exceeded what the couple was able to accomplish during their visit. In response to this initial visit to the Philippines, various volunteer agencies have since been established that are designed to provide assistance to some of the world's poorest countries in the management of cleft lips and cleft palates. Two of the better known agencies are **Operation Smile** and **Smile Train**. Trained surgeons and other members of a cleft palate team donate their time and services to travel to various countries and quickly treat a high number of cases in a one- to two-week period. The stated mission of these organizations is to provide free CL/P surgery for millions of poor children in developing countries—until there are no more children who need help, and the problems contributing to a CL/P have been completely eradicated.

CURRENT RESEARCH IN CLEFT LIP AND PALATE

Prenatal Diagnosis

Although there are approximately 7,000 babies born with a CL/P each year in the United States, the cause of the condition remains somewhat of a mystery. In the absence of a definitive cause for the condition, there is a need for greater emphasis on early diagnosis. The Cleft Palate Foundation notes that research regarding aspects of early investigation remains of paramount importance. The earlier the diagnosis, the more likely that services related to surgery and postnatal support services can be synchronized, resulting in better developmental outcomes for the child.

Fetal Surgery

Over 25 years ago, surgeons at the University of California (San Francisco) performed the first fetal surgery as a last-chance operation to save a dying baby. They partially removed the fetus from inside a pregnant woman's uterus, repaired a urinary obstruction, and then resealed the fetus into the mother's womb. Since then, fetal surgery has been performed on a number of occasions to repair a problem before a baby is born. Surgery before birth can be immediately life saving for a fetus at risk, or it may alter the course of physical development, resulting in a more favorable condition after birth. A major risk in this type of open surgery is that premature labor can be induced, thereby further threatening the life of the baby. The development of feto-endoscopic surgery is far less invasive and may ultimately serve as an approach to the treatment of CL/P (Papadopulos et al., 2005). Advantages of this fetal surgery are (1) scarless fetal wound healing and (2) better bone healing. At the moment, surgeons are not clinically ready to repair fetal CL/P, and the risks to the fetus and mother from the surgery are far too high.

Early Intervention

Over the years, much has been written about the communication problems associated with CL/P and the strategies that can be employed to remediate these problems. Traditionally, however, this research has focused on the voice and speech articulation problems demonstrated by preschool and school-age children. Past research assumed that CL/P did not affect the communication abilities of children until after they began producing meaningful speech. More recently, there has been a push to provide intervention to children at a much earlier age to lessen the impact of clefting on communication skills of children with CL/P (Hardin-Jones, Chapman, & Scherer, 2006). Intervention techniques for infants and toddlers with CL/P include a variety of approaches depending on the age and linguistic level, and the profile of communicative strengths and weaknesses of the child. The techniques combine early language intervention methods with speech production strategies to facilitate accurate voice and speech articulation skills.

CLEFT LIP AND PALATE ON THE WORLD WIDE WEB

Listed below are websites that provide further information on the topic of cleft lip and palate. At the time of publication, each website was freely accessible.

Cleft Palate Foundation
http://www.cleftline.org/

Smile Train
http://www.smiletrain.org

Operation Smile
http://www.operationsmile.org/

WebMD

http://www.webmd.com/
oral-health/guide/cleft-lip-
cleft-palate

Cleft Lip and Palate Videos

http://www.youtube.com/
watch?v=WGFBG94wZDc

http://on.aol.com/video/
help-for-cleft-palate-175540715

STUDY QUESTIONS

1. What are the milestones in face and lip/palate development?
2. What are the types of cleft lip and palate?
3. How has the historical treatment of CL/P changed over time?
4. List and describe the various areas that are assessed in a CL/P.
5. How is CL/P surgically treated?

REFERENCES

Bebout, L., & Arthur, B. (1997). Attitudes toward speech disorders: Sampling the views of Cantonese-speaking Americans. *Journal of Communication Disorders, 30*, 205–229.

Chan, R., McPherson, B., & Whitehill, T. (2006). Chinese attitudes toward cleft lip and palate: Effects of personal contact. *Cleft Palate–Craniofacial Journal, 43*, 731–739.

Hardin-Jones, M., Chapman, K., & Scherer, N. J. (2006, June). Early intervention in children with cleft palate. *ASHA Leader, 11*(8–9), 32.

Hunt, O., Burden, D., Hepper, P., & Johnston, C. (2005). The psychosocial effects of cleft lip and palate: A systematic review. *European Journal of Orthodontics, 27*, 274–285.

Loh, J., & Ascoli, M. (2011). Cross-cultural attitudes and perceptions towards cleft lip and palate deformities. *World Cultural Psychiatry Research Review, 6*, 127–134.

Meyerson, M. (1990). Cultural considerations in the treatment of Latinos with craniofacial malformations. *Cleft Palate Journal, 27*, 279–288.

Papadopulos, N.A., Papadopoulos, M.A., Kovacs, L., Zeilhofer, H., Henke, J., Boettcher, H., & Biemer, E. (2005). Foetal surgery and cleft lip and palate: Current status and new perspectives. *British Journal of Plastic Surgery, 58*, 593-607.

Peterson-Falzone, S., Hardin-Jones, M., & Karnell, M. (2009). *Cleft palate speech* (4th ed.). Maryland Heights, MO: Mosby Elsevier.

Rogers, B. (1971). History of cleft lip and palate treatment. In W. Grabb, S. Rosenstein, & K. Bzoch (Eds.), *Cleft lip and palate: Surgical, dental, and speech aspects* (pp. 371–390). Boston, MA: Little, Brown.

Slavkin, H. C. (1992). Incidence of cleft lips, palates rising. *Journal of the American Dental Association, 123*, 61–65.

SECTION 3

Acquired and Genetic Communication Disorders

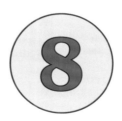

VOICE DISORDERS

INTRODUCTION

The use of voice is an integral part of communication. Dogs bark, growl, and howl. Cats purr and mew. Birds use different calls to warn other birds about threats or food. Each animal has a distinct voice, and all animal species have some form of set vocal patterns that they use to communicate. The use of voice allows animals to recognize each other and convey messages like "get away," "danger," and "that feels good." Humans also use voice to communicate basic needs and wants. Because humans have also developed the capacity to use language, our use of voice has become more specialized. When we open our mouths to speak, the voice we use is uniquely special to us. Our voice is one of the defining features of our individuality, and it shares a lot of information about you. Infants are able to recognize their caregivers on the basis of voice. Your voice tells others if you are happy or sad, healthy or unwell, young or old. Our voice can also reveal to others our background, such as the region of the world where we live, and even our social economic status. Although some people are expert at voice impersonations, our voice is what helps to define who we are. Indeed, many past and present celebrities are readily identifiable as a result of their voice. A list of some well-known voices is provided in Table 8–1. A "normal voice" is one that is pleasing to the ear, has a balance of sound through the mouth and nose, and matches a person's size, age, and sex. When a voice is produced that is perceived by others as unusual or strange and draws attention to the person who is speaking, it is quite likely the person is demonstrating a voice disorder.

Table 8–1. Unmistakable Voices of Well-Known and Some Not So Well-Known Celebrities

Humphrey Bogart	Actor
Bette Davis	Actor
Janeane Garofalo	Actor
Cary Grant	Actor
Arnold Schwarzenegger	Actor
Sylvester Stallone	Actor
Luciano Pavarotti	Singer
Elvis Presley	Singer
Justin Timberlake	Singer
Madonna	Singer
Kanye West	Singer
Bing Crosby	Singer
Barbra Streisand	Singer
Christopher Martin	Singer
Nat King Cole	Singer
Dan Castellaneta	Voice of Homer Simpson
James Earl Jones	Voice of Darth Vader
Andy Serkis	Voice of Gollum—Lord of the Rings
Frank Oz	Voice of Yoda—Star Wars
Mel Blanc	Voice of Looney Tunes cartoon characters
Don Pardo	Voice of Saturday Night Live introduction
Jim Henson	Voice of Kermit the Frog

Voice disorders occur in people of all ages. Voice disorders are also likely to be found among individuals whose occupation is dependent on having a healthy voice. These vocal performers work in a variety of settings such as the music industry, theatre, clergy, the courtroom, or the classroom. Voice disorders reflect a special form of communication disorder that involves a close working relationship between the patient, speech-language pathologist, and medical personnel. Amazingly, most instances of voice disorders are preventable by simply taking the proper precautionary steps. The fact that many voice disorders could be prevented also makes this form of communication disorder unique.

TERMINOLOGY AND DEFINITIONS

The key anatomical structures required for the production of voice can be found within the framework of the larynx. The **larynx** consists of a number of muscles and cartilages that work cooperatively to produce voice. To appreciate the nature of various voice disorders, it is necessary to reacquaint ourselves with the basic anatomy and physiology of the larynx that was covered in Chapter 3. The larynx is positioned between the base of the tongue and the top of the **trachea** (windpipe), the passageway to the lungs. The larynx is not designed for the daily wear and tear we place on

it for the production of voice. The key function of the larynx is to protect the breathing airway from foreign matter (i.e., food, liquid) that may be heading toward the lungs. The primary muscle involved in the generation of voice is the **thyroarytenoid muscle**, which is the formal term for the **vocal folds**. The thyroarytenoid muscle is composed of two bands of smooth muscle tissue that lie opposite each other and sit prominently over the trachea. One end of the muscle is inserted to the inside of the thyroid cartilage. The other end is attached to the arytenoid cartilages. When the vocal folds are **abducted** (open), a space forms between the two folds known as the **glottis**. During breathing, air flows in and out of the lungs and passes through the glottis. When the vocal folds are **adducted** (closed), the space (or glottis) disappears. During heavy duty activities such as lifting or pulling, as well as during moments of swallowing, the vocal folds are adducted. A depiction of the vocal folds in abducted and adducted positions is shown in Figure 8–1.

To produce voice, we exploit the structures of the larynx by adducting the vocal folds and causing them to vibrate. The technical term for the physiological process of generating voice is **phonation**. To produce voice, the brain precisely coordinates a series of events involving the three subsystems of voice: (1) respiration, (2) phonation, and (3) resonance. The respiratory system

---

FYI

A bird's larynx, called a **syrinx**, is anatomically simpler than that found in humans. Instead of being located at the top of the windpipe (trachea), it is located at the bottom, much closer to the lungs. This close proximity to the lungs is what allows very small birds to sing so loudly.

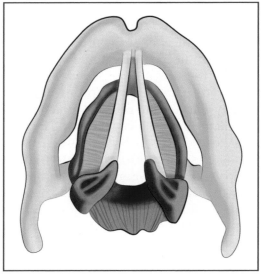 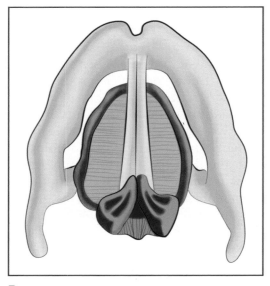

A   B

FIGURE 8–1. A superior (top-down) view of the larynx depicting abducted (open) vocal folds (**A**) and adducted (closed) vocal folds (**B**).

serves as the driving force of voice production. Without the forward (exhaled) flow of air from the lungs, we would not be able to produce voice smoothly. Upon exhalation of inspired air, the phonatory system is then responsible for closing the vocal folds in a deliberate but relaxed fashion. Once the vocal folds close, air from the lungs builds up underneath them until they are blown open, causing them to vibrate and produce sound. This sound then travels outward through the oral and nasal cavities, which serve to shape or resonate the sound quality as it leaves our mouth. The number of vocal fold vibrations per second determines the fundamental frequency (F0; or **pitch**) of our voice. A person's voice pitch can be high or low, variable (sing-song) or flat (monotonic). An individual might also demonstrate natural pitch breaks, such as the case when young males undergo puberty. These hormonal changes can affect voice production as a young male's voice pitch begins to lower with age.

FYI

A **castrato** is a male singer with an artificially created falsetto (high-pitched) voice, the result of castration in childhood that stunts the growth of the larynx. The combination of the larynx of a boy and the chest and lungs of a man produced a powerful voice of great range and unique sound. Castrati were especially popular in churches and opera in Europe during the 17th and 18th centuries.

Voice quality refers to the subjective aspect of voice that is perceived by listeners. The size and shape of the vocal folds, as well as the size and shape of the oral and nasal cavities, help to determine the quality of voice. Terms such as a **breathy voice** (i.e., excessive and audible air leakage), **hoarse voice** (i.e., a grating voice with pitch breaks), or **hyper/hyponasal voice** (e.g., too much or too little voice through the nasal cavity) are examples of qualitative descriptions of voice. Another aspect of voice quality is the dynamic range or **register of voice**. The term register was originally used to describe church pipe organs, where different regions of pipes combined to produce specific tones. A typical speaking voice has three registers that cover the low, middle, and high range of voice. The lowest register is called **pulse register** and refers to the pulse-like quality that is produced with a low pitch. The middle register is called **modal register** and is the region of our voice that is used during normal speaking behavior. The top range is called **falsetto** and is rarely used in daily speaking. This voice quality may come into play when laughing loudly or when singing a high note. Voice **loudness** is somewhat self-explanatory. A voice can be produced excessively soft or loud. The term **voiced sounds** encompasses all vowels, as well as approximately one half of all consonants.

A voice disorder is a condition whereby a person's voice pitch, quality, or loudness differs from that of people of the same sex, age, geographic region, or cultural background. **Dysphonation** refers to any type of impaired voice and includes a condition called **aphonia**, which is the inability to produce any sort of voice. The term **phonatory disorder** is synonymous with a voice disorder. **Edema** is a buildup of fluid in tissue that is a natural, protective reaction to trauma or misuse. The vocal folds are a delicate muscle that is prone to edema, even under the slightest instances of misuse. Edema may also develop in tissue as a side effect to certain drugs. **Hyperfunctional voice** refers to speaking with excessive muscular effort and force resulting in a tense, high-pitched voice. In contrast, **hypofunctional voice** reflects inadequate muscle tone of the laryngeal mechanism during the production of voice often resulting in a weak, low-pitched voice that may also sound breathy. An **otolaryngologist** is a surgeon who specializes in disorders of the ear, nose, and throat (i.e., ENT surgeon, or otolaryngology, head, and neck surgeon). These professionals provide the initial diagnosis of a voice disorder. Most recently, the physicist **Ingo Titze**, who is one of the world leaders in the scientific study of the human voice, coined the term **vocology** to reflect the clinical practice of voice rehabilitation (Figure 8–2).

FYI

Whistle register is the highest register of the human voice. The sound in this register resembles a flute. The ability to produce a voice in this register is believed to be rare. Minnie Riperton (1947–1979) was a famous vocalist of the 20th century who popularized whistle register. This style of singing is also used by the pop artist Mariah Carey.

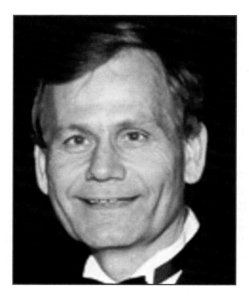

FIGURE 8–2. Ingo Titze, one of the world leaders in the scientific study of human voice. Permission granted by I. Titze.

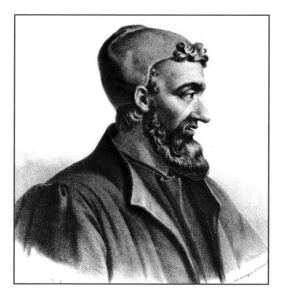

FIGURE 8–3. Claudius Galen, the founder of laryngology and voice science.

HISTORIC ASPECTS OF VOICE DISORDERS

Man has sung through the ages, and so it is not surprising to find accounts of normal or unusual voice production dating back many centuries. **Hippocrates** described the importance of the lungs, trachea, lips, and tongue in phonation in the early 5th century BC. In 350 BC, **Aristotle** was the first to mention the larynx in his book, *Historia Animalium*, in which he describes the neck as the part between the face and the chest. He noted that the larynx was located at the front of the neck, and it was through this structure that speech and breathing occurred.

Claudius Galen (129–200 AD) of Pergamum (Figure 8–3) was a physiologist considered the most important contributor to medicine following Hippocrates, and the founder of laryngology and voice science. Because dissections of human corpses were against Roman law in the second century, Galen uncovered information about laryngeal physiology and anatomy based on dissections of apes and pigs. Galen was the first to recognize that the larynx was the primary organ of voice, as well as for the regulation of breathing, and called it "an instrument of pneuma." Galen theorized that the larynx functioned similarly to a flute, where the vocal folds were the beak (mouthpiece) and the trachea was the body of the flute. Even though Galen learned much about the larynx, he had no ability to observe how it worked in a living person; therefore, knowledge regarding the specific aspects of voice production would not come about for many centuries.

Julio Casserius (1552–1616) was an Italian anatomist who made a major contribution to the study of voice with his 1600 publication of *The Anatomy of Voice* *and Hearing*. The book contained plates of the anatomy of the larynx in humans and mammals that were remarkably accurate from an artistic standpoint.

In 1741, a French anatomist **Antoine Ferrein** (1693–1769; Figure 8–4) concluded that the larynx functioned similarly to that of a stringed instrument, in which the loudness and variety of tones produced by the voice were a result of different degrees of tension and length. The concept of a vibrating string led Ferrein to develop the term vocal cords.

Henri Dutrochet (1776–1847; Figure 8–5) was a French botanist who was primarily interested in plant physiology. His research involved investigations of the mechanisms responsible for physical movement in plants that led to his discovery of cell biology. His interest in the natural biological movement of organisms also carried over to the examination of certain excitability responses in animals, namely the pro-

duction of voice. In 1806, he published *A New Theory of Voice* and theorized about the manner in which the vocal folds vibrated. His view was different from that of Ferrein—he recommended dropping the term vocal cords in favor of the term vocal folds because of the observation that the vocal ligaments of the larynx did not act as cords but like a reed of a clarinet.

In early days, the larynx was often times singled out as the root cause of various diseases. The primary symptom of many diseases such as diphtheria, typhus, and tuberculosis was a marked change in voice or coughing. Because the voice failed to function normally, considerable interest grew in examining the larynx from both a physiological and a clinical viewpoint. By the early part of the 19th century, there was an overwhelming curiosity to visualize the interior of the larynx through the development of various types of viewing

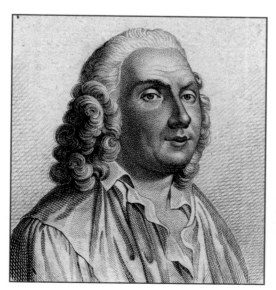

FIGURE 8–4. Antoine Ferrein, the 18th-century French anatomist who coined the term *vocal cords.*

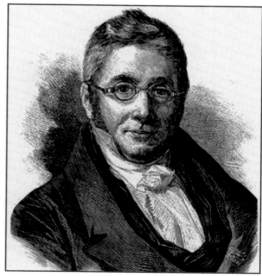

FIGURE 8–5. Henri Dutrochet theorized about the manner in which the vocal folds vibrated.

instruments. However, it was not until the Spaniard **Manuel García** (1805–1906) created the laryngeal mirror in 1855 that clear examinations of the larynx were possible. García was an opera singer who had a personal interest in the physiology of voice production. Using a dentist's mirror, he placed the mirror in the back of the throat, and by positioning it at a proper angle, he was able to see the reflection of his vocal folds in an opposing mirror (Figure 8–6). The procedure was originally referred to as auto-laryngoscopy but today is referred to as **indirect laryngoscopy**. García was hardly the first to look into the physiology of voice, but what made his work different was that he experimented on himself, seeking the cause of his own voice ailment.

Elizabeth Blackwell (1821–1910; Figure 8–7) was the first woman to obtain a medical degree in the United

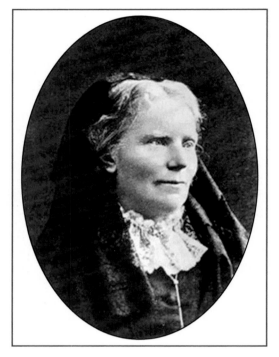

FIGURE 8–7. Elizabeth Blackwell. The first female physician in the United States.

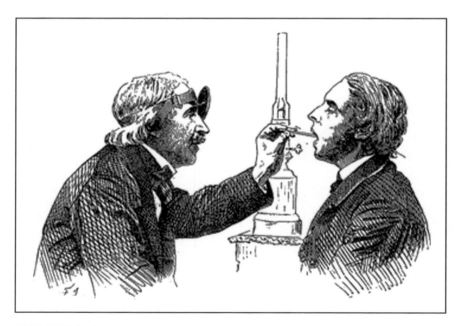

FIGURE 8–6. Manuel García performing an indirect laryngoscopy. Note that the light source is an oil lamp.

States by graduating at the top of her class from the Geneva Medical College of New York. Blackwell enabled many more women to follow in her footsteps, including one of the first female otolaryngologists, **Margaret F. Butler** (1861–1931). Dr. Butler initially decided to specialize in gynecology but recognized the need for her skills in otolaryngology. She was a clinical professor of laryngology and chief of the nose and throat department at the Woman's Medical College of Pennsylvania in 1906. She was the sole representative from the United States at the First International Congress of Rhinolaryngology held in Vienna in 1908. She invented a number of ENT surgical instruments, including a device to remove tonsils, called the Butler tonsil snare.

The assessment and management of voice disorders remained exclusively within the domain of otolaryngologists or singing teachers throughout the 19th century and the early 20th century. **Friedrich Brodnitz** (1899–1995) was a German physician who introduced the concept of **phoniatrics** (i.e., voice science) in the late 1930s (Figure 8–8). When he arrived in the United States in 1937, he was something of a novelty among ENT surgeons, having been

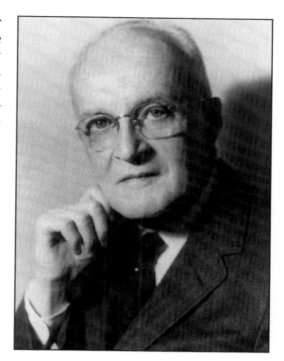

FIGURE 8–8. Friedrich Brodnitz, German physician who introduced the concept of *phoniatrics.*

trained in both otolaryngology and speech therapy. Prior to this time, there was little interest in the field of voice disorders among otolaryngologists. He established one of the first clinics in the United States for voice disorders and devoted his life to problems of the voice, especially if they interfered with the livelihood of opera singers, actors, or other professional voice users. Dr. Brodnitz was a pioneer in the so-called chewing method, which were exercises designed to strengthen and realign the throat muscles to produce less strain and better control of the vocal folds.

The development of the speech-language pathology profession served to greatly advance assessment and treatment approaches to voice disorders. Two textbooks were published

---

FYI

As late as 1947, there were 77 approved medical colleges in the United States with four still closed to women, including the world-renowned Harvard Medical College. Of the colleges that accepted both women and men during that time, most limited their enrollment of women to 5%.

in the 1930s that contained material concerning voice disorders that were specifically designed for use by speech-language pathologists in their clinical practice. The first of these books was *The Rehabilitation of Speech* (West, Kennedy, & Carr, 1937), followed by *Speech Correction: Principles and Methods* (Van Riper, 1939).

TYPES OF VOICE DISORDERS

It is rare for a voice problem to occur instantaneously; they do not occur overnight. Rather, it is likely for a voice disorder to result from daily lifestyle behaviors, including occupational or social demands on the voice, as well as issues related to overall health. Voice disorders are classified according to the causal basis of the disorder. Colton, Casper, and Leonard (2006) have organized voice disorders into three categories, those resulting from: (1) vocal misuse, (2) nervous system involvement, or (3) organic disease and trauma. Some of the more frequently encountered voice disorders found in each of these catego-

ries are highlighted below. A comprehensive list of the wide range of voice disorders can be found in Table 8–2.

Vocal Misuse

The first type of voice disorders are those related to vocal misuse. In these instances, the basic anatomy of the larynx is normal, but the manner in which the larynx is being used contributes to a voice disorder. Vocal misuse (also called **phonotrauma**) is any improper or inefficient speaking behavior that can damage the vocal folds and cause temporary or permanent changes in vocal function, voice quality, and possible loss of voice. Examples of vocal misuse include excessive talking, throat clearing, coughing, inhaling irritants, smoking, screaming, or yelling. The term **vocal misuse** is preferred over **vocal abuse** because "abuse" places blame for the disorder on the patient due to purposeful damaging actions. In reality, there are instances when the patient is simply using their voice incorrectly with little knowledge as to any vocal wrong doing. Disorders of vocal misuse are the most prevalent and preventable types of voice dis-

---

FYI

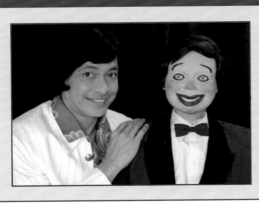

The term **ventriloquism** comes from Latin *venter* and *loqui*, which translates to "belly-speaking." It is not actually possible to throw your voice across the room. Rather, the effect used by ventriloquists is to disguise their voice to make it appear that it is coming from another voice (i.e., a dummy). This unusual manner of speaking can place strain on the voice.

Table 8–2. Types of Voice Disorders and the Vocal Quality Associated with Each Disorder

Classification	Type and Vocal Quality
Vocal Misuse/ Phonotrauma	*Nodules*—Breathiness and lowered pitch
	Polyps—Breathiness and lowered pitch
	Edema—Lowered pitch
	Laryngitis—Breathiness and lowered pitch
	Aphonia—Total loss of voice in spite of apparent normal vocal anatomy
	Puberphonia—Unusually high pitch in spite of normal vocal anatomy
Nervous System Involvement	*Parkinson Disease*—Monopitch and reduced loudness
	Myasthenia Gravis—Breathiness
	Spasmodic Dysphonia—Vocal strain/struggle
	Lesions of Peripheral Nerves—Breathiness
	Huntington Chorea—Hoarseness
	Motor Neuron Disease—Hoarseness or strain/struggle
	Multiple Sclerosis—Impaired loudness control and hoarseness
Organic Disease and Trauma	*Laryngeal Granuloma*—Hoarseness
	Contact Ulcer—Hoarseness
	Papilloma—Hoarseness
	Vocal Fold Hemorrhage (The table is a condensed version of the overall scale.)—Hoarseness and intermittent aphonia
	Laryngeal Web—Hoarseness
	Inhalation Trauma—Hoarseness
	Carcinoma—Hoarseness

Source: From Colton, Casper, & Leonard, 2006.

orders as people of all ages who use their voice excessively may experience phonotrauma. Young children, teachers, lawyers, cheerleaders, and professional voice users such as singers and actors are prone to voice disorders of this nature. Some disorders resulting from vocal misuse are laryngitis, vocal nodules, and vocal polyps. Each of these various dis- orders of vocal misuse represents a form of hyperfunctional voice disorder.

Laryngitis

Inflammation or swelling of the vocal folds results in **laryngitis** (Figure 8–9). Some symptoms associated with laryn- gitis are a sore throat and swallowing

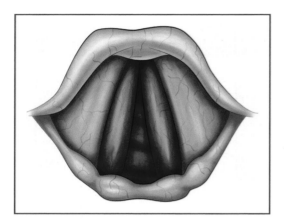

FIGURE 8–9. Example of laryngitis.

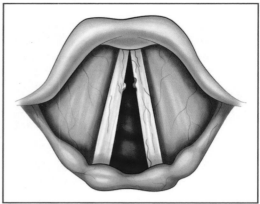

FIGURE 8–10. Example of vocal nodules.

difficulty. The condition may be caused by excessive use of the voice, bacterial or viral infections, or irritants, such as inhaled chemicals or the backup of stomach acid into the throat (i.e., **acid reflux**). The voice of someone with laryngitis will often sound breathy and hoarse. Laryngitis occurs in two forms: (1) acute, which lasts only a few days, and (2) chronic, which persists over a period of weeks or months. Chronic laryngitis can result in the development of a more severe and long-lasting voice disorder. In addition, children who experience severe forms of laryngitis can run the risk of breathing difficulty because inflamed vocal folds can serve to narrow the air passage leading to the lungs.

Vocal Nodules

Small, benign (noncancerous) callus-like bumps that form on the vocal folds are called **vocal nodules** (Figure 8–10). They can form on one or both of the folds, are located on the front one-third of the vocal folds, and range in size from a pinhead to a split pea. Nodules develop from irritation caused by repeated pressure on the same area of

the vocal folds, much like a callus forms on areas of a person's hands or feet following repeated physical activity. During normal voice production, the vocal folds should naturally meet together at a midline position. However, when a vocal nodule is present, the vocal folds are unable to close completely, resulting in excessive air escaping during the production of voice. Not surprisingly, the voice of a person who has vocal nodules usually sounds hoarse and slightly breathy. Voice pitch is also abnormally low as a result of the additional mass of the nodule on the vocal folds during vibration. Vocal nodules are a prevalent type of voice disorder resulting from vocal misuse. This condition is also referred to as "singer's nodes" because it is a frequent problem among professional singers. The inability to sing high notes is a hallmark feature of nodules. When the individual tries to sing in a high voice, there is a delay in the onset of the sound with an audible escape of air.

Vocal Polyp

A small, noncancerous growth on one or both of the vocal folds results in a **vocal**

polyp (also termed polypoid degeneration). Just as a vocal nodule is much like a hard callus, a vocal polyp is much like a soft blister (Figure 8–11). Symptoms of vocal polyps include abnormal voice quality, vocal fatigue, and the sensation of a lump in the throat that involves constant throat clearing. A polyp typically forms on only one vocal fold. Although polyps occur most often as a result of sudden vocal trauma, a specific type of polyp (known as Reinke's edema) results from long-term cigarette smoking, creating the well-known smoker's voice. People who develop a vocal polyp usually have a low-pitched, hoarse, breathy voice, similar to the voices of people who have vocal nodules.

Puberphonia

A fourth type of vocal misuse is **puberphonia**, also called mutational falsetto. Puberphonia refers to a condition in which an adult (usually an adolescent male) continues to speak with a high-pitched voice well after the age when a natural lowering in voice pitch should have occurred. The condition is rare and is believed to reflect a form of psy-

chogenic disorder. A psychogenic voice disorder is thought to result from an underlying psychological disturbance. In the case of puberphonia, there is no structural reason for the voice disorder. However, because the voice is not being used normally, a condition such as puberphonia is classified as a disorder of vocal misuse.

Nervous System Involvement

The nervous system consists of the brain, spinal cord, and an enormous network of sensory and motor nerves throughout the body. Malfunctions of the nervous system may result from disease, abnormal growths, or trauma. Nervous system damage can also impair normal voice production. Two particular conditions that reflect voice disorders having a nervous system origin are: (1) neurogenic disorders and (2) spasmodic dysphonia. These disorders are not related to trauma, as this forms the basis of organic voice disorders (see later section).

Neurogenic Voice Disorders

Two nervous system disorders that have an associated voice disorder are **Parkinson disease** and **Amyotrophic Lateral Sclerosis**, also known as motor neuron disease. The condition of Parkinson disease is a progressive neurological disorder affecting movements such as walking, talking, and writing. The disease generally affects people beyond the age of 40 years. The three main symptoms of Parkinson disease are tremor, stiffness, and bradykinesia (i.e., slowness of movement). These conditions can carry over into the production of voice, with approximately 50 to 80% of all patients with Parkinson disease demonstrating a

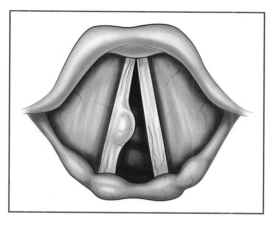

FIGURE 8–11. Example of vocal polyp.

voice disorder. The voice features found in Parkinson disease are **monotonic voice** and a low-pitched voice, as well as considerable variation in the loudness of voice. The condition of amyotrophic lateral sclerosis is a progressive chronic disease of the nerves that are responsible for supplying electrical stimulation to the muscles used for any and all movement. The disease causes gradual muscle weakness and wasting. The disease generally affects people over the age of 40 years, with a typical life span of less than three years from the date of diagnosis. The muscles responsible for the production of voice are not spared among individuals with amyotrophic lateral sclerosis. Early symptoms include a hoarse voice accompanied by vocal spasm. As the disease progresses, the voice becomes weaker and is characterized by breathiness and hypernasality. The increase in nasality results from weakness in the muscles responsible for closing off the nasal cavity from the oral cavity during normal voice production.

Spasmodic Dysphonia

A spasm is an involuntary and abnormal contraction of a muscle. In the case of **spasmodic dysphonia**, the particular voice disorder appears to be one of involuntary and abnormal functioning of the muscles responsible for voice production. Spasmodic dysphonia is perhaps the most mysterious of all voice disorders because we still do not know what causes it and how best to treat it. The disorder was originally thought to be a type of psychogenic condition, and because there was no identifiable physical cause to the problem, researchers believed it must result from some level of mental distress. This way of thinking is evident in use of the term hysterical dysphonia, which has since been dropped in favor of the term spasmodic dysphonia. Research over the past 30 years now indicates that the disorder probably reflects a motor disturbance deep in the brain.

There are two types of spasmodic dysphonia, based on whether the spasm affects the closing or opening phases of vocal fold vibration. **Adductor type** spasmodic dysphonia results in a severe hyperfunctional voice. The patient demonstrates obvious struggle in attempting to produce a clear voice. The vocal folds show intermittent spasms causing them to close and stiffen. Patients find it difficult, if not impossible, to shout, but surprisingly the spasms are usually absent while laughing, singing, or speaking on inhalation. **Abductor type** spasmodic dysphonia is more rare and essentially the opposite to that of the adductory type. In abductor spasmodic dysphonia, sudden involuntary muscle movements or spasms cause the vocal folds to open. The vocal folds are unable to vibrate when fully abducted causing periods of aphonia. The open position of the vocal folds also allows air to escape from the lungs during speech. As a result, the voices of these individuals sound weak and breathy. As with adductor spasmodic dysphonia, the spasms are often absent during activities such as laughing or singing. The prevalence of either type of spasmodic dysphonia in the general population is unknown. There is no difference in regard to its occurrence in men and women. The disorder is rarely found in children and young adults, with most cases occurring in middle-aged adults.

Organic Disease and Trauma

The third type of voice disorders are those that affect the structure of the vocal mechanism as a result of an organic disease or some form of physical trauma. Two voice disorders resulting from these conditions are: (1) papilloma and (2) cancer of the larynx.

Papilloma

Papillomas are benign epithelial (surface-level) tumors caused by infection with the human papilloma virus. The tumors can develop in various parts of the body, including the larynx. Laryngeal papillomas appear as numerous warty growths on the surface of the vocal folds (Figure 8–12). Laryngeal papillomas are most often found among children, and between 60 to 80% of cases occur in children, usually before the age of three. Although papillomas are benign, their rapid growth on the vocal folds can cause obstruction of the airway that could potentially lead to asphyxiation if not promptly treated. Like warts, papillomas are very stubborn lesions that tend to grow back no matter if they are completely removed. This is particularly the case among children. In adults, laryngeal papillomas tend to be less aggressive. Papillomas generally cause no physical pain with the most obvious symptom of the disorder being a hoarse-sounding voice.

Carcinoma

Cancer can develop in any part of the body, and the larynx is no exception (Figure 8–13). Laryngeal cancer composes approximately 5% of all forms of cancer. If allowed to develop without treatment, the condition can be life threatening. The primary cause of laryngeal cancer is smoking. In addition to laryngeal cancer, smoking is the major cause of cancers of the lungs, oral cavity, and esophagus. The ratio of men to women who develop laryngeal cancer is 5 to 1, although this ratio is rapidly decreasing with the rise in smoking among women. Smoking serves as an irritant to the vocal folds causing edema. It also decreases lung function, and without good lung power, more stress is placed upon the larynx when speaking or singing. This is why heavy, long-term smokers' voices are often hoarse and low in pitch. These voice features are also the prime symptoms or warning signs of laryngeal cancer.

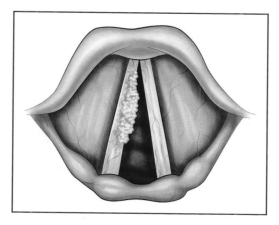

FIGURE 8–12. Example of vocal papilloma.

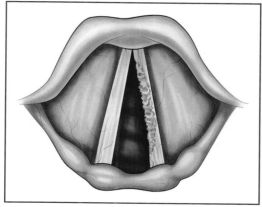

FIGURE 8–13. Example of vocal carcinoma.

CURRENT THEORIES OF VOICE DISORDERS

One of the earliest modern theories of normal voice production was proposed by the French scientist **Raoul Husson** in 1950, who sparked considerable debate as far as the physiology of the vibration of the vocal folds is concerned. In his **neurochronaxic theory**, he suggested that the frequency of vocal fold vibration was dependent on excitation of nerve cells from the laryngeal nerve (part of cranial nerve X). For example, if the vocal folds were to vibrate at a rate of 200 Hz, this theory suggests that 200 nerve impulses per second are sent to the thyroarytenoid (vocal fold) muscle. Husson's theory was eventually found to be invalid because we now know that nerves are unable to discharge at such high rates. This theory was eventually replaced by the **myoelastic aerodynamic theory of phonation** in 1959 by the Dutch scientist, **Janwillem van den Berg** (1926–1985; Figure 8–14). The title of the theory is self-explanatory in regard to the process of producing voice. The theory is that normal vocal fold vibration involves coordination of muscle tension and breath pressure. To produce voice, there needs to be air pressure and flow. Elastic muscular movement of the structures composing the vocal mechanism is also necessary, and the entire process is dynamic, involving movement and change. Over the past 50 years, the various intricate steps in vocal fold vibration have been more critically examined; however, the general concept of producing voice is still captured within the myoelastic aerodynamic theory of phonation.

More recently, Roy and Bless (2000) proposed a **personality and emotional**

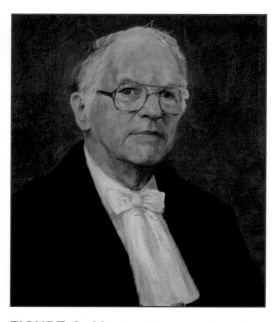

FIGURE 8–14. Janwillem van den Berg proposed the myoelastic aerodynamic theory of phonation.

adjustment theory of voice disorders. The premise of the theory is that an individual's personality and behavioral patterns may contribute to the eventual development of a voice disorder such as nodules. In turn, the subsequent voice disorder that develops creates further emotional problems and personality effects for the individual with the disorder. For example, a person with an impulsive, preservative personality who is misusing their voice may be unable to normally cease in misusing their voice, thereby contributing to a more long-lasting voice disorder. The role of personality and issues such as impulsivity have not been considered in previous theories concerning voice disorders. If personality issues are found to show a direct link to some voice disorders, advancements in the diagnosis and treatment of these disorders will likely occur.

ASSESSMENT OF VOICE DISORDERS

At any given time, approximately 6% of the general population experience a voice disorder, and a majority of these individuals tend to be female (Roy, Merrill, Gray, & Smith, 2005). Approximately 30% of the entire population will experience a form of voice disorder, either fleeting or long-term, at some point in their lives. Most instances of voice disorders occur in people between the ages of 40 to 60 years, although voice disorders are also found in children. Among children, there is a greater likelihood of voice disorders in boys compared with girls, with boys more often implicated in vocally abusive behaviors, such as shouting and screaming. Anyone who experiences vocal discomfort for more than two weeks should consider seeking an assessment of their voice. In some cases, the speech-language pathologist may be the first individual to encounter a patient complaining of a voice problem. The speech-language pathologist may perform an initial evaluation of the patient's voice; however, appropriate ethical practice requires the speech-language pathologist to immediately refer the patient to an otolaryngologist because of the possible underlying medical condition. The otolaryngologist will examine the individual's laryngeal mechanism and determine if a medical condition is indeed the root cause of the voice problem.

The assessment of voice disorders involves subjective and objective procedures. Both approaches are essential to obtaining the detail necessary to accurately diagnose the cause, type, and severity of voice disorder. A **subjective assessment** of voice entails listening and observing the patient while they are speaking, and the collection of a case history. When listening to the patient's voice, the speech-language pathologist will complete a rating of the patient's voice quality, which is based on having the patient prolong isolated vowels, read aloud, and speak in a conversational setting. This is where the speech-language pathologist may use terms such as "breathy" or "hoarse" to describe the patient's voice. The speech-language pathologist will also observe the patient's general body movements during speaking, in particular, examining for excessive neck tension and irregular breathing patterns. Obtaining a patient's case history provides the speech-language pathologist with background information that may hold relevance to diagnosing the voice disorder. The speech-language pathologist collects information about the patient's occupation, daily use of voice, onset and duration of the voice problem, and expectations for improving their voice. An example of a voice case history form is provided in Table 8–3.

Objective assessments involve use of instruments to examine the dynamic process of voice production. Two frequently employed instrumental approaches in voice diagnosis are indirect and direct laryngoscopy (Paparella & Shumrick, 1991). Both approaches are illustrated in Figure 8–15. The steps to performing an indirect laryngoscopy have changed little since the original method established by Manuel García in 1855. The patient is seated upright, and the otolaryngologist inserts a small hand mirror to the back of the throat. Prior to inserting the mirror, an anesthetic is sprayed in the back of the throat to prevent gagging. A light is projected into the throat and deflected off the

Table 8–3. Example of a Case History Form Used in the Assessment of Voice Disorders

Voice History Form

Name: _____ Age: _____ Sex: ☐ Female ☐ Male

Did concern over your voice begin with: ☐ Illness ☐ Trauma (injury) ☐ Surgery?

Voice History

Please list previous voice problems: _____

Please list previous voice treatments: _____

Current Status of Voice

Is your voice today typical of how it sounds since the voice problem began? ☐ Yes ☐ No

Does your voice vary with: ☐ Seasons/Weather? ☐ Time of day?

Do you ever experience voice loss where you are only able to whisper? ☐ Yes ☐ No

Medical History

Do you currently have or have you ever had any of the following conditions?

☐ Pain, tightness in throat ☐ Sinus ☐ Allergies ☐ Breathing difficulties

Please list current medications: _____

How much caffeine (coffee, tea, soft drinks, etc.) do you drink per day? Cups: _____

How much alcohol do you drink? _____

Do you smoke? ☐ Yes ☐ No How much? _____

Are you frequently in a situation where you are breathing noxious fumes? ☐ Yes ☐ No

Voice Use

How many hours do you spend?

- In conversation (friends, family, work, etc.): _____
- Talking in noise (work, machines, restaurants, taverns, crowds, etc.): _____
- Yelling (sporting events, coaching, etc.): _____
- Teaching, instructions, or training: _____
- Singing: _____

Are you using your voice less than usual because of the problem? ☐ Yes ☐ No

Table 8–3. *continued*

Self-Perception of Voice Concern

Please rate the importance of the following:

Use of voice for work: ☐ Unimportant ☐ Somewhat Important ☐ Very Important

Use of voice for socializing: ☐ Unimportant ☐ Somewhat Important ☐ Very Important

Please rate each of the following potential problems that most closely apply to you.
(1 = No problem, 2 = Slight problem, 3 = Moderate problem, 4 = Severe problem)

- My voice is not loud enough for people to hear me in some situations. _____
- My voice is too loud for some situations. _____
- My pitch is too high. _____
- My pitch is too low. _____
- My voice quality is not good. I sound harsh or hoarse. _____
- I'm bothered by the way people react to my voice. _____
- My voice gets tired and fatigued with talking. _____

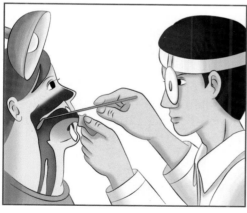
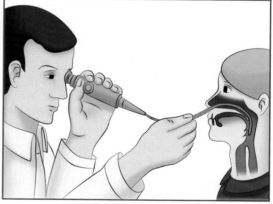

A   B

FIGURE 8–15. Examples of indirect and direct approaches to examining the larynx. **A.** An indirect examination of the larynx using a lamp and head mirror. **B.** Direct examination of the larynx using a flexible fiberoptic endoscope.

mirror toward the vocal folds to illuminate the area. The same mirror is also used to visualize the vocal folds. The patient is asked to sustain vowels ("say eee") during the examination. A **direct laryngoscopy** is most often performed after the indirect method to allow for viewing of a greater area of the larynx.

Direct laryngoscopy is easily accomplished using a flexible endoscope, which consists of hundreds of fiberoptic strands that serve as both a light source for illumination, as well as a camera for examination. The scope is inserted through one of the nostrils and is guided toward the back of the throat and rests slightly above the vocal folds. This particular view is valuable for direct examination of the surface of the vocal folds and any existing vocal pathology.

TREATMENT OF VOICE DISORDERS

The wide range of possible voice disorders and their occurrence in children and adults results in treatment programs varying from one patient to the next. The general goal of voice therapy is to restore the best voice possible. An acceptable voice is one that is functional for purposes of general communication. Ideally, the best form of treatment is one aimed at eliminating the vocal behavior that created the voice disorder in the first place. In the case of voice therapy with singers, therapy involves working on both the speaking and singing voice to achieve an easy natural voice without strain. When the healthiest possible voice is achieved, the speech-language pathologist may refer the patient to a singing teacher, whose role is to provide advice on singing style and technique. Four approaches to the management of voice disorders are: (1) indirect therapy, (2) direct therapy, (3) phonosurgery, and (4) prevention. These approaches seek to eliminate potentially harmful vocal behaviors, enhance vocal fold tissue healing following injury, and/or alter the manner of voice production.

Indirect Therapy

Techniques associated with indirect therapy include voice rest and patient education. **Voice rest** is the process of easing the strain placed on the vocal folds by not allowing any form of speaking, singing, or whispering for several days. Voice rest in itself is not a cure for most disorders. The purpose of voice rest is to hasten recovery time in conditions where the vocal folds have been traumatized. It is generally believed that if a person must absolutely speak during a prescribed period of vocal rest, regular phonation is preferred over whispering. The use of whispering does not allow the voice to rest. During whispering, the vocal muscles are still active. This action combined with air passing between the vocal folds actually has an irritating effect on the vocal folds. Patient education consists of informing the patient about laryngeal anatomy and the manner in which voice is produced. This might include a simplified interpretation of the myoelastic aerodynamic theory of phonation. As well, the patient is educated about the subsequent long-term vocal damage that may result from not producing voice normally.

Direct Therapy

The use of direct therapy involves alteration of a patient's existing speaking behavior in an attempt to increase vocal efficiency and improve voice quality. Four examples of direct therapy are: (1) vocal function exercises, (2) respiratory training, (3) use of confidential voice, and (4) the **Lee Silverman Voice Treatment**. **Vocal function** exercises are a form of calisthenics designed to strengthen and improve coordination of laryngeal musculature. Examples of vocal function exercises include maximum vowel prolongations and smoothly raising and lowering pitch along a musical scale. **Respiratory training** is one of the major methods for enhancing vocal function. Respiratory training focuses on coordinating muscles used for breathing and vocalizing. Professional singers are well aware of the importance of respiration in maintaining a normal healthy voice. **Confidential voice** therapy involves using a soft, breathy voice. The term is based on the concept of speaking softly with another individual so as to not be too obvious. This is not the same as using a whispered voice. From a physiological standpoint, speaking with soft voice reduces laryngeal muscle tension. Somewhat opposite to confidential voice therapy is Lee Silverman Voice Treatment (LSVT). The LSVT is a structured, programmatic approach to voice therapy. The premise of the approach is to encourage a full, loud speaking voice to improve overall voice quality as well as to improve aspects of speech clarity. The treatment has gained widespread acceptance for working with individuals with Parkinson disease (see also Chapter 9).

Phonosurgery

In some instances, indirect or direct therapy is not sufficient to improve one's voice. In these cases, an operation may be necessary to repair the vocal folds or remove growths from the vocal folds. The term **phonosurgery** denotes restoration of voice by using various surgical techniques. The term was original used by the otolaryngologist **Hans von Leden** (b. 1918) in the 1950s to describe any surgery performed specifically to improve voice. In most cases, some form of postoperative voice therapy is required following surgery. Two routine types of phonosurgeries performed by an otolaryngologist are: (1) phonomicrosurgery and (2) injection laryngoplasty. Both surgeries take place in an operating room with the patient asleep. **Phonomicrosurgery** involves use of a microscope to view the area of surgery, and the operation is carried out using special micro-instruments and lasers (Figure 8–16). Phonomicrosurgery is performed to remove vocal nodules and polyps. A guiding principle of this surgery is to maintain normal vocal function by only removing the growth found on the superficial tissue of the vocal folds. It is seldom performed on children's voices because nodules and polyps often reappear in developing children, so repeated phonosurgery would likely cause long-lasting damage to the vocal folds. Injection laryngoplasty entails use of a syringe to insert material (such as collagen) into one or both of the vocal folds to "plump up" the overall size and shape of the muscle. Injection laryngoplasty has been successfully used to treat vocal fold paralysis. An effective treatment for reducing the symptoms of spasmodic dysphonia is injections of very small amounts of botulinum toxin (Botox) directly into the affected muscles of the larynx. The toxin weakens muscles by blocking the nerve impulses to the muscle. Botox has gained widespread attention for its use as a form of cosmetic facial surgery. For treating spasmodic dysphonia the toxin blocks nerve activity to the vocal folds, thereby freeing up the muscle to vibrate in a more normal fashion. Botox injections improve the voice for a period of four months after which voice symptoms gradually return. This treatment

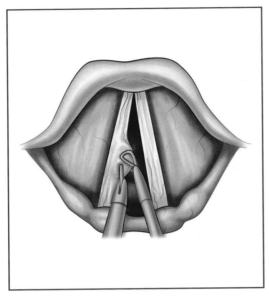

A

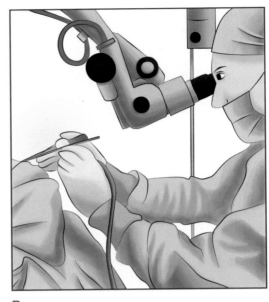

B

FIGURE 8–16. The process of phonosurgery. The surgeon uses delicate instruments to remove a growth from the vocal folds.

requires continual injections to maintain a good speaking voice.

A **laryngectomy** is the complete surgical removal of the larynx, most likely resulting from cancer of the larynx. In nearly all cases of laryngectomy, the individual was a cigarette (or cigar) smoker. A person who has undergone a laryngectomy no longer breathes through the nose or mouth, but through an opening in the neck called a **stoma**. The individual is incapable of producing a normal voice because the primary laryngeal structures needed to generate voice have been removed (Figure 8–17). Several alternative methods exist for producing **alaryngeal speech**. One of these methods involves use of a small handheld device known as an **electrolarynx** (see Figure 8–17). The device produces a buzzing sound that is transferred into the vocal tract by holding it firmly against the neck. The patient learns to modulate this sound by shaping the lips, tongue, and jaw as they normally would if they still had a larynx. The quality of the sound is unnatural, but many patients use the device for basic communication needs. Another method for producing speech is referred to as esophageal speech. **Esophageal speech** is a type of speaking in which air is purposely injected into the back of the esophagus in a manner similar to burping to create speech. This form of speaking is difficult to master. Although most of us are probably able to utter one or two words on a single burp, a skilled esophageal speaker is able to produce short phrases. A very popular method of speech used following laryngectomy is **tracheoesophageal speech**, which is similar to esophageal speech, but uses a device to redirect air from the trachea into the esophagus. This is done through a small shunt placed through an open-

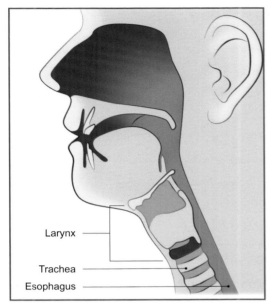

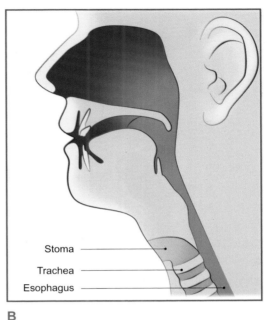

A   B

FIGURE 8–17. Depiction of vocal anatomy before (**A**) and after (**B**) a laryngectomy.

ing made between the trachea and esophagus called a tracheoesophageal puncture. A small one-way valve placed into this opening allows the patient to force air from their lungs into the mouth to create speech (Figure 8–18).

Prevention

Most voice disorders are preventable. Strategies that raise a person's awareness of inappropriate voice use and vocal health are essential to the prevention of voice disorders. **Vocal hygiene** refers to the healthy habits that patients should follow to take care of their voices. This includes being aware of how various speaking behaviors, as well as food and drinks, can have on one's voice and overall health. Vocal hygiene is analogous to taking care of your automobile. When you drive your car, you expect it to work perfectly at all times. For this to happen, you need to be aware of how the car works and the steps needed to keep the car mechanically sound. The same logic applies to using and taking care of your voice. Examples of good vocal hygiene are listed in Table 8–4. The various examples can be summarized using the acronym developed by voiceproblem.org, VOICE:

V = Value your voice through healthy diet and lifestyle.

O = Optimize your voice with vocal warm-ups before use.

I = Invest in your voice with training in proper voice technique.

C = Cherish your voice by avoiding voice misuse, overuse, and abuse.

E = Exercise your voice to increase endurance and power.

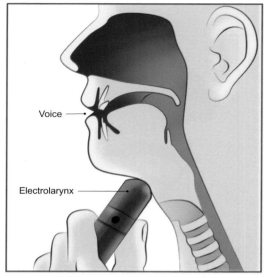
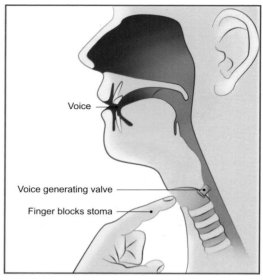

A   B

FIGURE 8–18. A. Use of an electrolarynx following a laryngectomy. **B.** Use of tracheo-esophageal speech.

Table 8–4. Examples of Good Vocal Hygiene
• Control the amount of shouting or yelling.
• Minimize or avoid using a whispered voice.
• Control the amount of caffeine and alcohol consumption.
• Reduce and avoid excessive coughing and throat clearing.
• Minimize grunting or vocalization during exercise.
• Limit the amount of talking in loud and noisy environments.
• Do not smoke and limit your exposure to second-hand smoke.
• Conserve your voice during periods of excessive fatigue and stress.
• Keep hydrated by drinking water every day.
• Maintain a healthy diet and minimize laryngopharyngeal reflux.
• Be aware of potentially traumatic vocal behaviors.

FYI

Each of us has a **habitual pitch**, or level at which we speak most frequently, and an **optimum pitch**, or the level at which we can produce our strongest voice with minimal effort. One way to determine your optimum pitch is through the yawn-sigh technique. Do just what the technique describes: yawn (or take a deep breath), and then sigh (usually we sigh, "ahh"). The pitch of the sigh is your optimum pitch.

CULTURAL CONSIDERATIONS AND VOICE DISORDERS

The occurrence of various types of voice disorders does not appear to differ significantly across racial and ethnic groups. However, a combination of social and cultural factors seems to influence voice and the subsequent development of voice disorders. For example, Japanese women tend to speak with a higher pitch (F_0) level than Western female counterparts. The high-pitch voice is assumed to project a vocal image associated with femininity. In contrast, Japanese men tend to use a lower pitch level compared with Western males that is used to emphasize masculinity. In both of these situations, the differences in F_0 are not due to anatomical differences in size of the larynx. Rather, the use of F_0 is altered due to sociocultural reasons. Presumably, this somewhat unnatural use of F_0 may place Japanese speakers at a higher risk for voice disorders due to possible misuse of the voice.

Society and culture also impact individuals who have undergone a sex change and require a subsequent change in speaking voice. Gender typically is demonstrated in a number of physical and behavioral ways, one of which is speaking voice. Transsexual individuals frequently undertake voice therapy as part of a female/male gender transition in order to make their voices sound appropriate and, therefore, facilitate their entrance (and acceptance) as females/males in society. **Voice feminization** is the desired goal of changing a perceived male sounding voice to a perceived female sounding voice. **Voice masculinization** is the opposite of voice feminization—the change of a voice from feminine to masculine. There is a greater likelihood of vocal misuse occurring in the process of voice feminization compared with masculinization due to the need to consistently maintain hyperadducted vocal fold behavior when speaking.

Other examples of society and culture influencing voice production can be found from the music industry and sporting events. A common anthem shared by today's youth is, "If it's too loud—you're too old." Examples of this perspective can be found in musical groups whose song lyrics tend to verge on shouting and yelling. Although this form of music may be accepted culturally and socially, there are clear risks of entertainers developing phonotrauma. Most sporting events consist of teams of athletes competing against each other, with the added sideline attraction of cheerleaders (both male and female). There is a cultural and social expectation that cheerleaders shout and yell as a means of supporting their team. Not

---

FYI

Adult men have a lower speaking voice (F_0) than adult women; however, among some elderly individuals, the reverse can be found. The raising of pitch among elderly men is attributed to a stiffening (calcification) of the vocal folds. The lowering in pitch among elderly women is attributed to a thinning and loss of elasticity (tension) of the vocal folds.

surprisingly, cheerleaders are at high risk of developing voice disorders due to vocal misuse.

CURRENT RESEARCH IN VOICE DISORDERS

Laryngeal Imaging

The ability to visualize the vocal folds is important in the diagnosis of a voice disorder, as well as monitoring progress in voice improvement. Technological advancements are taking place that are helping to improve visualization of the vocal folds (Hillman, 2013). One of these advancements is in the area of visual clarity provided by nasoendoscopes and videostroboscopes. Further improvements are found in the speed (or resolution) of the images provided by these scopes. It is now possible to visualize cycle-to-cycle movements of the vocal folds. Finally, the images are getting deeper, with advances in the development of multidimensional displays of the larynx.

Teachers

Approximately 10% of individuals rely on their voice as part of their profession. Perhaps foremost among these professionals are teachers. Vocal wear and tear is the greatest occupational hazard for teachers (Roy & Tanner, 2013). Teachers are required to speak for several hours each day, often in noisy and poorly soundproofed environments. A teacher's voice is put under a great deal of strain on a regular basis. Several studies completed in Australia, Europe, and the United States have shown that voice problems occur more frequently with teachers than with any other occupation. In the United States, for example, the prevalence of voice disorders among teachers is 12% compared with the 6% occurrence found in the general population (Roy et al., 2005). The occurrence of a voice disorder can trigger a whole series of problems including: (1) loss of the ability to communicate normally, (2) loss of employment, (3) loss of income, and subsequently, (4) loss of professional identity.

Spasmodic Dysphonia

The precise cause of spasmodic dysphonia remains unknown. The mystery surrounding this unusual voice disorder is of high research interest. The search for a specific gene linked to spasmodic dysphonia has been elusive. This is primarily due to the rarity of the disorder and the difficulty in finding family members with a history of spasmodic dysphonia. In 2009, the National Institutes of Health (Office of Rare Diseases Research) started a five-year study designed to improve the diagnosis of the disorder. Research centers across the United States are using (1) questionnaires, (2) clinical examinations, and (3) laryngeal endoscopic examinations in attempt to identify the most important indicators of spasmodic dysphonia. So in spite of the difficulties in pinpointing the cause for spasmodic dysphonia, steps are being taken to improve the accurate diagnosis of the condition.

VOICE DISORDERS ON THE WORLD WIDE WEB

Listed below are websites that provide further information on the topic of voice disorders. At the time of publication, each website was freely accessible.

Index of Voice Disorders Videos
http://www.fauquierent.net/voice.htm

The Voice Foundation
http://www.voicefoundation.org/

The Voice and Swallowing Center Video
http://www.entandallergy.com/vas/media.php

The Voice Problem Website
http://www.voiceproblem.org/

Voice Disorders Resources
http://www.voicedoctor.net/media/videos

STUDY QUESTIONS

1. What are the major structures of the larynx, and how is voice produced?
2. What are the classifications and types of voice disorders?
3. What are the similarities and differences in indirect and direct laryngoscopy?
4. List and describe the four examples of direct voice therapy.
5. What are the various types of phonosurgery?

REFERENCES

Colton, R. H., Casper, J., & Leonard, R. (2006). *Understanding voice problems: A physiological perspective for diagnosis and treatment* (3rd ed.). Philadelphia, PA: Lippincott Williams & Wilkins.

Hillman, R. (2003, January). Laryngeal imaging goes sharper, faster, deeper. *ASHA Leader*, 39.

Paparella, M. M., & Shumrick, D. A. (1991). *Otolaryngology* (3rd ed.). Philadelphia, PA: Saunders.

Roy, N., & Bless, D. M. (2000). Personality traits and psychological factors in voice pathology: A foundation for future research. *Journal of Speech, Language, and Hearing Research, 43*, 737–748.

Roy, N., Merrill, R. M., Gray, S. D., & Smith, E. M. (2005). Voice disorders in the general population: Prevalence, risk factors, and occupational impact. *Laryngoscope, 115*, 1988–1995.

Roy, N., & Tanner, K. (2013, March). All talked out. *ASHA Leader*, 37–40.

Van Riper, C. (1939). *Speech correction: Principles and methods.* New York, NY: Prentice-Hall.

West, R., Kennedy, L., & Carr, A. (1937). *The rehabilitation of speech: A textbook of diagnostic and corrective procedures.* New York, NY: Harper and Bros.

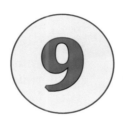

NEUROGENIC COMMUNICATION DISORDERS

INTRODUCTION

Individuals who have a neurogenic communication disorder are frequent clients of speech-language pathologists who work in a health care setting, ranging from acute care hospitals to long-term (nursing home) settings. The term **neurogenic** refers to having its origin or starting with the nervous system. Therefore, a neurogenic communication disorder is usually a brain-based disorder. Although the brain is likely to be involved in nearly all types of communication disorders, neurogenic disorders represent a special set of communication difficulties that are attributed to disease or damage of the nervous system, of which the brain is a major component. These particular disorders can affect speech sound articulation and/or language formulation and production. Neurogenic communication disorders typically are acquired disorders. That is, they reflect a disorder that occurred later in life and following a period of normal communication behavior. Although neurogenic communication disorders can be found in children, the majority of cases tend to be adults.

TERMINOLOGY AND DEFINITIONS

When the nervous system is compromised due to developmental abnormalities, acquired damage, or illness, communication is often compromised as well. To fully appreciate the nature of neurogenic communication disorders, understanding the anatomy and physiology of the nervous system is essential.

The detail of the human nervous system is immense and cannot be adequately covered in an introductory textbook on communication disorders; therefore, the terminology covered in this section is somewhat abbreviated and simplified.

The human nervous system can be grossly divided into two parts: the **central nervous system** and the **peripheral nervous system**. An illustration of the basic division of the nervous system is shown in Figure 9–1. The central nervous system is made up of the cerebrum, brainstem, cerebellum, and spinal cord. The **cerebrum**, which is most commonly referred to as the brain, is a major landmark of the central nervous system. The brain allows humans to engage in high-level functions such as thinking and learning. The brain has specialized areas that are designed for purposes of receiving, organizing, and producing language. The surface of the cerebrum is called the **cortex**, which has a variety of ridges and grooves. The ridges are called **gyri**, and the grooves are referred to as either a **sulcus** (i.e., a shallow groove) or a **fissure** (i.e., a deep groove), depending on the depth of the groove. On the basis of the grooves along the surface of the cortex, the cerebrum can be divided into two halves, known as the left and right **hemispheres**. The grooves in each hemisphere serve to further subdivide the cerebrum into four parts, or lobes. Each of these lobes is found in both the left and right hemispheres of the cerebrum.

The **frontal lobes**, as aptly named, are found in the front of the cerebrum and play a major role in the planning of physical (i.e., motor) movement for all parts of the body. An important language feature of the frontal lobe is **Broca's area**, which is located in the left hemisphere only. As detailed below, Broca's area plays a pivotal role in the

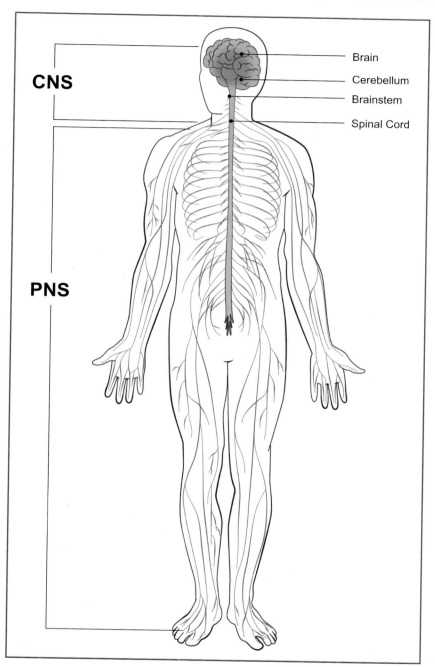

FIGURE 9–1. Illustration of the nervous system consisting of the central nervous system (CNS) and the peripheral nervous system (PNS).

expression of speech and language. The left and right **parietal lobes** are located at the top of the cerebrum, behind the frontal lobes. The role of the parietal lobes is to process incoming sensory information (e.g., the mental sensation of touching something hot or cold). The **temporal lobes** are located along the side of the cerebrum. There are two important landmarks in the temporal lobes that are relevant to communication. The first of these is the **primary auditory center** (also called Heschl's gyrus) found in both left and right temporal lobes. This is the endpoint location in the brain responsible for hearing. Sound, initially entering the ears, travels along a specific nervous system pathway and terminates in the primary auditory center. Further information regarding the anatomy and physiology of hearing can be found in Chapter 3. The second landmark of the temporal lobe is **Wernicke's area**. As noted below, Wernicke's area is only found in the left temporal lobe and is responsible for the understanding (or comprehension) of language. The fourth lobes are the **occipital lobes** and are found at the back of the cerebrum. A major function of the occipital lobes is the processing of incoming visual information. Deep within the cerebrum is an area known as the **limbic system** (or lobe) that includes part of most of the other lobes (i.e., frontal, parieta, and temporal). The limbic system is involved in affective behaviors such as emotion and motivation. An illustration of the lobes of the cerebrum is provided in Figure 9–2.

The remaining parts of the central nervous system include the brainstem, spinal cord, and cerebellum. These structures contain bundles of nerve fibers (or pathways) that transmit sensory and motor information. Sensory pathways are those that carry information from the periphery toward the cerebrum. Motor pathways carry information away from the cerebrum toward the peripheral regions of the body. Damage to these structures can have an adverse impact on speech and language because these pathways either originate or terminate in the brain.

The peripheral nervous system consists of all of the remaining nerves that lie outside the cerebrum, brainstem, and spinal cord. The peripheral nervous system connects the brain to the outside world. Foremost among these nerves are a collection of **spinal nerves** and **cranial nerves**. There are 31 pairs of spinal nerves that are connected to the spinal cord and pass into the central nervous system where neural signals

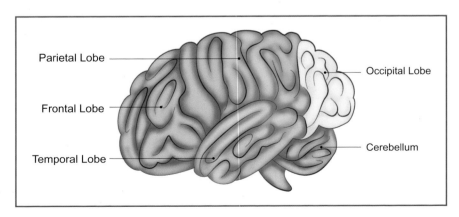

FIGURE 9–2. Depiction of the four lobes of the left hemisphere of the cortex. The location of the cerebellum is also shown.

are processed. There are 12 pairs of cranial nerves that emerge from the base of the brain and are commonly identified by the Roman numerals I through XII. Several cranial nerves are involved in various aspects of speech, hearing, and swallowing, particularly CNV, CNVII, CNVIII, CNIX, CNX, CNXI, and CNXII (Table 9–1). So, damage to any of these cranial nerves could have a negative effect on communication and swallowing.

There are a wide range of conditions that can contribute to neurogenic communication disorders. These conditions result from damage to either the central nervous system or the peripheral nervous system, and sometimes both. Foremost among these damaging conditions is a **cerebrovascular accident**, or what used to be called apoplexy. The term apoplexy is a Greek word meaning "struck down," so this was a condition that would strike an otherwise healthy person at random. Physicians now commonly refer to this condition as a **stroke**. A stroke is an injury to blood vessels in the brain (not the heart), usually in the form of a clot or hemorrhage (i.e., bleeding). Because blood is the means by which oxygen is transferred to the brain, injury to blood vessels results in a lack of oxygen to brain cells that can lead to brain cell death within only a few minutes. There are two types of blood clots: (1) **thrombosis**, which is a stationary blood clot, and (2) **embolism**, which is a blood clot that is carried to

Table 9–1. The 12 Cranial Nerves Composing the Peripheral Nervous System (The primary function associated with each nerve is shown.)

Cranial Nerve	Function
Olfactory (I)	Smell
Optic (II)	Vision
Oculomotor (III)	Eye movement (opening)
Trochlear (IV)	Eye movement (closing)
Trigeminal (V)	Facial sensation and chewing
Abducent (VI)	Eye movement
Facial (VII)	Facial expression and taste
Auditory (VIII)	Balance and hearing
Glossopharyngeal (IX)	Taste and salivation
Vagus (X)	Swallowing and talking Taste and respiration
Accessory (XI)	Pharynx/larynx muscles Neck and shoulder movement
Hypoglossal (XII)	Tongue movement

a brain artery where it lodges permanently. Approximately 80% of strokes result from a blood clot. A **hemorrhage** is a condition where a blood vessel bursts, resulting in internal bleeding in the brain. This condition makes up 20% of all strokes. The occurrence rates for stroke show that men are at a slightly higher risk than women. The occurrence of stroke increases with age—approximately 75% of all strokes occur in people over the age of 65 years. Stroke is the second single most common cause of mortality worldwide. Strokes are typically unilateral, affecting only one side of the brain. There is no difference in the frequency of occurrence of left-hemisphere and right-hemisphere strokes. When a stroke is not fatal, it leaves people physically impaired (Figure 9–3).

Aside from strokes, there are various diseases affecting the nervous sys-

---

FYI

Many famous people have died from stroke including Carol Barnes (newsreader), Winston Churchill (politician), Charles Dickens (writer), Catherine the Great (Empress of Russia), Rob Guest (entertainer), Isaac Hayes (singer), Curly Howard (one of the Three Stooges), Judy Mazel (author), Kirby Puckett (baseball star), Franklin Roosevelt (politician), Joseph Stalin (politician), and Luther Vandross (singer).

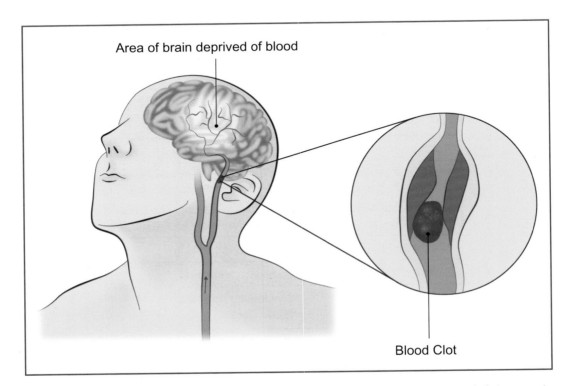

FIGURE 9–3. Illustration of a cerebrovascular accident (i.e., stroke). A blood clot prevents the flow of blood and oxygen to the brain.

tem that contribute to communication disorders. **Parkinson disease** causes a progressive loss of nerve cell function in the part of the brain that controls muscle movement. The disease is the most common later-life degenerative disease that affects around 1 to 2% of people aged 60 years and beyond. Degenerative means that the effects of this disease worsen over time. The four primary symptoms of Parkinson disease are: (1) limb and facial tremor, (2) stiffness of the limbs and trunk (3) **bradykinesia** (i.e., slowness of movement), and (4) postural instability, or impaired balance and coordination. As these symptoms become more pronounced, patients may have difficulty walking and talking.

Alzheimer disease is a frequent form of dementia among older people. **Dementia** is a brain disorder that seriously affects a person's ability to carry out daily activities. The disease begins slowly and initially involves the parts of the brain that control thought, memory, attention, and language. Over time, symptoms get worse, and people may not recognize family members or have trouble speaking, reading, or writing. An estimated five million Americans has Alzheimer disease, most of whom are older than 65 years of age. The disease is the sixth leading cause of death in the United States.

Multiple sclerosis is a nervous system disease of the brain and spinal cord that is a result of damage to the **myelin sheath**, the material that surrounds and protects nerve cells. This damage slows down or blocks electrical impulses between the brain and body. The condition is characterized by sporadic episodes of symptoms that may last for weeks or months and then periods where symptoms diminish or disappear (i.e., remissions). There are approximately 2.5 million people worldwide with multiple sclerosis. The disease occurs most often among women between the ages of 20 to 40 years. There are a variety of symptoms of multiple sclerosis due to the different ways it can affect the central nervous system, including lack of energy, fatigue, clumsiness, vision problems, and speech difficulties such as slurred speech.

Amyotrophic lateral sclerosis, also referred to as motor neuron disease or Lou Gehrig disease (because it affected this well-known American baseball player), is a nervous system disease that attacks nerve cells that transmit messages from the brain and spinal cord to voluntary muscles such as the arms and legs. The disease generally appears between the ages of 40 to 60 years and affects males more often than females. The disease occurs in four to six individuals per 100,000, as seen across the United States, United Kingdom, Australia, and New Zealand. The disease leads to severe impairments in all motor

---

FYI

Cerebral palsy is a form of brain damage that occurs at birth. The damage affects the ability to perform voluntary motor movements. This condition is often accompanied by involuntary spasms. Dysarthria is a common feature of cerebral palsy. The severity of the speech disorder is dependent on the degree of motor damage. Cerebral palsy occurs in roughly 2.5 out of every 1,000 births.

activities including walking, writing, and speaking. The disease is fatal and, on average, runs its full course between three to five years following diagnosis. The disease eventually affects breathing ability, leading to respiratory failure. It is estimated that approximately 30,000 Americans have the disease at any given time.

Traumatic brain injury, also called a head injury, occurs when a sudden blow to the head causes damage to the brain. Traumatic brain injury can result when the head suddenly and violently hits an object, or when an object pierces the skull and enters brain tissue. Most traumatic brain injuries are caused by motor vehicle accidents; falls and assaults account for the remaining cases. Symptoms of a traumatic brain injury can be mild, moderate, or severe, depending on the extent of the damage to the brain. If various centers of the brain that affect speech, language, or hearing are affected by trauma, it is likely that a communication disorder will occur. Traumatic brain injury has been referred to as a silent epidemic because the condition does not receive much public attention, and the results are not visible to the naked eye. Yet traumatic brain injury is a major public health problem and is a leading cause of disability among children and young adults, particularly males because they tend to be higher risk takers than fe-

males, leading to sometimes devastating consequences. Many face lasting impairments that affect their independence and daily lives. Each year the number of new cases of traumatic brain injury is approximately 1.7 million in the United States and 60,000 in the United Kingdom.

HISTORIC ASPECTS OF NEUROGENIC COMMUNICATION DISORDERS

The history of neurogenic communication disorders has its origins in the discipline of neuroscience. A key issue in the historical developments of neuroscience was the debate over the functioning of the brain, particularly, whether areas of the brain had specific functions (**localism theory**) or whether the brain functioned as a single organ (**holism theory**). **Franz Joseph Gall** (1758–1828) was a German anatomist and an early advocate of localism (Figure 9–4). He developed a theory in 1800 known as **phrenology**, in which he claimed that character and personality traits, as well as criminal intentions, could be determined based on the shape of the head. That is, a person's mental characteristics were physically engraved in the brain and were signified by bumps on

---

FYI

Long-term alcohol consumption could possibly lead to the development of a cognitive communication disorder. Brain damage is a common and potentially severe consequence of regular alcohol consumption. Even mild-to-moderate drinking can adversely affect cognitive functioning, including memory loss and various language processes.

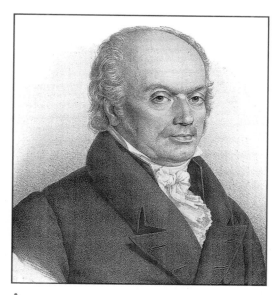

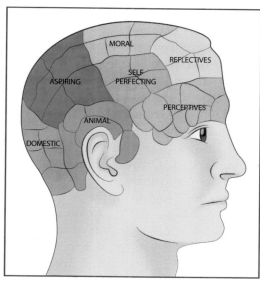

A

B

FIGURE 9–4. **A.** Franz Joseph Gall. **B.** Gall's model of phrenology.

the surface of the head. Reportedly, Gall was jealous of a friend who showed outstanding memory skills and language proficiency. Because this friend had big bulging eyes, Gall thought the brain was particularly large at this location in the head, thus the brain functions for language and memory must be located behind the eyes. Gall's theory was very popular in the 19th century. A phrenology example is provided in Figure 9–4.

Paul Broca (1824–1880) was a French neurologist and surgeon who also believed that the brain functioned in a localized matter; however, he rejected phrenology (Figure 9–5) and instead was part of a group of scholars who thought there were specific centers within the brain responsible for specific motoric functions. This perspective was referred to as cortical localization. Broca became convinced of localization based on observations of two of his patients. The first was a 30-year-old who had progressive neurological problems.

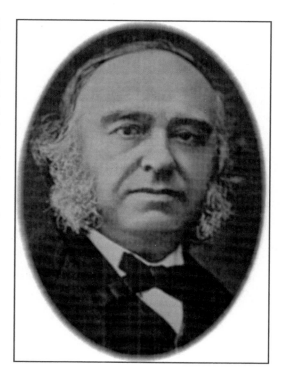

FIGURE 9–5. Paul Broca identified a region in the frontal lobe of the left hemisphere responsible for language formulation and production.

Near the time of his death, at the age of 51, the man was only able to utter the word, "tan." The second patient was an 84-year-old who lost his speech after falling down a flight of stairs (most likely due to the sudden occurrence of a stroke). After the accident, the individual could only utter four words, "yes," "no," "always," and "three." Upon each person's death, Broca performed an autopsy of the brain and found specific damage to a region of the frontal lobe on the left hemisphere. Broca deduced that this particular region of the brain, which was later termed Broca's area, must be responsible for the production of speech.

Karl Wernicke (1848–1905) was a German neurologist (Figure 9–6). In 1873,

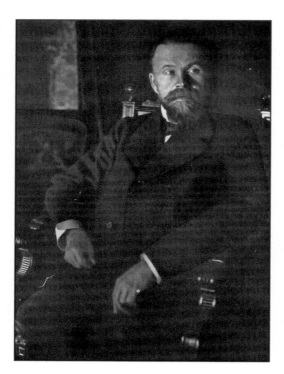

FIGURE 9–6. Karl Wernicke identified a region in the temporal lobe of the left hemisphere responsible for language comprehension.

Wernicke examined a patient who had suffered a stroke. Although the man was able to speak, he showed considerable difficulty understanding what was said to him. He also showed difficulty understanding written language. When the man died, Wernicke performed an autopsy of his brain and found a lesion in the temporal lobe of the left hemisphere. Wernicke deduced that this particular region in the brain must be localized for understanding language. This unique and highly specialized area of the brain was later termed Wernicke's area.

Korbinian Brodmann (1868–1918) was a German neurologist who supported the theory of localism. By staining tissues in various parts of the brain, he was able to show that different cell types (i.e., the histology) of various brain regions differed. In total, he was able to categorize the brain into 52 distinct areas (now referred to as **Brodmann's areas**) based on the cellular organization of the cortex. The notation system developed by Brodmann is still in use today. A map of Brodmann's areas is shown in Figure 9–7. Brodmann's research career was influenced by his close working relationship with another German neurologist, **Alois Alzheimer** (1864–1915) who is credited with publishing the first case of senile dementia (later known as Alzheimer disease).

Augusta Déjerine-Klumpke (1859–1927) was a renowned American neurologist, neuroanatomist, and an eminent physician of her time (Figure 9–8). She was a pioneer of rehabilitation therapy after spinal cord injuries and contributed much to our current knowledge of spinal cord diseases. She distinguished herself as being the first woman allowed to practice in the hospitals of Paris.

Karl Lashley (1890–1958) was an American psychologist who believed

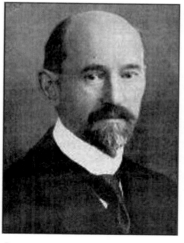

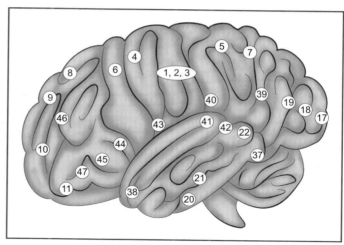

A   B

FIGURE 9–7. **A.** Korbinian Brodmann. **B.** An illustration of the Brodmann numbering system for various brain functions.

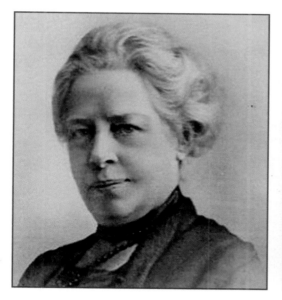

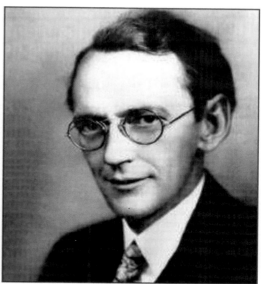

FIGURE 9–8. Augusta Déjerine-Klumpke, eminent neurologist who was a pioneer of rehabilitation therapy resulting from spinal cord injury.

FIGURE 9–9. Karl Lahsley, American psychologist who believed that certain types of brain functioning involved holistic brain activity.

that certain parts of the brain were indeed holistic based on his search for the location in the brain responsible for memory (Figure 9–9). From work with rats, he reasoned that memory is not found in a specific location within the brain but rather the sum of many locations throughout the brain.

Hildred Schuell (1906–1970) received her PhD from the University of Iowa in 1946. Shortly after she graduated, she joined the Minneapolis veteran's hospital where she worked for most of her professional life. She was interested in both the evaluation and treatment of aphasia, and over her career, she became known worldwide for her research in the area of aphasia. She published *Differential Diagnosis of Aphasia with the Minnesota Test*, portions of which are still used today. Schuell was reputed to be a skilled clinician, working with many war veterans who had experienced aphasia. Her philosophy was that most individuals with aphasia could make progress in their communication abilities under the right conditions.

Finally, **Wilder Penfield** (1891–1976) was an American neurosurgeon who was an expert in the area of epilepsy (i.e., a brain disorder involving recurrent seizures). While performing brain surgery in a number of patients in a wide-awake state, Penfield would stimulate different sections of their cerebrum. He found that by stimulating very specific regions of the brain, the patients would provide a very specific response. Based on this very direct brain stimulation, he provided compelling support for the view of brain localism (Figure 9–10).

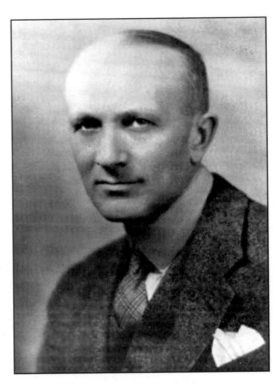

FIGURE 9–10. Wilder Penfield, neurosurgeon who provided compelling support for the view of brain localism.

The debate over brain localism and holism has long since subsided. With advances in technology, we are now able to identify and visualize many aspects of brain functioning. The results have shown that it is incorrect to assume a one-to-one mapping between brain structure and function. The preferred term regarding the functions of the brain is now **connectionism**. This view essentially supports a mix of both localized and holistic functions in the brain. Lower level or primary sensory and motoric functions seem to be strongly localized, but higher level functions, such as memory and language, are the result of interconnections between brain areas.

TYPES OF NEUROGENIC COMMUNICATION DISORDERS

Neurogenic communication disorders can affect speech and/or language components of communication. Two disorders that reflect impairments in speech sound production are **dysarthria** and **apraxia**. These particular conditions are sometimes referred to as **motor speech**

disorders. Two disorders that reflect impairments in language are **aphasia** and **cognitive-communication disorder**. There are also a collection of disorders that have a neurogenic basis but are less well-defined. The general distribution of the various neurogenic communication disorders is displayed in Figure 9–11 (Duffy, 2005).

Dysarthria

The disorder of dysarthria is an impairment of the motor control for speech caused by weakness, paralysis, slowness, or incoordination of the muscles responsible for producing speech sounds. Dysarthria is not a language disorder; however, a language disorder often may coexist with this condition. Individuals with dysarthria understand language and know what they want to say, but may have trouble moving the muscles necessary to clearly produce

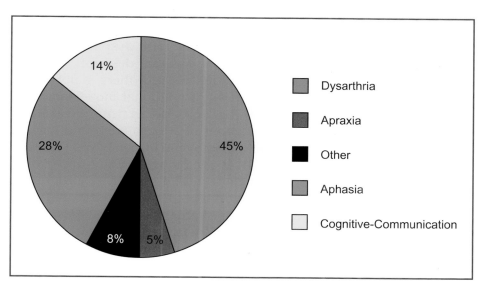

FIGURE 9–11. Distribution of neurogenic communication disorders.

FYI

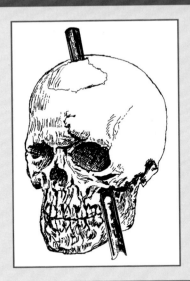

Phineas Gage is by far the most famous case demonstrating the alteration of *personality* via brain injury. Gage was a railway worker in Vermont. On September 13, 1848, an accidental explosion of a charge he had set blew a three-foot iron upward through his palate and exited out of his left frontal skull region. Amazingly, he recovered from this massive open-head wound, but something had changed. Over a course of time, Phineas's personality changed from his old friendly self to an impulsive, crude-mouthed individual. This case further solidified the belief that regions of the brain were dedicated to specific human functions and attributes.

vowels and consonants. At least six different types of dysarthria have been reported in the research literature. Each type of dysarthria reflects an impairment of a specific location in the nervous system. A detailed description of the various types of dysarthria is shown in Table 9–2. The most frequently seen form of dysarthria is **mixed dysarthria**, resulting from more diffuse damage of the nervous system compared with other forms of dysarthria. Collectively, the six types of dysarthria account for approximately 45% of all neurogenic communication disorders. Common speech problems found in dysarthria are slow and sluggish speech that is often slurred and may be accompanied by drooling. There is reduced vocal loudness and a lack of intonation (i.e., monotone). Three nervous system diseases that show dysarthria are Parkinson disease, multiple sclerosis, and amyotrophic lateral sclerosis.

Apraxia

The term apraxia is derived from the Greek word *praxis,* which means to work or perform. The condition of apraxia, therefore, refers to an inability to voluntarily perform skilled motor movements that are not a result of muscle weakness. The term dyspraxia is probably a more accurate description of the condition because there is not a complete loss of volitional movement, as might be expected in true apraxia. Conditions of apraxia are found for a variety of movement behaviors such as hand and leg movements. Apraxia of speech is a motor speech disorder resulting from impairment in the ability to mentally organize the speech muscles and articulators for volitional production of speech sounds. There are two types of speech apraxia: developmental and acquired. Developmental apraxia of speech occurs in children and is present

Table 9–2. The Six Types of Dysarthria

Type of Dysarthria	Cause and Features
Hyperkinetic	• Results from damage to the basal ganglia (deep in the brain). • Problems with involuntary movement.
Hypokinetic	• Results from damage to the substantia nigra (a small region in the brainstem). • Condition most often associated with Parkinson disease.
Spastic	• Results from damage to the pyramidal (motor) tract of the nervous system. • Problems with executing fine motor movements.
Flaccid	• Results from damage to the cranial nerves involved in speech. • Problems with vocal fold movement (paralysis).
Ataxic	• Results from damage to the cerebellum. • Problems regulating the force, timing, rhythm, speed, and overall coordination of movement.
Mixed	• Results from simultaneous damage to two or more motor components of the nervous system. • Condition most often associated with motor degenerative diseases such as Lou Gehrig disease.

from birth for most affected individuals. Further details concerning developmental (childhood) apraxia of speech can be found in Chapter 5.

Acquired apraxia is typically found in adults and results from an identifiable neurological impairment. Acquired apraxia of speech accounts for approximately 5% of all neurogenic communication disorders. The condition often co-occurs with language problems among individuals who have a form of nonfluent aphasia (to be discussed in a following section). The condition is also apparent in degenerative diseases of the central nervous system, such as amyotrophic lateral sclerosis or Creutzfeld-Jacob ("mad cow") disease. Individuals with speech apraxia will report that

they know the words they want to say, but they will not come out the right way. A primary feature of speech apraxia is inconsistent and variable speech sound misarticulations. In some instances, a person may clearly articulate words, whereas in other instances, there is a breakdown in speech articulation. The articulatory breakdowns show up as substituting one consonant for another or completely deleting consonants. Correct articulation of multisyllabic words are more troublesome then monosyllabic words. Apraxic speakers "grope" for the correct word. They may make several attempts at a word before they are able to accurately articulate the word. Individuals may also show oral (i.e., nonverbal) apraxia. This condition is characterized by an inability to imitate or follow commands to perform volitional movements of the speech structures. For example, a patient may have difficulty whistling, coughing, or blowing-out a match upon request. Minutes later, when not consciously thinking of the task, a patient may naturally cough to clear his or her throat.

Aphasia

Aphasia is a language disorder associated with brain injury, usually a stroke. Aphasia refers to a collection of clinically diverse disorders that affect the production and comprehension of language and the ability to read, write, or calculate. This disorder accounts for roughly one quarter of all neurogenic communication impairments. There are four primary types of aphasia, each of which involves damage to the left hemisphere of the cerebrum and are categorized according to the fluency of language expression (Table 9–3). People with **fluent aphasia** have major problems understanding spoken and written language, although their language expression seemingly appears to be within normal limits. **Wernicke's aphasia** and **anomic aphasia** are examples of fluent aphasia. People with **nonfluent aphasia** have difficulty expressing themselves when speaking or writing, although their ability to understand language seems to remain relatively intact. **Broca's Aphasia** and **mixed (or global) aphasia** are examples of nonfluent aphasia.

Table 9–3. Various Types of Aphasia

Type of Aphasia	Language Examples
Fluent Aphasia: Wernicke	• May say words that make little sense. • May use made-up words such as "frangle" and are not aware of doing so. • May produce a full-length sentence that has no meaning. It sounds like a sentence, but there is no content to what is being spoken.
Fluent Aphasia: Anomia	• May have difficulties naming certain words. • Patients tend to produce grammatically correct, yet empty, speech. • Language comprehension tends to be preserved.
Nonfluent Aphasia: Broca	• May struggle to say words and form a sentence. • Affected people often omit small words such as "is," "and," and "the." • Often aware of their difficulties and can become easily frustrated by their speaking.
Nonfluent Aphasia: Mixed (or Global)	• May be totally nonverbal and/or only use facial expressions and gestures to communicate. • May understand some words.

Wernicke's aphasia is so named because of the location in the brain where damage has occurred. Wernicke's area is found in the temporal lobe of the left hemisphere at Brodmann area 22 (see Figures 9–7 and 9–12). The lesion does not damage the frontal region of the brain, which is responsible for all motor behavior. Therefore, one obvious feature of Wernicke's aphasia is that there are no signs of body paralysis. The condition is characterized by fluent language expression but impaired language comprehen-

sion. To a naïve listener, the individual with Wernicke's aphasia may seem to have no expressive language difficulty because the speech is effortless. However, when listening closely, it becomes evident that the content of what is being spoken about may be impaired. Anomic aphasia generally results from damage to a very isolated region in Wernicke's area of the brain. Similar to Wernicke's aphasia, there are no obvious signs of body paralysis. This particular communication disorder is characterized by

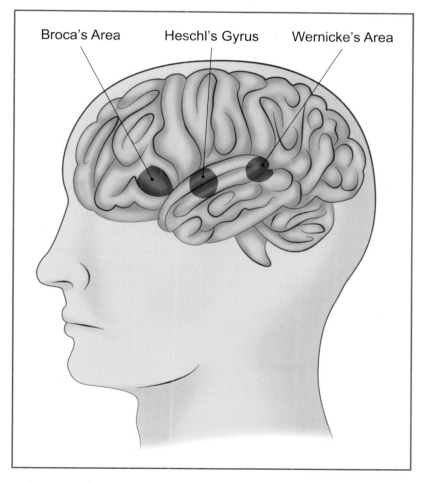

Broca's Area   Heschl's Gyrus   Wernicke's Area

FIGURE 9–12. Location of Broca's area, Heschl's gyrus, and Wernicke's area. Broca's area and Wernicke's area are found only in the left hemisphere of the brain.

difficulty in word retrieval. The patient's speech is essentially fluent; however, there are high instances of **circumlocutions** (i.e., roundabout talking) due to word-finding problems.

Broca's aphasia results from a lesion to Broca's area, which is in the left frontal lobe at Brodmann area 44 (see Figures 9–7 and 9–12). The lesion is accompanied by some sort of one-sided body weakness or paralysis (i.e., **hemiparesis**). This particular type of aphasia is characterized primarily by fairly intact language comprehension skills but nonfluent expressive language. The nature of the expressive language is confined to short utterances of approximately four words or less, and speech articulation is likely to be slow and labored as a result of dysarthria co-occurring. Mixed aphasia and global aphasia are nonfluent forms of aphasia that relate more to the severity of the brain lesion rather than the distinctive communication disorder. The lesion is usually deep and covers portions of both Wernicke's and Broca's areas. In mixed aphasia, the problems with expressive and receptive language are generally no more than moderate in severity. Global aphasia reflects a severe to profound communication disorder due to a massive brain lesion. In mixed and global aphasias, speech dysarthria is likely to be present as well.

Cognitive-Communication Disorders

The term **cognitive-communication disorder** is used to describe a broad range of communication problems that are caused by damage to the frontal lobe regions of the brain. Along with controlling motor movement, this region of the brain also controls our ability to think (i.e., cognition). Damage to this part of the brain results in impairment in the ability to transform thoughts into meaningful expressive language. The impairment is also found in a person's ability to use gestures and writing. This language disorder should not be confused with aphasia. ASHA (2004) defines cognitive-communication disorders as problems with attention/concentration, memory, organization, reasoning, and social skills that impact communication. A cognitive-communication disorder can result from damage to the right hemisphere, as well as the left hemisphere. They compose approximately 14% of all neurogenic communication disorders.

Symptoms of cognitive-communication disorders vary widely depending on the type and cause of brain damage, and the communication problems can range from minor to severe. Individuals who have experienced a traumatic brain injury are at a high risk for developing a cognitive-communication disorder. Injury to the frontal lobes can occur in a number of ways, including: (1) laceration, (2) concussion, and (3) contrecoup. A **laceration** is a wound or cut to the brain that involves direct tearing of brain tissue. A **concussion** is a direct blow to the head that may result from violent shaking of the head, or a whiplash type of injury. A **contrecoup** injury involves a secondary injury that is opposite to the primary injury, whereby the brain essentially rocks back and forth. Examples of the types of traumatic brain injury are illustrated in Figure 9–13. Individuals with Alzheimer disease or those with a history of drug and/or alcohol abuse can also develop a cognitive-communication disorder.

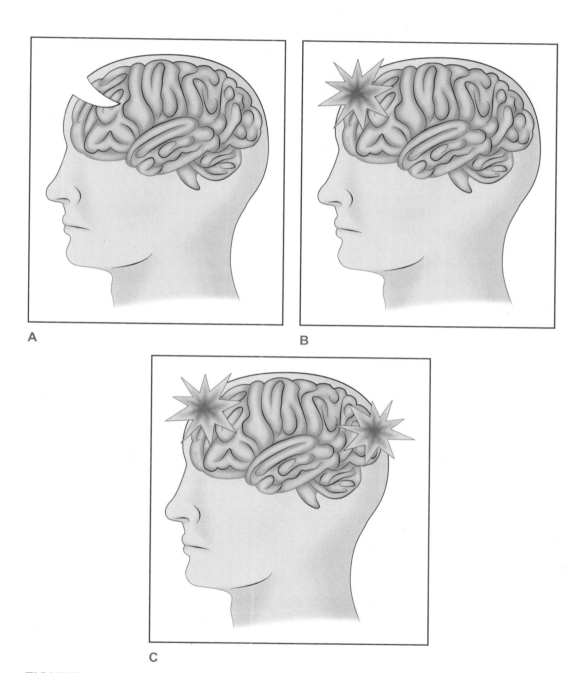

FIGURE 9–13. Types of traumatic brain injury including: laceration (**A**), concussion (**B**), and contrecoup (**C**).

CURRENT THEORIES REGARDING NEUROGENIC COMMUNICATION DISORDERS

One unique aspect of brain injury relates to a concept known as **spontaneous recovery**. This concept concerns a patient's natural reestablishment of skills that initially were lost immediately following the brain injury. Spontaneous recovery is not specific to just communication but for motor and sensory abilities as well. All patients are expected to show some level of spontaneous recovery as a result of brain healing (e.g., reduction in swelling). Yet no two patients are alike as to the amount of their spontaneous recovery. Patients may fully recover their communication abilities, a portion of their abilities, or show very minimal recovery. In addition, the time span of spontaneous recovery varies, ranging from a few days to several years post-injury. The investigation of spontaneous recovery is linked to a fascinating area of neurobiological research known as neuroplasticity (Cappa, 2000). **Neuroplasticity** refers to the changes that occur in the organization of the brain as a result of trauma. A dedicated area in the brain associated with a given function can transfer to a different location in the brain as a consequence of brain damage or recovery. In regard to aphasia, researchers are intrigued as to why and how recovery from aphasia takes place. One of the earliest hypotheses about neuroplasticity was that due to damage to the left hemisphere (e.g., stroke), the right hemisphere simply takes over all linguistic functions that normally would have occurred in the left hemisphere. The **right hemisphere theory of recovery** is still a popular theory, and with advances in functional imaging of the brain, the specific role of the right hemisphere as part of spontaneous recovery can be examined more directly.

There are numerous theories as to the cause of acquired apraxia of speech. Because of the inconsistency in speech sound misarticulations, and the tendency for these misarticulations to occur on words containing multiple syllables, the disorder is assumed to be related to difficulty sequencing the speech articulators (e.g., lips, tongue, jaw). The prevailing theory is that acquired apraxia is a **phonetic-motoric disorder**. The manner in which speech sounds/words are organized in the brain prior to saying them is intact. The disorder occurs as a result of the actual execution of speech. The motor system governing our speech

---

FYI

An individual who experiences a stroke in the right hemisphere can acquire a condition known as **left neglect**. This is a type of attention disorder where the individual no longer acknowledges the left side of the body, or any environmental space that is in the person's left visual field. The person may not shave the left side of their face, or avoid eating food on the left side of the plate. The neglect is also found in their reading behavior.

articulators is thought to have its own "cognitive architecture" that is activated and monitored in part by the language system (Ballard, Granier, & Robin, 2000). In the case of apraxia of speech, this cognitive architecture is faulty.

ASSESSMENT OF NEUROGENIC COMMUNICATION DISORDERS

Dysarthria

Evaluation of the patient's speech sound articulation is a major component in the assessment of dysarthria. The examination includes evaluation of speech **intelligibility** at a variety of levels including: (a) individual speech sounds, (b) single word production, (c) reading aloud, and (d) conversational speech. Because of the obvious physical and motoric impairments associated with this condition, a number of neuromuscular features that may influence speech sound production are examined. These include assessments of oral-motor strength, speed of articulator movement, and accuracy and steadiness of voice pitch. If possible, speech-language pathologists may use various forms of equipment to assist in the assessment of dysarthria. For example, aerodynamic testing can be performed to examine the patient's respiratory abilities, in particular breath support for producing speech. Measurement of muscle activity through the use of **electromyographic** recording also can inform the speech-language pathologist as to the role of various muscles in the production of speech.

Apraxia

There is no single factor or test that can be used to diagnose apraxia of speech. In addition, speech-language pathologists do not fully agree about which specific symptoms must exist to confirm the diagnosis of an apraxia condition. The speech-language pathologist looks for the presence of a group of symptoms, including those described above. Ruling out other contributing factors, such as muscle weakness or language-comprehension problems, also can help with the diagnosis. To diagnose acquired apraxia, the speech-language pathologist may ask the person to perform speech tasks like repeating a particular word several times or repeating a list of words of increasing syllable length (e.g., wreck, reckless, recklessly). In the event of a motor sequencing problem (apraxia), it is likely that breakdowns in speech articulation would occur in the words of longer length. The patient also may be asked to engage in conversation, during which time the speech-language pathologist would note any inconsistent speech misarticulations. Aspects of nonspeech oral apraxia are also tested by having the patient perform volitional movements of the speech structures, such as whistling, coughing, or blowing. If available, use of instruments to directly image the brain is especially useful to help distinguish acquired apraxia of speech from other communication disorders in people who have experienced brain damage.

Aphasia

Assessment of aphasia is a problem-solving activity. The speech-language pathologist must first determine whether the patient actually demonstrates aphasic symptoms. If so, the speech-language pathologist will try to determine the nature or type of aphasia (e.g., fluent, nonfluent). Next, the speech-language pathologist should appraise the patient's existing functional communication abilities. The assessment occurs in two stages. The first stage is the **initial assessment**, which happens at the patient's bedside while she or he is still a hospital inpatient. During this initial assessment, the speech-language pathologist obtains a sample of the patient's spoken language and also assesses general language comprehension abilities. Within approximately one week following the initial assessment, the patient should have regained enough strength to sit at a table and tolerate the demands of a more sustained interaction. The **primary assessment** occurs at this time, and the patient's language expression and comprehension are fully evaluated, as well as reading and writing abilities.

A dilemma when performing a language assessment in a person with aphasia is that often there is no baseline record of the person's language abilities prior to the brain injury (i.e., the **premorbid state**). Information regarding the person's prior vocabulary and reading abilities, as well as general loquaciousness would be useful to the speech-language pathologist in determining the severity of aphasia. The most logical source of this information would be to consider the person's prior vocation and educational background, or to simply ask the patient's family members. Those individuals closest to the patient may be at a loss as to how best to communicate with their loved one following a brain injury. Some common approaches to communication with people with aphasia have been developed by the National Aphasia Association and are shown in Table 9–4.

Cognitive-Communication Disorders

A cognitive-communication disorder encompasses difficulty with any aspect of communication that is affected by disruption of cognition (ASHA, 2004).

Table 9–4. Some Tips for Communicating with People Who Have Aphasia

- Praise and accept all attempts to speak.
- Avoid talking "down" to the person. Communicate to the person as an adult.
- Avoid speaking in the presence of excessive background noise.
- Allow time for the person to talk and permit a reasonable amount of time for the person to respond.
- Keep your communication simple so as ensure its understanding.
- Augment your speech with gestures and visual aids whenever possible.
- If needed, repeat a statement.
- Make sure you have the person's attention before communicating.

Therefore, an assessment of this disorder should involve examination of all aspects of communication, particularly listening, speaking, gesturing, reading, and writing. The assessment also needs to include close inspection of the individual's cognitive abilities, including behaviors like attention, memory, and organization. An important consideration in the evaluation of individuals who may have a cognitive-communication disorder is to consider the impact of the disorder on overall functioning. Therefore, the assessment incorporates observations of the individual in his or her home/daily environment and includes interviews with caregivers and other frequent communication partners (Hopper, 2005).

TREATMENT OF NEUROGENIC COMMUNICATION DISORDERS

Dysarthria

The treatment of dysarthria focuses on improvement of speech clarity and speech naturalness. Specific goals for therapy are targeted toward altering speaking rate and increasing breath support, as well as muscle strengthening exercises designed to increase mouth, tongue, and lip movement. The speech-language pathologist can help the person's caregivers or family learn to adapt to the environment so they can understand the person better. Among individuals with mild to moderate dysarthria, particularly those with Parkinson disease, a popular treatment approach known as the **Lee Silverman Voice Treatment** is in widespread use.

The Lee Silverman Voice Treatment technique emphasizes high-effort loud phonation to improve respiratory, laryngeal, and articulatory functions during speech (Ramig, Fox, & Sapir, 2004; see also Chapter 8).

Apraxia

Treatment approaches for apraxia of speech depend on the severity of the impairment. In some cases, people with acquired apraxia of speech recover some or all of their speech abilities on their own. Individuals with mild apraxia might be taught strategies to help them correctly articulate multisyllabic words that tend to give them trouble. People with moderate to severe apraxia usually need frequent and intensive therapy sessions with a speech-language pathologist. One approach to therapy is to work on **sound-sequencing** skills. In this approach, a word to be spoken is dissected into individual consonants and vowels. The patient is asked to say the individual sounds in a controlled, deliberate fashion, while also thinking about how the lips and tongue should be positioned for speaking. Sometimes tapping or clapping out the rhythm of speech helps patients to speak more clearly. An alternative approach to having the patient produce individual speech sounds is to work on more complex forms of articulation first, such as two- and three-element consonant clusters (e.g., stop, street). The logic behind this approach is to help the patient gain control over more challenging forms of speech sound-sequencing first, which will have a trickle-down effect of naturally stabilizing the articulation of less complex (individual) speech sounds (Maas, Barlow, Robin, & Shapiro, 2002).

Aphasia

Patients who experience a brain injury resulting in aphasia may spontaneously recover their original communication abilities. Although some level of natural recovery might be expected in most patients with aphasia, speech-language therapy is still an important facet in the patient's recovery. The goal of therapy for patients with aphasia is to: (1) maximize recovery of impaired function, (2) assist in the development of communication strategies, and (3) help the patient adjust to the residual deficits of the brain injury. It is unlikely that any two patients with aphasia will experience an identical stroke, and patients do not come from identical backgrounds. So the treatment program for each patient is unique (Wambaugh, Duffy, McNeil, Robin, & Rogers, 2006).

Approaches to treating aphasia include: (1) stimulation, (2) memorization, and (3) inhibition. **Stimulation** involves encouraging the patient to use all modalities of communication to foster the return of language abilities that are impaired but appear to have the potential to be regained. For example, the patient may be asked to verbally "echo" language models provided by the speech-language pathologist. The patient could be encouraged to read lips, attempt writing symbols/shapes, and read single words. In essence, the patient is asked to try everything in regards to expression of language.

Working on a patient's **memory** skills is thought to assist with the development of new neural pathways in the brain, which can lead to learning how to speak again. Memory tasks can include imitating/recalling motor sequences or repetition of phrases and sentences. Some individuals who have experienced a brain injury could show difficulty with **inhibiting** their emotion, especially those emotions that are generally suppressed. Patients might demonstrate uncontrollable laughing/crying or may become sexual aroused. This aspect of therapy attempts to assist the patient to recognize when these emotions are evident and to help extinguish them. For example, the speech-language pathologist could ask the patient to purposely pretend to laugh uncontrollably and to have them halt doing so on the basis of a visual or verbal prompt. This contrived activity can serve to heighten the patient's awareness and subsequent ability to control his emotions.

Cognitive-Communication Disorders

Patients with this disorder typically have some level of intellectual impairment (e.g., dementia) that affects language, attention, memory, and personality. The goal of therapy is to assist patients in increasing their reliance on more intact cognitive abilities to compensate for those abilities that have become impaired. Hopper (2005) recommends a variety of treatment approaches to working with a patient with a cognitive-communication disorder. These approaches include: (1) validation therapy, (2) graphic cues, (3) Montessori techniques, and (4) caregiver training. **Validation therapy** is a technique used to confirm (through words and gestures) what the person with dementia says, regardless of accuracy or basis in fact, rather than correcting or reorienting the person. **Graphic cuing** involves providing written factual information and/or familiar photographs to facilitate communication. This approach capitalizes on the patient's recognition memory and the ability to read aloud. **Montessori-**

based interventions involve the development of structured activities that are appropriate to an individual's cognitive abilities that take place in the context of social interaction. Finally, when working with a patient with a cognitive-communication disorder, it is important to incorporate the patient's caregivers in the treatment program. Each letter in the acronym FOCUSED stands for a particular communication technique to be used by caregivers (Ripich & Ziol, 1998). The goal is to teach the patient a functional piece of information or behavior that can be used in everyday situations. A summary of the FOCUSED program is found in Table 9–5.

Alternative or Augmentative Communication

In cases of significant neurological impairment, some individuals may not have the physical capacity to produce speech that is understandable. These individuals may also have severe motor impairments affecting other parts of their body that prevents them from using other forms of communication such as sign language. Severe communication impairment can result from conditions like cerebral palsy or some types of neurodegenerative disorders (e.g., amyotrophic lateral sclerosis). In these cases, it is unlikely the patient's speech clarity will improve with traditional treatment approaches. The speech-language pathologist may recommend using somewhat nontraditional approaches to facilitate communication, known as **alternative or augmentative communication**. The term alternative or augmentative communication refers to any mode of communication other than speech. The goal of alternative or augmentative communication is to achieve the most effective communication possible

Table 9–5. Summary of the FOCUSED Approach to Caregiver Training for Patients with Cognitive-Communicative Impairments

F = Face	Face the person directly. Call his or her name. Touch the person. Maintain eye contact.
O = Orient	Orient the person to the topic by repeating key words. Repeat phrases. Use nouns and specific names.
C = Continue	Continue the same topic of conversation as long as possible. Restate the topic throughout the conversation.
U = Unstick	Help the person become "unstuck" when she or he uses a word incorrectly by suggesting the intended word.
S = Structured	Structure your questions so that the person can recognize and repeat a response. Provide two simple choices at a time. Use yes or no questions.
E = Exchange	Keep up the normal exchange of ideas used in everyday conversation. Give the person clues as to how to answer questions.
D = Direct	Keep sentences short, simple, and direct. Put the subject of the sentences first. Use hand signals, pictures, and facial expressions.

for the individual using a set of tools and strategies to solve everyday communicative challenges.

The communication can take many forms such as eye gazing/blinking, typing, facial expressions, symbols, pictures, and speech generating devices. The use of communication devices is a frequently used alternative or augmentative communication approach. The construction of these devices and their use can range from basic to sophisticated. An example of a basic or low-technology device would be an alphabet or picture board (Figure 9–14). The patient with a severe dysarthria would simply point to letters or pictures on the board to express words and messages rather than attempting to verbally say the words. A sophisticated or high-technology device might include a computer that has an artificial voice output. The theoretical physicist Stephen Hawking, who has amyotrophic lateral sclerosis, uses an alternative or augmentative communication device to communicate.

The form of communication is tailored around the person's cognitive and motoric abilities. The inability to speak can be frustrating and emotionally devastating. The general theory behind alternative or augmentative communication is that the form of communication is less important than the successful understanding of the message. For many individuals, they will use a combination of alternative or augmentative communication strategies as part of their daily communication, depending on their communicative situation. The combined use of approaches used by an individual is known as their particular alternative or augmentative communication system.

CULTURAL CONSIDERATIONS AND NEUROGENIC COMMUNICATION DISORDERS

A range of multicultural factors interact with neurogenic communication disorders. For example, **race** and **ethnicity**

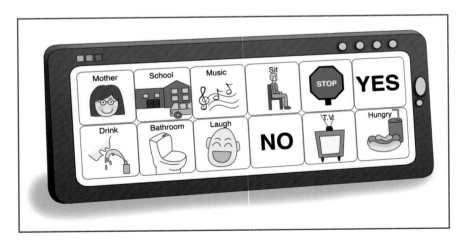

FIGURE 9–14. Simplified example of an alternative communication device for use by individuals who are unable to use speech as a sole means of communication.

are predisposing factors for a number of neurological conditions that can lead to a communication disorder. In the United States, African Americans and Hispanics are at greater risk for dementia than other cultural groups (Qualls & Muñoz, 2005). African Americans, Hispanics, Native Americans, as well as Pacific Islanders are at particularly high risk for Type 2 (adult onset) diabetes, thus making these groups at greater risk for heart disease and stroke. Also, African Americans have the highest death rate from traumatic brain injury, and long-term disability following traumatic brain injury tends to be more severe for African Americans than other racial groups (Thurman, Alverson, Dunn, Guerrero, & Sniezek, 1999).

The occurrence of various nervous system diseases, such as multiple sclerosis, differs according to **geographic region**. People living beyond the 40-degree latitude mark north or south of the equator are far more likely to develop multiple sclerosis than those living in warmer climates near the equator. This is especially true for people in North America, Europe, and New Zealand, whereas Asia continues to have a low incidence of multiple sclerosis. Caucasians are far more likely to develop multiple sclerosis than those of African heritage.

A person's **socioeconomic status** is also a consideration in neurogenic communication disorders. Individuals coming from a low socioeconomic status background are less likely to have access to appropriate health care than middle socioeconomic status and high socioeconomic status individuals. Lack of access to health care places these individuals at greater risk for later appearing conditions (e.g., hypertension, diabetes) that are precursors to some neurological conditions (e.g., stroke, dementia). Also,

the diet of low socioeconomic status individuals can lead to nutritional deficiencies that affect neurological growth and development, as well as the risk of and response to neurological impairment (Qualls & Muñoz, 2005).

The bilingual speaker who has experienced a brain injury resulting in language impairment presents a unique challenge for the speech-language pathologist, not only from a multicultural perspective but from a neurological perspective. The languages of a bilingual speaker are stored in the left hemisphere, similar to monolingual speakers; however, the languages may not completely overlap in cortical and subcortical regions in the brain (Roberts, 2001). This can result in quite different abilities in the two languages following the injury. It is important for the speech-language pathologist to recognize the likelihood of an uneven language profile in these patients.

CURRENT RESEARCH IN NEUROGENIC COMMUNICATION DISORDERS

Practice Makes Perfect

The adage, *practice makes perfect* applies to most physical activities, such as learning to dance or engaging in sports. The same can be said for learning (or relearning) to produce speech. Recent neuroplasticity research has shown that synapses are constantly being recreated or removed according to how they are used. Repeated movements of a speech task can serve to reinforce these synaptic connections. The electropalatograph is a tool that displays and records tongue contact against the palate. The wearer of the device is provided with visual biofeedback concerning the accuracy of their speech articulation. The use of this device, along with repeated practice, is proving to be a promising treatment approach for individuals with acquired apraxia of speech (Mauszycki, 2013).

Direct Brain Stimulation

The use of brain stimulation techniques to treat neurologically based communication disorders is gaining widespread attention. Two of these approaches are **deep brain stimulation** and **transcranial direct current stimulation**. Individuals with Parkinson disease are often prescribed medications to help alleviate muscle stiffness and restricted range of movement. These drugs eventually prove to be ineffective as the severity of the disease progresses. As an alternative to drug therapy, deep brain stimulation has been attempted by directly stimulating parts of the brain to help reduce disordered movement patterns. The procedure involves inserting electrodes via a hair-thin wire through the skull into the area of the brain that controls movement (Figure 9–15). The patient is able to control the device with a neurotransmitter that sends electrical impulses down the wire into the brain. The person can turn the deep brain stimulation on when needed and turn it off during sleep (when the motor disturbance is minimal). Currently, there is research taking place in both the northern and southern hemisphere testing the safety and effectiveness of the procedure (Silberstein et al., 2009).

The transcranial direct current stimulation procedure involves plac-

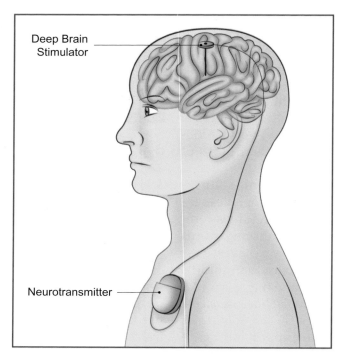

FIGURE 9–15. Illustration of deep brain stimulation.

ing electrodes on a person's scalp and inducing low electrical current. Depending on the location of the electrodes, the stimulation provided to the brain can either excite or inhibit brain function. Research has shown that by targeting regions of the left side of the brain that remain intact following a left-hemisphere stroke, it is possible to increase language performance in aphasic individuals (Fridriksson, Richardson, Baker, & Rorden, 2011). These researchers feel that transcranial direct current stimulation is most useful as a supplement to behavioral aphasia therapy rather than a stand-alone treatment approach.

International Classification of Functioning Framework

When considering assessment of neurogenic communication disorders, it is important to recognize that a brain injury can have a devastating, life-changing impact on a patient's everyday existence. Therefore, it is imperative to consider the patient's overall lifestyle and to take steps to reduce any barriers to everyday functioning. The **International Classification of Functioning** (ICF) framework was developed by the World Health Organization (2001) as a model of practice for rehabilitation clinicians. The WHO ICF model shifts the concept of disability from one that focuses on impairments to one that focuses on the individual. Using an ICF perspective, a patient's disability can be assessed according to two factors: (1) functioning and disability and (2) contextual factors. Functioning and disability includes: (a) body functions and structures, which describes the actual anatomy/physiology and psychology of the human body and

---

———— FYI ————

Advances in research are likely to lead to new ideas about the neurogenic bases of a variety of communication disorders, particularly those that currently have no identifiable cause, such as stuttering and specific language impairment.

(b) activity and participation, which describes the person's functional status, including communication, mobility, interpersonal interactions, self-care, learning, and applying knowledge. Contextual factors include: (a) environmental factors, which are those factors that are not within the person's control, such as family, work, government agencies, laws, and cultural beliefs, and (b) personal factors, which include race, gender, age, educational level, and coping styles. The characteristics of the ICF make it attractive to speech-language pathologists for the holistic treatment of patients with a communication disorder. Although the ICF is not a formal assessment tool, it provides a framework to identify the key issues that may impact a patient's overall rehabilitation. Research using the ICF is providing encouraging results for addressing various neurogenic communication disorders such as apraxia of speech and traumatic brain injury (Eden & Larkins, 2007; Wambaugh & Mauszycki, 2010).

Stem Cells

Stem cells are found in bone marrow and blood vessels in human embryos. They are the "starter" cells that have the ability to grow into adult tissue.

Research has shown that stem cells, taken from embryos that are just a few days old, can turn into any of the 300 different types of cells that make up the adult body (Wu, Boyd, & Wood, 2007). An important line of research in this area concerns the muscle cells that are affected in neuromuscular disorders. This may lead to new therapies that treat diseases such as amyotrophic lateral sclerosis (Umbach et al., 2012). Although this research is still considered controversial and highly restrictive in some countries, the U.S. National Institute on Deafness and Other Communication Disorders identifies the use of stem cells as a possible approach to improving communication disorders resulting from impaired or decreased nerve cells.

NEUROGENIC COMMUNICATION DISORDERS ON THE WORLD WIDE WEB

Listed below are websites that provide further information on the topic of neurogenic communication disorders. At the time of publication, each website was freely accessible.

Aphasia Institute Video
http://www.aphasia.ca/?s=video

Components of a Neurological Examination Video
http://www.neuroexam.com

Traumatic Brain Injury Video Library
http://www.traumaticbrain injury.com

Dysarthria Videos
http://www.stroke4carers .org/?p=5409

http://library.med.utah.edu/ neurologicexam/html/mental status_resources.html

AAC Video
http://www.youtube.com/channel/ HCxyNDj6hqVrc

STUDY QUESTIONS

1. What are the essential anatomical features of the nervous system and their role in communication disorders?
2. What are the various types of dsyarthria?
3. What are the various types of aphasia?
4. How are neurogenic communication disorders assessed?
5. How are neurogenic communication disorders treated?

REFERENCES

American Speech-Language-Hearing Association. (2004). Roles of speech-language pathologists in the identification, diagnosis, and treatment of individuals with cognitive-communication disorders. Practice guidelines and policies. *ASHA, Supplement 24.*

Ballard, K., Granier, J., & Robin, D. (2000). Understanding the nature of apraxia of speech: Theory, analysis, and treatment. *Aphasiology, 14,* 969–995.

Cappa, S. (2000). Recovery from aphasia: Why and how? *Brain and Language, 71,* 39–41.

Duffy, J. (2005). *Motor speech disorders: Substrates, differential diagnosis, and management*. St. Louis, MO: Mosby.

Eden, D., & Larkins, B. (2007). The application of the International Classification of Functioning Disability and Health (ICF) in speech-language therapy: A case example of a client with aphasia following stroke. *New Zealand Journal of Speech-Language Therapy, 62*, 20–28.

Fridriksson, J., Richardson, J. D., Baker, J. M., & Rorden, C. (2011). Transcranial direct current stimulation improves naming reaction time in fluent aphasia: A double-blind, sham-controlled study. *Stroke, 42*, 819–821.

Hopper, T. (2005, November). Assessment and treatment of cognitive-communication disorders in individuals with dementia. *ASHA Leader*, 10–11.

Maas, E., Barlow, J., Robin, D., & Shapiro, L. (2002). Treatment of sound errors in aphasia and apraxia of speech: Effects of phonological complexity. *Aphasiology, 16*, 609–622.

Mauszycki, S. (2013, January). Biofeedback for acquired apraxia of speech. *ASHA Leader, 40*.

Qualls, C. D., & Muñoz, M. L. (2005). Race ethnicity, socioeconomic status, and cognitive-communicative functioning in individuals with neurogenic communication disorders: Clinical implications and research directions. *ECHO: E-Journal for Black and Other Ethnic Group Research and Practices in Communication Sciences and Disorders, 1*(1), 30–39.

Ramig, L. O., Fox, C., & Sapir, S. (2004). Parkinson's disease: Speech and voice disorders and their treatment with the Lee Silverman Voice Treatment. *Seminars in Speech and Language, 25*, 169–180.

Ripich, D., & Ziol, E. (1998). Dementia: A review for the speech-language pathologist. In A. Johnson & B. Jacobson (Eds.), *Medical speech-language pathology: A practitioner's guide* (pp. 467–496). New York, NY: Thieme.

Roberts, P. (2001). Aphasia assessment and treatment for bilingual and culturally diverse patients. In R. Chapey (Ed.), *Language intervention strategies in adult aphasia* (5th ed., pp. 208–232). Philadelphia, PA: Lippincott Williams & Wilkins.

Silberstein, P., Bittar, R. G., Boyl, R., Cook, R., Coyne, T., O'Sullivan, D., . . . Watson, P. (2009). Deep brain stimulation for Parkinson's disease: Australian referral guidelines. *Journal of Clinical Neuroscience, 16*, 1001–1008.

Thurman, D., Alverson, C., Dunn, K., Guerrero, J., & Sniezek, J. (1999). Traumatic brain injury in the United States: A public health perspective. *Journal of Head Trauma and Rehabilitation, 14*, 602–615.

Umbach, J. A., Adams, K. L., Gundersen, C. B., & Novitch, B. G. (2012). Functional neuromuscular junctions formed by embryonic stem cell-derived motor neurons. *PLoS ONE, 7*(5), e36049.

Wambaugh, J. L., Duffy, J. R., McNeil, M. R., Robin, D. A., & Rogers, M. A. (2006). Treatment guidelines for acquired apraxia of speech: Treatment descriptions and recommendations. *Journal of Medical Speech Language Pathology, 14*, 283–299.

Wambaugh, J. L., & Mauszycki, S. C. (2010). Application of the WHO ICF to management of acquired apraxia of speech. *Journal of Medical Speech-Language Pathology, 18*, 133–140

World Health Organization. (2001). *International classification of functioning, disability, and health*. Geneva, Switzerland: Author.

Wu, D. C., Boyd, A. S., & Wood, K. J. (2007). Embryonic stem cell transplantation: Potential applicability in cell replacement therapy and regenerative medicine. *Frontiers in Bioscience, 12*, 4525–4535.

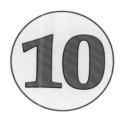

DYSPHAGIA

OBJECTIVES

After reading this chapter, the student should be able to:

■ Describe the basic anatomical and neuromuscular systems involved in swallowing.

■ Demonstrate understanding of bedside methods of dysphagia assessment.

■ Demonstrate understanding of instrumentation for the assessment and treatment of swallowing functions.

■ Demonstrate knowledge of swallowing disorders including their etiologies.

■ Describe current surgical techniques related to communicative and swallowing functions, and prosthetics.

■ Describe various nonsurgical techniques related to the management of dysphagia.

■ Describe multicultural considerations in the assessment and management of dysphagia.

INTRODUCTION

People swallow a thousand times or more each day. Swallowing begins at the lips and ends at the stomach. Swallowing is an activity that we tend to take for granted and perform easily. Yet the process of normal swallowing actually is a highly complex activity. Approximately 30 to 40 pairs of muscles, and at least six pairs of nerves, are involved in moving food from the lips to the stomach. To add to this complexity, these structures must perform in sequence with our breathing patterns to ensure the material being swallowed is directed toward the stomach rather than the lungs.

Among some disabled children and adults, there is a breakdown in coordination of swallowing. This breakdown may be due to the person's: (1) wakefulness or awareness (2) brain functioning, and/or (3) muscular strength. The medical term for swallowing difficulty is called **dysphagia** ("dis fay ja" or "dis fah ja"). Dysphagia is one of the newest specialty areas in the speech-language pathologist profession. Speech-language pathologists are called upon tens of thousands of times every day to evaluate swallowing in the estimated 18 million adults suffering from dysphagia in the United States and many millions more internationally. Dysphagia can severely affect an individual's quality of life and can also require a person to be dependent on others to be fed. Aside from these social issues, disordered swallowing may be life threatening. A person can run the risk of choking or having the airway blocked. Malnutrition, weight loss, and increased chances of dehydration are possible outcomes of prolonged periods of swallowing

---

FYI

Most people believe they chew their food thoroughly before swallowing, but this may not be the case. It is recommended that, on average, we should chew food between 20 and 30 times before swallowing. The more we chew, the more saliva we generate that helps break down food and facilitate the digestion process.

---

difficulties. Dysphagia also could pose a threat for respiratory infections resulting from food entering the lungs rather than the stomach. What is generally considered an automatic and even pleasurable experience can be one of discomfort and worry.

TERMINOLOGY AND DEFINITIONS

There are a variety of terms associated with normal and disordered swallowing. To begin, the formal term used to describe the act of normal swallowing is **deglutition**. We swallow for two reasons. The first reason is maintenance. This type of swallowing is used to remove the natural buildup of saliva in the oral cavity. **Maintenance** swallowing tends to occur subconsciously and happens even when we sleep. Maintenance swallowing also has been observed in infants prior to birth. Although, in most cases, this type of swallowing occurs automatically, we also can swallow deliberately whenever we feel like clearing our throats. The second reason we swallow is for **ingestion**. This type of swallowing is for the consumption of liquids and foods. Ingestive swallowing of **per oral** (p.o.) nutrition (i.e., food taken by mouth) requires that we are awake and cognizant of the presence of food or fluid in the mouth. Typically, the process of swallowing food involves chewing. The technical term for chewing is **mastication**. When we chew, the food inside the mouth is turned into a soft mass referred to as a **bolus**. During deglutition, the bolus moves through the tubes of the digestive system in waves of alternating contraction and

relaxation (i.e., snakelike movement) known as **peristalsis**.

The term dysphagia is a combination of the prefix *dys* (disordered) and the Greek word *phagein* (eat). Dysphagia can occur at locations anywhere from the lips to the stomach and is found in approximately 7% of the general population. Among people aged 50 years or older, the occurrence of dysphagia ranges anywhere from 15% to 30% and may be as high as 60% in acute hospital wards and nursing homes. The frequency of occurrence of dysphagia does not differ between females and males. A primary indicator of dysphagia is coughing moments after swallowing. This can lead to **aspiration**, which refers to the situation where food or liquid inadvertently enters the breathing airway (trachea) before, during, or after the swallow (Figure 10–1). Among individuals who experience a stroke, it is not uncommon for them to be susceptible to aspiration during the

---

FYI

We swallow during our sleep; however, much less so compared with when we are awake. On average, we swallow approximately once per hour.

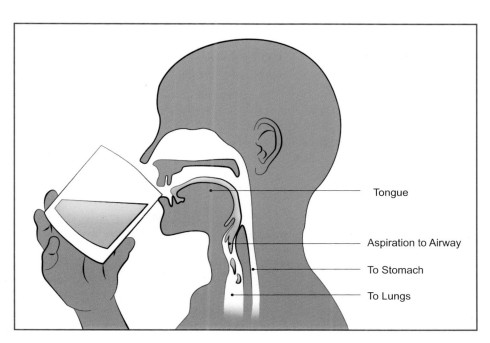

FIGURE 10–1. Illustration of aspiration.

Tongue

Aspiration to Airway

To Stomach

To Lungs

earliest days of recovery. A condition known as **reflux** is also indicative of dysphagia. Reflux is a backward flow of food or liquid. Esophageal reflux is a condition in which the stomach contents flow backward into the esophagus.

Because of the obvious anatomical and physiological processes underpin-ning swallowing behavior, it is impor-tant to be familiar with some of the pri-mary physical structures involved in swallowing. Most of the key structures were covered in Chapter 3. A summary of these structures and their function in regard to swallowing is provided in Table 10–1. A corresponding illustration

Table 10–1. Primary Anatomical Structures Involved in Swallowing	
Structure	*Description*
Oral Cavity	
Lips	Are responsible for sealing the oral cavity for preparation of swallowing.
Tongue	Is responsible for pushing food toward the hard palate and back toward the pharynx.
Teeth	Are required for mastication (chewing).
Saliva	A special digestive enzyme for softening and moistening food. Glands are located in cheeks, underside of tongue, and underside of mandible.
Nasal Cavity	
Velum	The soft palate muscles that raise during swallowing to close off the nasal cavity from the oral cavity.
Pharynx	
Muscles	A series of overlapping muscles in the throat cavity. The cavity extends from the back of the nasal cavity to the top of the larynx.
Epiglottis	A leaf-shaped cartilage that protects the vocal folds from collecting foreign matter and diverts the bolus around the airway.
Valleculae	The space between the base of the tongue and the epiglottis. The collection of residue in this space indicates a problem with tongue movement during swallowing.
Upper Esophageal Sphincter	A specialized muscle that separates the pharyngeal and esophageal cavities.
Trachea	
Cartilage	A series of cartilaginous rings that form the wind pipe. The trachea branches off from the base of the pharynx and leads to a series of smaller tubes composing the lungs
Esophagus	
Muscle	A long muscular tube that branches off from the pharynx and sits behind the trachea. This is the "food tube" that serves as the conduit to the stomach. The esophagus normally is collapsed and only opens during swallowing.

of the major structures used for swallowing and their anatomical location is provided in Figure 10–2.

From start to finish, normal swallowing is an almost instantaneous activity, taking around two minutes to accomplish. Although the action of swallowing is relatively quick and automatic, the process of moving liquid or food toward the stomach is extremely complicated. To conceptualize swallowing, it is useful to think of the process as occurring in a series of three sequential stages: (1) oral, (2) pharyngeal, and (3) esophageal. Each stage represents specific physiological activity in the progression of moving material from the mouth to the stomach. These three stages are illustrated in Figure 10–3.

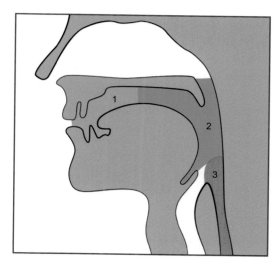

FIGURE 10–3. The three stages of swallowing, including the oral (transfer), pharyngeal (transport), and esophageal (entrance) stages.

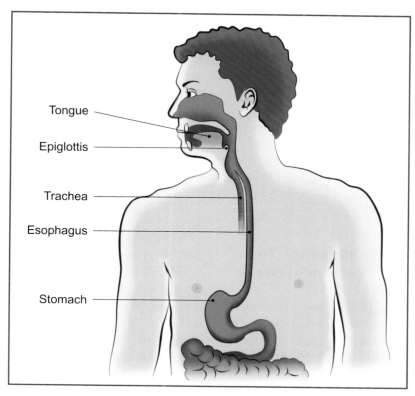

FIGURE 10–2. Swallowing anatomy.

Stage 1 of Swallowing: The Oral (Transfer) Stage

The **oral stage** begins when we first take food or drink into our mouths. Once material is placed in the mouth, the lips are sealed. The tongue then moves the material around the mouth for mastication. Saliva helps to soften and moisten food to create a bolus that is easy to swallow. This stage is one of preparation for swallowing by transferring the food or drink to the back of the mouth. We maintain normal nasal breathing during this stage.

Stage 2 of Swallowing: The Pharyngeal (Transport) Stage

The **pharyngeal stage** begins once the tongue transfers the food or liquid bolus to the back of the throat. Once the bolus reaches the back of the mouth, a reflex automatically occurs that transports the bolus through the pharynx. During this stage of the swallow, the nasal cavity is closed off from the oral cavity to prevent food from going through the nose. Muscles of the throat serve to shorten the pharynx and push the food toward the esophagus. The vocal folds close tightly and breathing stops to prevent food or liquid from entering the lungs.

Stage 3 of Swallowing: The Esophageal (Entrance) Stage

The **esophageal stage** begins when the bolus is directed away from the trachea and enters the esophagus (or gullet), which is the canal that carries food and liquid to the stomach. The esophagus is separated from the pharynx by a sphinc-ter muscle that relaxes and is pulled open by muscles of the throat. After the bolus exits the pharynx, the normally collapsed esophagus is pushed open by the propelling bolus. During this process of the swallow, peristalsis occurs to move the bolus through the esophagus into the stomach. Once the bolus is fully in the esophagus and the sphincter is again closed, the airway is reopened and normal breathing resumes.

HISTORIC ASPECTS OF DYSPHAGIA

To an outsider, a speech-language pathologist may not seem to be the most qualified individual to deal with swallowing difficulties. By the very nature of their professional title, a speech-language pathologist supposedly works exclusively with speech and language problems. Yet some speech-language pathologists have been indirectly treating aspects of dysphagia since the early 1930s. This early work was focused primarily on young children with oral-motor disorders such as cerebral palsy, as well as head and neck surgery patients. One of the core features in the educational curriculum of a speech-language pathologist student has always been knowledge of the anatomy and physiology of the head, neck, and respiratory system. This coursework, along with extensive clinical education with clients who have disordered function of the oral, pharyngeal, and laryngeal systems, made speech-language pathologists the prime candidates for assessing and treating dysphagia. Prior to the involvement by the speech-language pathologist profession, no other health

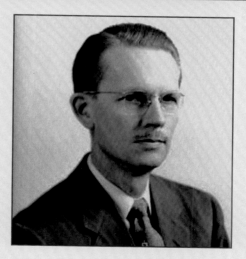

One of the pioneers of speech-language pathology, Dr. Grant Fairbanks (1910–1964) died by asphyxiation, as a result of choking on a piece of food that had lodged in his throat. Dr. Fairbanks died tragically while onboard an airplane in 1964 traveling from San Francisco to Chicago (see also Chapter 5).

he found that most speech-language pathologists tended to address only speech difficulties, leaving the swallowing difficulties to either go unaddressed or be dealt with by some other health profession (e.g., neurologist, otolaryngologist, nurse, physiotherapist, occupational therapist). Larsen believed that a patient who showed both speech and swallowing problems was the result of a similar nervous system disturbance. Therefore, by working on swallowing, it would be expected that improvements in speech production would follow. Although this was not found to be the case, Larsen is credited with establishing a range of therapeutic techniques to help individuals regain the ability to swallow. His approach to the evaluation, management, and treatment of swallowing difficulties was considered artistic and intuitive (Miller & Groher, 1993).

The next major advancement in dysphagia was made by **Jeri A. Logemann** who completed a PhD from the Department of Communication Disorders at Northwestern University, Illinois, in the early 1970s with particular emphasis in dysphagia (Figure 10–4). Logemann applied a more rigorous scientific methodology to assessing and treating dysphagia compared with Larsen by undertaking controlled examinations of swallowing physiology and treatment efficacy. Logemann also made major contributions in regard to outlining the essential educational and clinical training required of speech-language pathologists dealing with dysphagia. Education in dysphagia is now a standard component among all speech-language pathology university programs worldwide.

It is important for speech-language pathologists to recognize that due to the complex medical issues involved in

professions specifically included dysphagia as part of their scope of practice.

Two individuals from the United States are often given credit for advancing the profession in regard to helping people with swallowing problems. The first is **George L. Larsen**, who in the early 1960s developed the speech-language pathology clinical services program at the Seattle Veterans Administration Hospital. Because of Larsen's employment in a hospital setting, he was aware of a large number of people who experienced difficulties with both speech and swallowing. To his dismay,

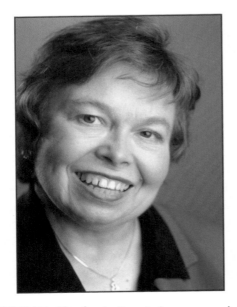

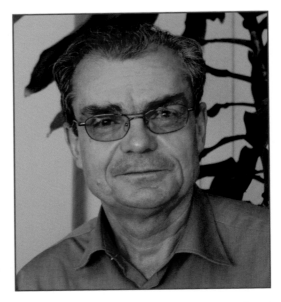

FIGURE 10–4. Jerilyn A. Logemann has made important clinical contributions to the field of dysphagia. Permission granted by J. Logemann.

FIGURE 10–5. Andre Jean has examined the role of the brainstem in normal and disordered swallowing. Permission granted by A. Jean.

management of the dysphagic patient, this area of clinical practice is by necessity and design of an interdisciplinary clinical field. Appropriate management includes input from a variety of health professionals, including but not limited to neurology, otolaryngology, radiology, and dietetics. Indeed substantial research that guides our understanding of swallowing comes from outside of speech language pathology. One such example involves the research of the French physiologist **Andre Jean** (Figure 10–5). Over the past 25 years, Professor Jean has been instrumental in defining the role of the brainstem in normal and disordered swallowing.

There has been a dramatic growth of involvement by speech-language pathologists in the field of dysphagia both in regard to service delivery and research. More than one-third of present-day speech-language pathologists deal with dysphagia as part of their annual caseload. For speech-language pathologists working in a health care setting, dysphagia can often exceed 80% of the total caseload. In 1986, a research journal entitled *Dysphagia* was created. This is an interdisciplinary journal dedicated exclusively to the many aspects of normal and disordered swallowing.

TYPES OF DYSPHAGIA

There are three generally agreed-on types of dysphagia: (1) oropharyngeal dysphagia, (2) esophageal dysphagia, and (3) functional dysphagia. The first two types are related to known anatomical or physiological difficulties with swallowing. The third type is a form of dysphagia with no known causal factors.

Oropharyngeal Dysphagia

Oropharyngeal dysphagia is the most common type of dysphagia. The anatomical description of this form of dysphagia indicates that the condition affects the transfer of liquid or food from the mouth and pharynx into the esophagus. This type of dysphagia results from abnormalities of muscles, nerves, or structures of the oral cavity and pharynx. Attempts to swallow food may be misdirected upward toward the nasal cavity. Many patients choke or cough when swallowing and may have food or fluids enter the trachea instead of the esophagus. This can allow harmful bacteria to grow in the lungs or bronchial tubes, resulting in a condition known as **aspiration pneumonia** (Figure 10–6). Patients often complain of difficulty chewing and swallowing both liquids and foods. They appear to have a hoarse or wet-sounding voice that may be accompanied by bad breath.

Esophageal Dysphagia

Esophageal dysphagia is less common than oropharyngeal dysphagia and arises during the latter stages of the swallowing sequence. Patients with esophageal dysphagia have difficulty passing a bolus of food from the esophagus to the stomach. Patients usually complain of swallowing only solid foods, as opposed to both solid foods and liquids. Their swallowing difficulty is due to either an obstruction or stricture (i.e., narrowing) of the esophagus or else problems with peristalsis (i.e., a motility problem). Patients report that it feels like food is stuck in the base of their

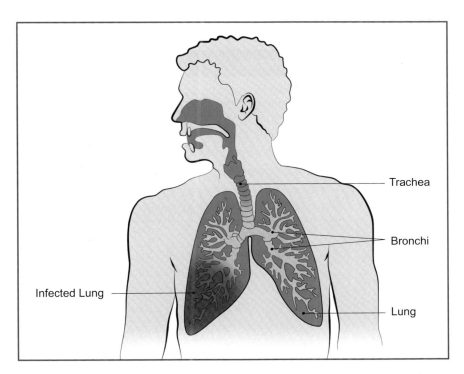

FIGURE 10–6. Illustration of lung infection that can result from aspiration.

throat or in the chest. Patients generally point to their neck as the primary region of the problem, indicating that the site is at or below this region.

Functional Dysphagia

The least frequently occurring type of dysphagia is known as **functional dysphagia**. This form of dysphagia is poorly understood, primarily because there is no identifiable anatomical cause. Examples of functional dysphagia include difficulty in swallowing pills and a condition known as **globus**, which is the sensation of having a lump in one's throat. The International Foundation for Gastrointestinal Disorders defines functional dysphagia as the sensation of solid and/or liquid foods sticking, lodging, or passing abnormally through the esophagus. Functional dysphagia is diagnosed based on symptoms present for at least three months and not associated with anatomical abnormalities such as reflux (Galmiche et al., 2006).

CAUSES OF DYSPHAGIA

Although there are three primary types of dysphagia, the causes of dysphagia are numerous. Swallowing requires healthy functioning of many different oral structures, muscles, and nerves, so a wide range of medical and even dental conditions can cause dysphagia. Dysphagia actually is a symptom of an underlying condition. A list of likely causes associated with the three types of dysphagia is provided in Table 10–2. A common cause of oropharyngeal dysphagia is a **cerebrovascular accident** (i.e., stroke). Dysphagia can result from strokes that affect the area of the brain

Table 10–2. Some Likely Causes of Various Types of Dysphagia

Type	Cause
Oropharyngeal dysphagia	Stroke
	Parkinson disease
	Muscular dystrophy
	Cleft palate
	Tumors of mouth or pharynx
	Drug- or radiation-induced dry mouth (xerostomia)
Esophageal dysphagia	Esophageal spasms
	Tumors of the esophagus
	Age-related changes of motor function of the esophagus
	Lack of involuntary esophageal peristalsis (achalasia)
	Pill-induced inflammation of the esophagus
	Esophagitis due to gastroesophageal reflux disease
	Narrowing of lower esophageal ring (Schatzki's ring)
Functional dysphagia	Stress

that controls motor actions, particularly the frontal lobes of the cerebrum. Strokes that affect the area of the brain that houses the **swallowing center** also can lead to dysphagia. The swallowing center is made up of a network of neurons in the brainstem that are responsible for the reflexive act of swallowing. About one-half of all stroke victims experience some degree of dysphagia during the earliest days following the stroke. In most cases, normal or near-normal swallowing function returns within one week poststroke, although dysphagia and aspiration will persist in some. Additionally, people with disorders of the nervous system, such as cerebral palsy or Parkinson disease, could experience oropharyngeal dysphagia. Traumatic brain injury and progressive neurologic diseases like multiple sclerosis and amyotrophic lateral sclerosis (motor neuron disease) may cause oropharyngeal dysphagia. Any number of cancers affecting the head and neck also can lead to oropharyngeal dysphagia. These various conditions may affect the coordination of the swallowing muscles or limit sensation in the mouth and throat. To compound matters, sometimes the preferred treatment for various types of cancers (e.g., radiation or drugs) has side effects that can cause dysphagia.

A frequent cause of esophageal dysphagia is a structural problem that creates a blockage within the esophagus. The blockage prevents food and liquid from moving toward the stomach. The most common structural problems are esophageal cancer, strictures, and narrowing of the lower region of the esophagus (called Schatzki's rings). An infection or irritation can also cause narrowing of the esophagus, resulting in a condition known as **esophagitis**. One type of irritation is **gastroesophageal**

FYI

The term **odynophagia** refers to the feeling of pain or a burning sensation upon swallowing. Such pain may be a symptom of a serious medical condition.

---

reflux disease. Gastroesophageal reflux disease (or acid reflux), is a condition in which acid, bile, and partially digested food in the stomach back up into the esophagus. Partially digested food contains a strong acid that can inflame and damage the lining of the esophagus. Many people think that heartburn (or acid indigestion) is a separate disease. It actually is one symptom of gastroesophageal reflux disease. Heartburn is an unpleasant burning sensation behind the breastbone that usually occurs after a meal.

The absence of a clear anatomical reason for the occurrence of functional dysphagia leads most experts to speculate that the cause of this condition is a combination of physiological and psychosocial problems (Galmiche et al., 2006). Anecdotal information has been reported that individuals who show functional dysphagia may show significantly higher instances of anxiety and depression compared with those who do not have this form of dysphagia (Clouse, Richter, Heading, Janssens, & Wilson, 1999).

Finally, dysphagia is not limited to adults. Young children can experience difficulties with swallowing. **Pediatric dysphagia** is not simply an adult problem on a smaller scale. As previously pointed out in Chapter 3, the anatomical configuration of a young child's vocal tract is quite different from a fully grown adult vocal tract. These developmental differences in pharyngeal and laryngeal anatomy also can influence the manner of swallowing in children compared with adults. Normal adult swallowing is a complicated process, but because the underlying swallowing anatomy is fully mature, the process of swallowing is quite stable. In children, ongoing physical growth and development of motor coordination create a situation whereby swallowing behavior changes "in step" with anatomical changes (Kramer & Eicher, 1993). In pediatric populations, dysphagia may be present in babies who are born prematurely, or who have genetic syndromes (e.g., Down syndrome) or maxillofacial deformities. Infants who are born with a cleft lip and palate are unable to suck properly, which complicates nursing and drinking from a regular baby bottle. Swallowing difficulties have been reported to occur in as many as 25% of all children, with greater prevalence in children with physical disabilities, medical illness, and prematurity (Manikam & Perman, 2000).

ASSESSMENT OF DYSPHAGIA

All of us at some time have experienced difficulty swallowing. Perhaps it was that time when you were taking a drink and someone made you laugh so hard that fluid went through your nose. Or perhaps you once choked on a piece of food. For most of us, these events are fleeting; however, for some individuals, swallowing difficulties occur more often. There are a number of symptoms that require evaluation for a possible swallowing problem. A list of some of the warning signs for dysphagia is provided in Table 10–3.

The procedures used for assessing the presence of dysphagia fall into two general categories: (1) clinical assessment and (2) instrumental assessment. **Clinical assessment** is an approach

Table 10–3. Some Warning Signs of Dysphagia

- Coughing
- Drooling
- Choking
- Food or fluid coming out of the nose
- Gurgling voice quality
- Wet-sounding breathing
- Spillage of food or liquid from the mouth
- Frequent throat clearing
- Low grade fever
- Progressively slower rate of food intake
- Difficulty initiating a swallow
- Pain upon swallowing
- Food or liquid left in the mouth after a swallow
- Difficulty manipulating food or liquid in the mouth
- Weight loss

commonly used for the initial screening of swallowing dysfunction, and as the term suggests, typically occurs while a patient is in a clinic setting. Sometimes this may involve assessing a patient sitting upright in a hospital bed. The approach is designed to determine a patient's cognitive abilities, language abilities, and readiness to eat or swallow (Sitoh, Lee, Phua, Lieu, & Chan, 2000). Clinical assessments have been criticized for being too general and lacking in necessary precision to detect pharyngeal pathophysiology or moments of aspiration. Yet most speech-language pathologists would agree there is a need for a simple bedside assessment that would at least identify patients who are "at risk" for aspiration. Detection of dysphagia at a patient's beside mandates the speech-language pathologist to be highly suspicious of swallowing difficulties, and have a clear understanding of the mechanisms of swallowing. An important feature of a bedside assessment requires the patient to ingest fluids and foods of different textures when seated in an upright position. While the patient is swallowing, the speech-language pathologist observes whether: (1) swallowing occurred in a natural, automatic fashion, (2) there was drooling during the swallow, (3) the patient coughed during swallowing, and (4) the patient's voice sounded hoarse. Based on the bedside swallowing assessment, a patient would be diagnosed by the speech-language pathologist to have *possible* dysphagia if any one of these four observations were present.

Another rather novel bedside approach to evaluating normal swallowing involves a procedure known as **cervical** (neck) **auscultation**. The process of auscultation is the diagnostic listening of sounds. Physicians perform this diagnostic test frequently by using a stethoscope to listen to heart and lung sounds. In the case of cervical auscultation, a stethoscope is placed in the region of the neck, and the patient is asked to swallow. Based on listening to the swallow, the speech-language pathologist makes a perceptual judgment as to the functioning of the swallow based on the perceived "crispness" of the signal. Some experts believe there is a distinct acoustic pattern of normal swallowing that can be used as a backdrop to evaluate disordered swallowing (Huckabee, Coombe, & Robb, 2005); however, application of cervical auscultation as a standard clinical measure has not received widespread support.

Use of instrumentation to determine the existence of dysphagia provides a more in-depth form of assessment compared with the bedside approach. In most cases, the instruments employed by the speech-language pathologist allow for visualization of the different stages of swallowing. Although this may seem the logical choice for determining the existence of swallowing difficulties, there are drawbacks associated with the various instrumental techniques. Some of the most common instrumental assessment techniques are: (1) videofluoroscopic swallowing study, (2) fiberoptic endoscopic evaluation of swallowing, (3) ultrasound, and (4) electromyography.

Videofluoroscopic Swallowing Study

The **videofluoroscopic swallowing study** approach to determining the existence of dysphagia involves an imaging technique known as **videofluoroscopy**. Fluoroscopy is a procedure that allows for a dynamic x-ray to be taken of a person's bodily organs as they are actually moving. Because swallowing is a form of bodily movement, fluoroscopy is amenable to the visualization of swallowing. The most common anatomical view is a cross-section (side view) of the entire vocal tract to allow for examination of swallowing from start to finish. A typical fluoroscopic image of the vocal tract is shown in Figure 10–7. The videofluoroscopic swallowing study procedure is usually completed under the direction of a speech-language pathologist, while working with a radiologist. The radiologist operates the videofluoroscopy equipment and, along with the speech-language pathologist, provides an interpretation of the radiographic images. To visualize swallowing behavior, the patient is required to swallow a radiopaque substance known as **barium**, which can easily be detected using an x-ray. As the patient swallows the barium substance, the movements of the swallow are videorecorded for later analysis. This x-ray helps the speech-language pathologist determine what types of food and drink are safe to swallow and what type of dysphagia therapy might be appropriate. A primary drawback with the videofluoroscopic swallowing study approach is that the x-ray beams directed into the body for visualization expose the patient to mild levels of radiation. Such radiation is cumulative on the body and is not dissipated. Therefore, it is advisable to perform this procedure as infrequently as possible. The use of the videofluoroscopic swallowing study has proven to be an effective instrumental approach to evaluating the swallowing function and will likely continue to be performed regularly for years to come.

Fiberoptic Endoscopic Evaluation of Swallowing

Although use of the videofluoroscopic swallowing study is widely considered the "gold standard" examination for oral and pharyngeal dysphagia, another instrumental approach known as **fiberoptic endoscopic evaluation of swallowing (FEES)** is gaining widespread appeal. The fiberoptic endoscopic evaluation of swallowing procedure involves use of a flexible endoscope to visualize the pharyngeal and laryngeal structures involved in swallowing. An endoscope is a thin, flexible tube that contains both a light source and a camera lens that provides an image on a computer monitor. This tube can be inserted into bodily orifices that are typically difficult to visually examine (stomach, larynx, ear canal), thus providing an opportunity to assess both structure and function. Langmore, Schatz, and Olsen (1988) were the first group of researchers to describe the fiberoptic endoscopic evaluation of swallowing technique for evaluating oropharyngeal dysphagia. Fiberoptic endoscopic evaluation of swallowing originally was conceived to be used as a backup, or secondary procedure, performed only when the videofluoroscopic swallowing study was not available or convenient. For example, use of the videofluoroscopic swallowing study is not feasible for patients in an intensive care unit, or in a nursing home, or for patients who are extremely obese. The fiberoptic endoscopic evaluation of swallowing procedure involves the insertion of a flexible endoscope into the nose to visualize the pharynx and larynx immediately before and after eating and drinking foods and liquids of different consistencies (Figure 10–8).

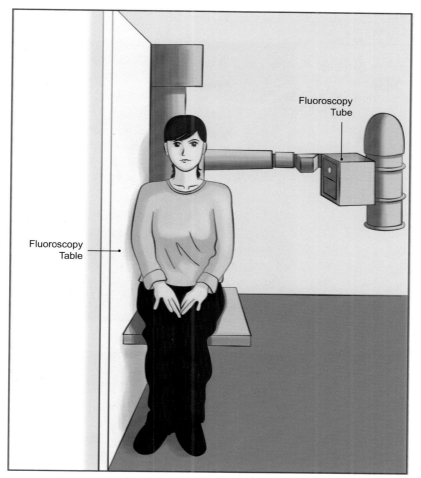

A

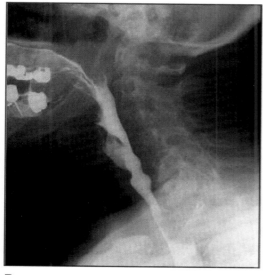

B

FIGURE 10–7. Fluoroscopic examination of swallowing. **A**. The general procedures of the examination are shown. **B**. The resultant image of the vocal tract is shown. The white substance in the vocal tract is a radiopaque substance known as barium.

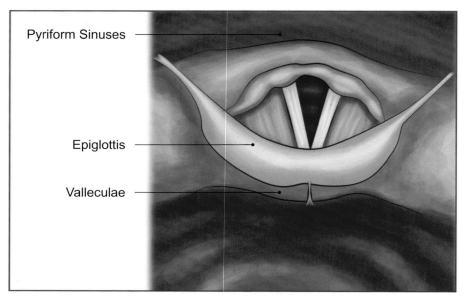

Pyriform Sinuses

Epiglottis

Valleculae

A

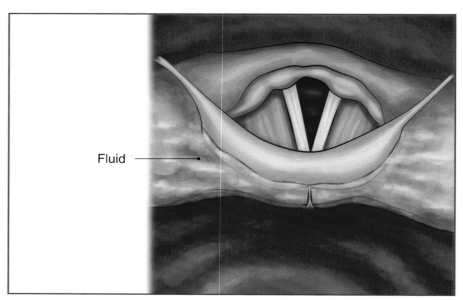

Fluid

B

FIGURE 10–8. View of pharyngeal area during a fiberoptic endoscopic examination of swallowing procedure. **A**. A normal swallow. **B**. A disordered swallow as indicated by pooling of fluid in the valleculae.

Depending on the laws established for various countries (and states), the approach can be done exclusively by the speech-language pathologist or may require additional medical personnel. During the actual swallow, the video image on the computer monitor becomes momentarily obliterated (i.e., a whiteout). The image is restored upon completion of the swallow. A telltale sign of dysphagia is the observation of any pooling of fluid that accumulates in the valleculae or piriform sinuses in the pharynx either before or after the swallow. Although the view provided by fiberoptic endoscopic evaluation of swallowing is not as dynamic as the videofluoroscopic swallowing study, it is far less damaging to the patient. The patient does not need to ingest barium, but rather food (milk, pudding) that is dyed either blue or green to make for better visualization. Fiberoptic endoscopic evaluation of swallowing has the advantage of being free from radiation, so patients undergoing this test can be examined for longer time intervals or at repeated intervals. A disadvantage of the fiberoptic endoscopic evaluation of swallowing is that aspiration may not be noted as reliably as the videofluoroscopic swallowing study, as the whiteout phenomenon at the height of the swallowing is often when aspiration occurs.

Ultrasound

Ultrasound has been used to image the human body for at least 50 years. It is one of the most widely used diagnostic tools in modern medicine. Health care professionals use ultrasound to view the heart, blood vessels, kidneys, liver, and other organs. Ultrasound is commonly used during pregnancy to examine the developing fetus (see also Chapter 11). During an ultrasound test, a special technician or doctor moves a device called a transducer over a specific body part. The transducer sends out high-frequency sound waves, which bounce off the tissues inside the body, and the same transducer captures the sound waves that bounce back. These sound waves are then translated and assembled into a visual image on a computer monitor. This same technology can be used to track tongue movement during a swallow. The procedure works by holding a transducer under the patient's chin and high-frequency sound waves travel through the tissues in the neck and are reflected off the tongue to create an image. Because the approach is exclusive to the tongue's role in swallowing, only the oral stage of swallowing can be evaluated; however, the approach is far less invasive than the videofluoroscopic swallowing study and the fiberoptic endoscopic evaluation of swallowing approaches. An example of the ultrasound approach to evaluating swallowing is shown in Figure 10–9.

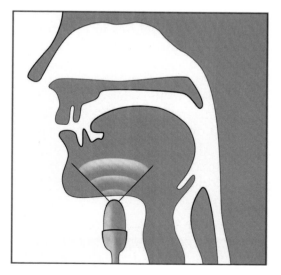

FIGURE 10–9. Illustration of an ultrasound examination of the tongue during the oral stage of swallowing.

Electromyography

When a muscle is used (i.e., contracts), it generates a very small electrical signal, which can be detected with an antenna (i.e., an electrode). This instrumental procedure is known as **electromyography**. When a very thin wire electrode is inserted directly into a muscle, the activity of the muscle can be viewed and recorded. There also are less invasive disc electrodes that can simply be taped to the surface of the skin. In regard to swallowing, a variety of muscles in the region of the mouth, larynx, and pharynx can be examined using the electromyography approach. A muscle that is not working correctly will emit an electrical signal that is different from a normal functioning muscle. In an extreme case where a muscle is paralyzed, it is possible that no electrical activity would be emitted. Examples of electromyography signals found in normal and disordered swallowing are presented in Figure 10–10. A drawback with this approach is that the procedure can be highly invasive, requiring insertion of an electrode directly into the muscle. The use of a surface electrode may also be problematic because these electrodes are attached to the surface of the skin, and the electromyography signal can be obscured due to multiple muscles overlapping. This form of instrumental swallowing assessment is not routinely used in a clinical setting. Rather, it is used more often in research settings (Perlman, 1993).

TREATMENT OF DYSPHAGIA

Successful management of dysphagia requires a team of various health specialists such as speech-language pathologists, occupational and physical therapists, otolaryngologists, neurologists, gastroenterologists, as well as a dieticians. Once the cause of the dysphagia is found, there are a number of treatment approaches to consider, including: (1) swallowing therapy, (2) lifestyle changes, (3) drugs, and (4) surgery.

Swallowing Therapy

The speech-language pathologist could be called on to test the person's ability to eat and drink and may teach the person new ways to swallow. The therapy program established for the patient is tailored to suit her or his medical condition. Treatment may involve rehabilitation exercises to strengthen weak oral and pharyngeal muscles or to improve coordination of the overall swallowing musculature. For others, treatment may involve learning compensatory swallowing strategies. For example, some people might have to eat and drink with their head turned to one side or looking straight ahead. Preparing food in a certain way or avoiding certain foods can help other people. Some fluids that might normally be easily aspirated can be altered by adding a thickening agent.

FYI

Acid reflux is a warning sign of dysphagia. In addition, acid reflux can serve to impair our speaking voice. In extreme cases of reflux, acidic juices may back up from the stomach and irritate the laryngeal mechanism, including the vocal folds.

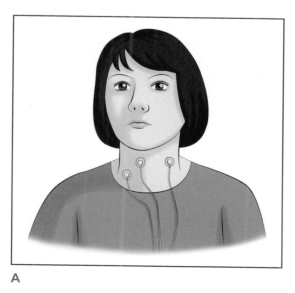

A

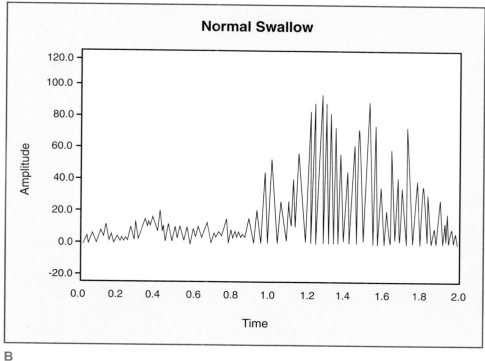

B

FIGURE 10–10. **A.** An illustration showing surface electrode placement for electromyographic recording of swallowing. **B.** An idealized electromyographic recording reflecting normal muscle functioning during a swallow. *continues*

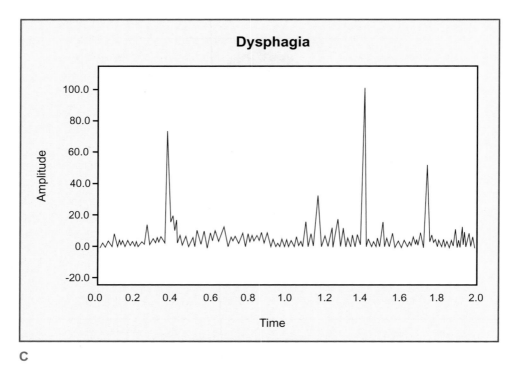

C

FIGURE 10–10. *continued* **C.** An impaired muscle functioning during a swallow.

The patient may be discouraged from swallowing hot or cold items if they are particularly sensitive to reflux.

Lifestyle Changes

As noted earlier, acid reflux is a dysphagic condition that can have serious consequences on health and quality of life. There are a number of steps people can take to greatly reduce the likelihood of reflux disease. These steps involve changes in lifestyle such as increased exercise and diet modification. Some common recommendations include:

- Eat smaller, more frequent meals
- Eat a bland diet
- Avoid alcohol and caffeine
- Lose weight
- Reduce stress

- Avoid eating three hours before bedtime
- Slightly elevate your head while sleeping

Drugs

The prescription of drugs to treat dysphagia typically has been dictated on the basis of the particular medical condition contributing to the disorder. Because of the wide range of causes that could contribute to dysphagia, there presently is no "magic pill" that can cure dysphagia. In many cases, drugs serve to relieve some of the symptoms of dysphagia, primarily those associated with esophageal dysphagia. The types of medications found to be useful include over-the-counter antacids that are taken before or after eating. There also are prescription medications known as proton-pump inhibitors, which substantially reduce acid production in the stomach.

Surgery

A typical surgical treatment of dysphagia involves muscle incisions to release muscle tension or to stretch/dilate an unusually narrow stricture. For some, however, consuming foods and liquids by mouth may not be possible in the immediate future. These individuals must use other methods to nourish their bodies. Usually, this involves surgical intervention to create a new feeding system, such as a **feeding tube**, that bypasses the part of the swallowing mechanism that is not working normally. It is common to have a feeding tube inserted during the early stages of severe dysphagia to reduce the risk of aspiration pneumonia. The tube also helps ensure that the person's nutrition and hydration is adequate. These tubes can be easily removed if and/or when the dysphagia diminishes. Two main types of feeding tubes are used: (1) parenteral tubes and (2) enteral tubes.

A **parenteral tube** (or IV tube) is administered through either a central or peripheral heart vein (Figure 10–11). The tube is essentially a catheter that

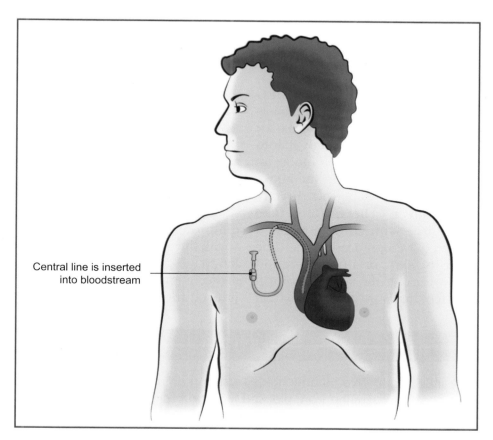

Central line is inserted into bloodstream

FIGURE 10–11. Parenteral tube—nutrients are delivered directly into the bloodstream for patients who are unable to swallow.

provides micronutrients directly into the bloodstream. It is only appropriate for individuals whose stomach and intestines are not working properly. The tube allows for the digestive tract to heal after surgery to the stomach or bowel and is kept in place with a stitch. Use of a parenteral tube typically is a very costly surgical procedure.

Enteral tubes involve providing nutrition directly into the stomach or small intestine. There are two general types of enteral tubes: (1) nasogastric and (2) gastrostomy. A **nasogastric tube** (or NG tube) is used on a short-term basis and entails passing a tube through the nose, pharynx, and esophagus directly into the stomach. Once the tube is correctly positioned, it is taped to the patient's nose or cheek to keep it in place. Food passes through the tube into the stomach.

A **gastronomy tube** (or percutaneous endoscopic gastrostomy—PEG tube) is used on a longer term basis or for indefinite time periods. Like an NG tube, food passes through it into the stomach, but unlike an NG tube, an external opening is made in the abdomen, and the tube is placed directly into the stomach. The feeding tube is held in place with either a stitch, a small inflated balloon around the tube just under the skin, or a flange around the tube just under the skin. This form of enteral feeding is more invasive than NG tubes. Examples of the two types of enteral feeding tubes are shown in Figure 10–12.

CULTURAL CONSIDERATIONS AND DYSPHAGIA

The speech-language pathologist who works with patients who have dysphagia may encounter a unique set of social and cultural issues that need to be considered as part of the overall treatment plan. Riquelme (2007) has identified four particular factors that, if not considered, may hinder speech-language pathologists' effectiveness in treating dysphagia. These factors include: (1) language barriers, (2) physical space, (3) ageism, and (4) food and nutrition.

Language Barriers

Based on the introductory material presented in this chapter, it is evident that a large and unique vocabulary is used when dealing with the disorder of dysphagia. These terms are, in many cases, quite foreign even for someone who may speak the same language as the speech-language pathologist, so speaking the same language may not ensure there is a cultural connection between the

---

FYI

The Heimlich maneuver is a technique used in emergency situations to prevent suffocation resulting from blocked food or foreign matter. The approach involves placing your arms around the choking individual (from behind) and delivering a series of five thrusts into the abdomen to dislodge the blockage. The maneuver was developed by Dr. Henry Heimlich in 1974.

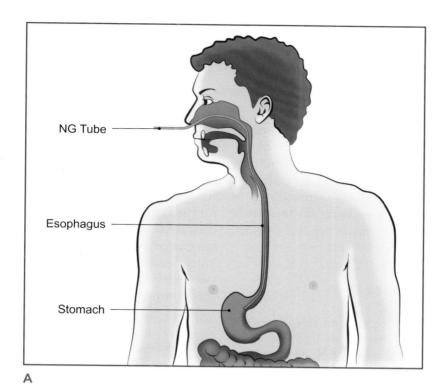

A

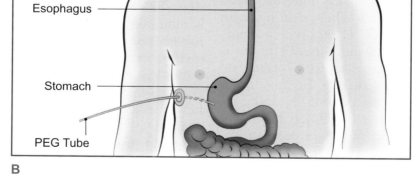

B

FIGURE 10–12. Examples of enteral tubes for patients to consume food and liquid if unable to swallow. **A.** A nasogastric (NG) tube, gastronomy tube. **B.** A percutaneous endoscopic gastrostomy.

clinician and client. In cases where the client speaks English as a second language, the speech-language pathologist may need to use an interpreter to communicate with the patient, and if so, great care should be taken in monitoring how the translated information is presented. Sensitivity to a patient's knowledge of medical terminology is important. Not everyone understands terms such as *no foods per oral/mouth, aspiration,* or *reflux.*

Physical Space

One aspect of assessing and treating dysphagia that is not found in most areas of speech-language pathology is the literal hands-on approach to assisting the patient. Any sort of touching used by the speech-language pathologist needs to be clarified with the patient beforehand. There may be times when adjusting the patient's posture or palpating the patient's throat during swallowing could be inappropriate. The speech-language pathologist should not assume the patient understands all of the procedures involved in an examination and subsequent treatment. In addition to matters concerning physical proximity, the clinical setting may also need to be considered when dealing with dysphagia. Lyon (1997) recommends that working in the patient's home is the best environment for working on dysphagia because it is the most natural setting for the patient. By doing so, there is a greater likelihood of patient compliance and carryover of treatment recommendations.

Ageism

In most cases, the dysphagic patient is elderly, and the speech-language pathol-

ogist is not. The age difference between client and clinician can impact overall interactions and patient compliance, both of which are critical to effective treatment outcomes (Riquelme, 2007). For many ethnic groups, elderly people are treated with great overt respect, and these individuals hold high social status within the immediate and extended family. This needs to be acknowledged during clinical interactions. The speech-language pathologist-patient relationship needs to be equalized or at least balanced to effectively provide culturally competent care.

Food and Nutrition

Issues concerning food and nutrition for the dysphagic patient can be particularly challenging in a multicultural population. Eating a meal with others is an enjoyable and highly social activity, and in some cultures, eating implies a sense of community. The U.S. holiday of Thanksgiving is just one example of how food can be linked to culture. If the patient with dysphagia has difficulty partaking in food consumption, yet his or her culture places high importance on food, steps need to be taken to ensure that a balance between food and culture is maintained. When selecting types of foods, the speech-language pathologist may encounter difficulty with the patient due to their prior history and culture of eating. Therefore, it is important to seek input from a nutritionist. For example, when establishing a diet that does not recommend solid foods (due to increased risk of aspiration), some patients may report they "are not able to do without fish." So when selecting specific foods, it is important to provide a patient with choices that reflect cultural preferences. For instance, the choice of pureed plantains versus potatoes may be quite important to a Latino patient who normally does not have potatoes in his or her diet (Riquelme, 2007).

CURRENT RESEARCH IN DYSPHAGIA

Scientists are conducting research that is designed to improve the ability of physicians and speech-language pathologists to evaluate and treat swallowing disorders. Much of this research focuses on the various stages of the swallowing process. Research involves examining people of all ages, including those who do not have dysphagia. Some of the current areas of rehabilitation research being explored are: (1) transcranial magnetic stimulation, (2) effortful swallowing, and (3) neural plasticity.

Transcranial Magnetic Stimulation

Transcranial magnetic stimulation is a noninvasive method of stimulating regions in the brain by either depolarizing or hyperpolarizing neurons. Transcranial magnetic stimulation involves applying a weak current in the form of electromagnetic pulses over specific regions of the head (brain) thought to be involved in particular motor movements. The device is now being used in research related to disordered swallowing. Preliminary results would appear to indicate that application of transcranial magnetic stimulation can help to improve the motor function/coordination of swallowing in individuals with Parkinson disease, brain injury, and stroke (Kim, Chun, Kim, & Lee, 2011).

Effortful Swallowing

This particular exercise of **effortful swallowing** is exactly what the name implies—to swallow hard (i.e., with effort). The idea behind this approach is that the best practice for impaired swallowing is to practice swallowing. By doing so in an effortful fashion, it is possible that more motor neurons are called upon, which can serve to strengthen the swallow. Recent research has shown that effortful swallowing specifically modifies the hyoid bone movement and increases the activation of muscles under the chin (submental muscle group), and these movements are believed to be especially important for swallowing (Park, Kim, Oh, & Lee, 2012)

Neural Plasticity

Dysphagia rehabilitation historically has focused on teaching the patient alternative ways of swallowing to prevent aspiration and improve swallowing efficiency. The patient also is provided with strengthening exercises to improve overall swallowing behavior. However, there is little documented evidence as to the best approach (or exercises) to improve swallowing. Recently, there has been research exploring the role of **neural plasticity** and dysphagia (Robbins et al., 2008). Neural plasticity refers to the ability of the brain and/or certain parts of the nervous system to change in order to adapt to new conditions, such as an injury (see also Chapter 9). In many ways, the rehabilitative techniques used by physiotherapists rely heavily on the notion of neural plasticity. These therapists will not simply tell a stroke patient to stand up and walk—they first work on strengthening muscles of interest and discrete movements until patients can stand and take a few steps. They start with the components of a movement and then ultimately train the movement of interest, which in this case would be walking. By working on discrete physical movements, the therapist is working to strengthen the overall neuromuscular patterns associated with walking. The same logic is now being applied to the treatment of dysphagia. By starting with the first stage of the swallowing process, the patient is taught to consciously move toward task-specific exercises and more challenging levels of swallowing (Burkhead, Sapienza, & Rosenbek, 2007). As research progresses in this area, the most optimum approaches to treating dysphagia may be discovered.

DYSPHAGIA ON THE WORLD WIDE WEB

Listed below are websites that provide further information on the topic of dysphagia. At the time of publication, each website was freely accessible.

Swallowing Videos

http://www.swallowingdisorderfoundation.com/swallow-a-documentary/

http://www.nlm.nih.gov/medlineplus/ency/anatomyvideos/000126.htm

Dysphagia Online
http://www.dysphagiaonline.com

Dysphagia Resource Center
http://dysphagia.com/

Oropharyngeal Dysphagia Video
http://www.nature.com/gimo/contents/pt1/fig_tab/gimo82_V1.html

The Voice and Swallowing Center Video
http://www.entandallergy.com/vas/galleries/swallowing_gallery

STUDY QUESTIONS

1. What are the primary anatomical structures involved in swallowing, and how are they involved in the three stages of swallowing?
2. List and describe the three types of dysphagia.
3. What are some of the likely causes of dysphagia?
4. What are the four approaches to assessing dysphagia?
5. What are the four approaches to treating dysphagia?

REFERENCES

Burkhead, L., Sapienza, C., & Rosenbek, J. (2007). Strength-training exercise in dysphagia rehabilitation: Principles, procedures, and directions for future research. *Dysphagia, 22*, 251–265.

Clouse, R., Richter, J., Heading, R., Janssens, J., & Wilson, J. (1999). Functional esophageal disorders. *Gut, 45*(Suppl.), II31–II36.

Galmiche, J., Clouse, R., Balint, A., Cook, I., Kahrilas, P., Paterson, W., & Smout, A. (2006). Functional esophageal disorders. *Gastroenterology, 130*, 1459–1465.

Huckabee, M. L., Coombe, T., & Robb, M. (2005). Repeatability of the acoustic swallowing pattern in normal adults. *Journal of Medical Speech-Language Pathology, 13*, 213–221.

Kim, L., Chun, M., Kim, B., & Lee, S. (2011). Effect of repetitive transcranial magnetic stimulation on patients with brain injury and dysphagia. *Annals of Rehabilitation Medicine, 35,* 765–771.

Kramer, S., & Eicher, P. (1993). The evaluation of pediatric feeding abnormalities. *Dysphagia, 8,* 215–224.

Langmore, S. E., Schatz, K., & Olsen, N. (1988). Fiberoptic endoscopic examination of swallowing safety: A new procedure. *Dysphagia, 2,* 216–219.

Lyon, J. (1997). Optimizing communication and participation in life for aphasic adults and their prime care givers. In G. Wallace (Ed.), *Multicultural neurogenics* (pp. 137–159). San Antonio, TX: Communication Skill Builders.

Manikam, R., & Perman, J. A. (2000). Pediatric feeding disorders. *Journal of Clinical Gastroenterology, 30,* 34–46.

Miller, R., & Groher, M. (1993). Speech-language pathology and dysphagia: A brief historical perspective. *Dysphagia, 8,* 180–184.

Park, J., Kim, Y., Oh, J., & Lee, H. (2012).

Effortful swallowing training combined with electrical stimulation in post-stroke dysphagia: A randomized controlled study. *Dysphagia, 27,* 521–527.

Perlman, A. (1993). Electromyography and the study of oropharyngeal swallowing. *Dysphagia, 8,* 351–355.

Riquelme, L. (2007). The role of cultural competence in providing services to persons with dysphagia. *Topics in Geriatric Rehabilitation, 23,* 228–239.

Robbins, J., Butler, S., Daniels, S., Gross, R., Langmore, S., Lazarus, C. L., . . . Rosenbek, J. (2008). Swallowing and dysphagia rehabilitation: Translating principles of neural plasticity into clinically oriented evidence. *Journal of Speech, Language, and Hearing Research, 51,* S276–S300.

Sitoh, Y., Lee, A., Phua, S., Lieu, P., & Chan, S. (2000). Bedside assessment of swallowing: A useful screening tool for dysphagia in an acute geriatric ward. *Singapore Medical Journal, 41,* 376–381.

GENETICS AND SYNDROMES

OBJECTIVES

After reading this chapter, the student should be able to demonstrate:

- Knowledge of the biological aspects of genetics that impact the process of normal human development.

- Knowledge of the terminology pertaining to genetics.

- Understanding of the historical aspects of genetics.

- Knowledge of various genetic and chromosomal syndromes, and the respective impacts on various aspects of hearing and speech-language development.

- Knowledge related to genetic counseling and genetic testing.

- Knowledge of various forms of treatment for genetic conditions.

- Understanding of the relationship between ethnicity and genetic disorders.

INTRODUCTION

Genetics refers to "life" or the "beginning." The field of human genetics is concerned with inheritance of traits. We often see family traits in various generations of family, such as facial features or body shape and size. By closely studying these traits, particularly those that may impact normal healthy functioning, we are able to answer questions about human nature, understand various diseases, and develop effective treatments for diseases. Aside from disorders resulting from physical injury, most communication disorders are genetically based. Many functional (or idiopathic) communication disorders are thought to have some form of genetic basis. Most hearing impairments have a genetic origin, and approximately 50% of all cases of newborn deafness are due to faulty genetics. It is important for audiologists and speech-language pathologists to understand the rules of inheritance and the means of preventing genetic disorders (Gerber, 1990).

A **syndrome** refers to a distinct group of symptoms that together are characteristic of a specific disorder or disease. For example, the common cold is a familiar syndrome, having symptoms such as a runny nose, cough, and fever (Gerber, 1990). A wide range of syndromes have a communication disorder as a prevailing symptom. These syndromes are linked to a genetic abnormality. Although speech-language pathologists and audiologists are not qualified to render a genetic diagnosis, they are required to diagnose the type of speech problem or exact nature of hearing loss. Therefore, these professionals need to be aware of the manner in which various genetic conditions can affect features of speech and hearing. The purpose of this chapter is to provide an introduction to the field of genetics and the influence of genetic-based syndromes on communication disorders. There is a long list of syndromes showing speech, language, hearing, and cognitive impairments, some of which are quite rare. The focus of this chapter is on a selective few of syndromes that an audiologist or speech-language pathologist may encounter during their professional careers.

TERMINOLOGY AND DEFINITIONS

Prior to presenting features of various syndromes, it is necessary to provide a refresher on the terms and concepts related to human genetics. Life begins with a **cell**, which is the smallest unit of living matter. The human body comprises 100 trillion cells in many shapes and sizes. Inside the body of the cell sits the **nucleus**, which is a vast storehouse of biochemical information. Within the nucleus reside **chromosomes**. The term chromosome means "colored body from *chroma* (meaning color) and *soma* (meaning body)." The term originated from the observation by the German anatomist, **Wilhelm Waldeyer** (1836–1921) who in 1888, found that the material composing chromosomes could be observed in clear detail following staining for microscopic examination (Figure 11–1). Chromosomes are found in every cell of the body except for red blood cells, which do not contain a nucleus. Red blood cells are specially adapted to carry oxygen around the body. Each chromosome contains two very long coiled strings of

DNA (deoxyribonucleic acid). Genes are located on these DNA strings. They are the functional units of heredity that occupy a very specific place on a chromosome and have two functions: (1) they contain the basic set of instructions for putting together an organism and (2) they regulate the function, growth, and development of an organism after birth. Genes carry information for making all the proteins required by all organisms. These proteins determine, among other things, how the organism looks, how well its body metabolizes food or fights infection, and sometimes even how it behaves. There are approximately 20,000 genes distributed among the chromosomes of the human body. Amazingly, only 2% of the DNA string contains genes. The remaining 98% of the material composing the string was once referred to as "junk DNA" because it appeared to consist of meaningless sequences. However, research is slowly unraveling the function of this remaining DNA. The basic genetic template of a cell is shown in Figure 11–2.

Normal human cells contain 46 chromosomes that exist in 23 pairs. Not all species have the same number of chromosomes. For example, cats have 38 chromosomes and fish have 78 chromosomes. Among the 46 chromosomes found in humans, 23 chromosomes are received from each parent. The number assigned to the first 22 pairs is related to chromosome length. Chromosome pair 1 is longest and contains the most genetic material. Chromosome pair 22 is the shortest. Chromosome 23 designates sex. Among females, the 23rd chromosome pairing is known as XX. The male body contains two types of sex

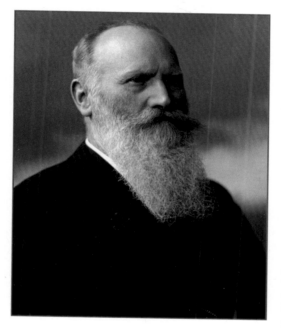

FIGURE 11–1. Wilhelm Waldeyer, German anatomist who discovered chromosomes.

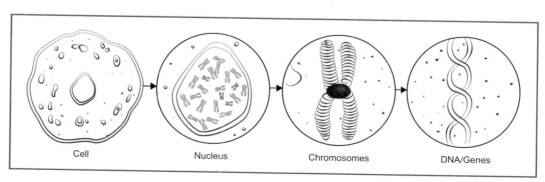

Cell Nucleus Chromosomes DNA/Genes

FIGURE 11–2. Genetic template of a cell.

chromosomes known as XY. The Y chromosome of the 23rd chromosome, although designating the male sex, is also found to contain the least amount of genetic material across the entire set of 46 chromosomes. Males produce both X- and Y-bearing sperm. Sex is determined by the father, depending on whether an X-bearing sperm or Y-bearing sperm joins with the female X chromosome. When the egg and sperm join at the time of conception, they form the first cell of the baby.

Each chromosome consists of two strands that resemble an "X" in structural appearance. The point at which the two strands cross is called the **centromere**. An individual chromosome can be further described with regard to the location of the centromere. A **metacentric chromosome** has a centromere in the approximate center, a **submetacentric chromosome** has a centromere that is slightly off center, and an **acrocentric chromosome** has a centromere that is near the tip of the chromosome. The top two arms of each chromosome are called the short arms or the p-arms. The letter "p" is in reference to the word *petite*, which is the French word for small. The

---

FYI

The number of chromosomes varies considerably across living organisms. Among animals, the mosquito is low on the list with 6 in total, whereas the hermit crab tops in at 254. Among plants, hawkweed has 8 chromosomes per cell and ferns have 1,200 chromosomes.

---

lower two arms are called the long arms or q-arms. The letter "q" is in reference to the word *queue*, which is the word meaning a long line of people. Examples of various chromosome shapes are displayed in Figure 11–3.

The entire DNA of an organism, including its genes, is called the **genome**. Knowledge about the effects of DNA variations among individuals can lead to new ways to diagnose, treat, and even prevent thousands of genetic disorders. Begun formally in 1990, the **Human Genome Project** was a 13-year effort coordinated by the U.S. Department of Energy and the National Institutes of Health. Additional contributions

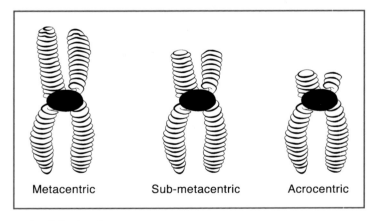

| Metacentric | Sub-metacentric | Acrocentric |

FIGURE 11–3. The various shapes of chromosomes.

to the Human Genome Project came from China, England, France, Germany, and Japan. The international effort to sequence the 3 billion DNA letters in the human genome is considered by many to have been the most ambitious scientific undertaking of all time, even compared with splitting the atom or landing on the moon. The project was expected to take 15 years to complete, but rapid technological advances pushed forward the completion date to 2003. The goal of the project was to identify all of the genes in human DNA. Originally, it was assumed the human body consisted of 60,000 to 100,000 genes. It was discovered that humans are made up of approximately 20,000 genes. In the years since completion of the Human Genome Project, the human genome database has enabled identification of a number of genes that are associated with disease. As a result, more objective and accurate diagnoses are being made for various genetic conditions even before overt clinical symptoms are observed.

Heredity is the genetic transmission of characteristics from parent to offspring. The term **genotype** refers to the genetic variation that separates one individual from another. No two individuals have the exact same genotype. But, you might ask, do identical twins have the same genotype? The answer is a resounding yes and no. The answer is yes, if we consider that identical twins have the same DNA because they came from a fertilized egg cell (zygote) that gets split in half. But the answer is also no, because even though identical twins may have the same DNA, their genes are in different bodies. Alone, DNA does nothing—it is like a book sitting on a shelf. It sits there until someone (or something, like a protein) comes along to read it and assemble the informa-

tion (i.e., to create a person). The way a protein interprets the gene can vary, which is why identical twins may have different fingerprints, and even look different. This is because their bodies are taking the same DNA and using it in different ways. The physical expression of genetic variation (i.e., traits) is referred to as **phenotype**. The complete set of chromosomes for an individual is referred to as the **karyotype**. An example of the karyotype for a female and male is provided in Figure 11–4. Note that the most obvious difference in karyotype is in regard to chromosome 23, which is the sex chromosome.

HISTORIC ASPECTS OF GENETICS

A time line of major events that shaped the field of genetics is displayed in Table 11–1. Some of the more profound events are detailed below. From the earliest recorded history, ancient civilizations observed patterns in reproduction. Animals bore offspring of the same species, children resembled their parents, and plants gave rise to similar plants. Some of the earliest ideas about reproduction, heredity, and the transmission of information from parent to child were the **particulate theories** developed in ancient Greece during the fourth century BC. These theories posited that information from each part of the parent had to be somehow transmitted to create the corresponding body part in the offspring. For example, the particulate theories held that information from the parent's heart, lungs, and limbs was transmitted directly from these body parts to create the offspring's heart, lungs, and limbs.

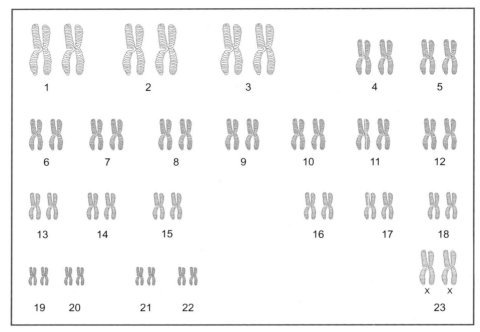

A

B

FIGURE 11–4. A female (**A**) and male (**B**) karyotype. Note the obvious difference in regard to pairing of the 23rd (sex) chromosomes.

Table 11–1. Some Milestones in the Field of Genetics

Year	Event
1590	The microscope is invented by Zaccharias Janssen.
1858	Charles Darwin announces the theory of natural selection.
1863	Studying peas, Gregor Mendel discovers that traits are transmitted from parents to progeny by discrete, independent units, later known as genes. His observations lay the groundwork for the field of genetics.
1869	Johann Friedrich Miescher discovers DNA in human white blood cells and in the sperm of trout.
1879	Walther Fleming discovers chromatin, the rod-like structures inside the cell nucleus that are later named chromosomes.
1905	Nettie Stevens and Edmund Wilson independently describe the behavior of sex chromosomes.
1907	Thomas Hunt Morgan's work on *Drosophila* (i.e., the fruit fly) leads to further understanding of genetics.
1953	James Watson and Francis Crick publish their findings describing the double helical structure of DNA, marking the beginning of the modern era of genetics.
1972	The DNA composition of humans is found to be 99% similar to that of chimpanzees and gorillas.
1983	The first artificial chromosome is synthesized.
1983	James Gusella uses blood samples to demonstrate that the Huntington disease gene is on chromosome 4.
1984	The DNA fingerprinting technique is developed.
1990	The first federally approved gene therapy treatment is performed on a four-year-old girl with an immune disorder.
1996	Discovery of a gene associated with Parkinson disease provides insight as to its cause and potential treatment.
1997	Scottish scientists report cloning a sheep, named Dolly, using DNA from adult sheep cells.
2000	The Human Genome Project presents its preliminary results.

One reason particulate theories were inaccurate was that they relied on observations unaided by the microscope. The microscope was invented around 1600 by a Dutch spectacle maker, **Zaccharias Janssen** (1580–1538). The English naturalist **Robert Hooke** (1635–1703) was the first to use this device to identify plant cells, specifically the cell walls in cork tissue. Hooke coined the term *cells*. The boxlike shape of cells in cork reminded him of the cells of a monastery. Over the next century, improvements in microscopy and the increasing study of cytology (i.e., the formation, structure, and function of cells) enabled scientists to identify parts of the cell.

One of the most important developments in the study of hereditary processes came in 1858, when **Charles Darwin** (1809–1882) and **Alfred Wallace** (1823–1913) announced the theory of natural selection (see also Chapter 1). The premise of this theory was that members of a population who are better adapted to their environment will be the ones most likely to survive and pass their traits on to the next generation. Darwin published this theory in 1859 in the classic text, *On the Origin of Species by Means of Natural Selection*. At the time of publication, Darwin's work was not viewed favorably. Religious leaders believed the theory refuted the biblical interpretation of how life on Earth began. To this day, debate continues regarding evolution and creationism.

During the period of 1856 to 1863, the Austrian **Gregor Mendel** (1822–1884) conducted carefully designed genetic experiments with nearly 30,000 pea plants (Figure 11–5). Mendel was an Augustinian monk who taught natural science to high school students. He cultivated pea plants in the monastery garden and chose to study them because they had distinct, identifiable characteristics that could not be confused. His experiments were designed to test the inheritance of a specific trait from one generation to the next. For example, to test inheritance of the characteristic of plant height, Mendel self-pollinated by hand several short pea plants, and the seeds they produced grew into short plants.

In 1907, the American **Thomas Hunt Morgan** (1866–1945) studied *Drosophila*

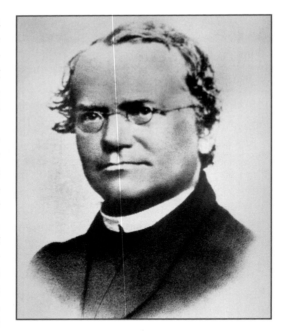

FIGURE 11–5. Gregor Mendel's genetic experiments with pea plants were designed to test the inheritance of specific traits.

(i.e., the fruit fly) as a means of understanding genetic traits (Figure 11–6). This research revolutionized the study of genetics because the fly's rapid life cycle and minute size enabled Morgan to undertake a large number of experiments over a short period of time. Contrast the whole year required between generations of peas with the two weeks needed for the life span of a fruit fly. Morgan was able to study hundreds of fruit fly characteristics. In addition, he identified gene mutations, such as discovery of some fruit flies having a white-eyed mutation.

Nettie Maria Stevens (1861–1912) was an American biologist and geneticist who studied under the guidance of Thomas Hunt Morgan (Figure 11–7). Based on research with beetles, she helped prove that chromosomes determine the sex of an organism. Prior to this discovery, researchers assumed that the sex of an organism was influenced by food and temperature conditions during the early stages of an organism's development.

The discovery in 1953 of the double-helix structure of DNA marked the beginning of the modern era of genet-ics. The American anthropologist **James Watson** (b. 1928) and British physi-cist **Francis Crick** (1916–2004) worked together at the University of Cambridge (Figure 11–8). Many of their findings were based on examination of x-ray

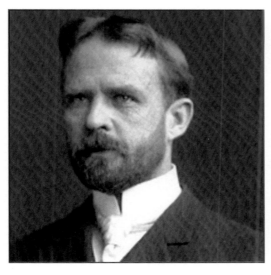

FIGURE 11–6. Thomas Hunt Morgan stud-ied fruit flies as a means of understanding genetic traits.

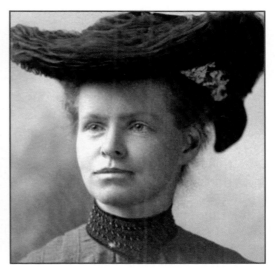

FIGURE 11–7. Nettie Maria Stevens, Amer-ican biologist who helped prove that chromo-somes determine the sex of an organism.

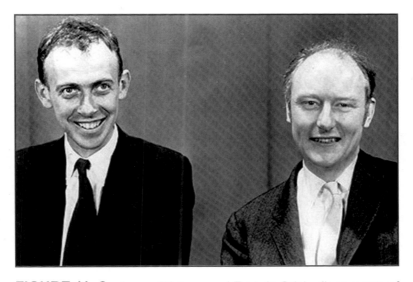

FIGURE 11–8. James Watson and Francis Crick, discoverers of the double-helix structure of DNA.

diffraction photographs. In 1988, Watson was later appointed as head of the Human Genome Project at the National Institutes of Health.

TYPES OF SYNDROMES

Use of the term birth defect is a generalized description of any genetic or nongenetic condition that occurs at birth. The term is not entirely accurate because: (1) Some abnormalities may not be present at birth and are evident only after the child begins to mature (such as dentition), and (2) the term does not take into account abnormalities of behavior. A more accurate description of these conditions is a **congenital anomaly**. An example in which both physical and behavioral anomalies may not surface until later in a child's development is fetal alcohol syndrome. The characteristics of fetal alcohol syndrome are described later in this chapter.

Syndromes can be broadly classified into two types: (1) chromosomal syndromes and (2) genetic syndromes. **Chromosomal syndromes** involve visible changes in the chromosomal structure (i.e., karyotype) of the individual. These types of syndromes typically result in rather severe anomalies such

---

FYI

Gene splicing is a technique used to join segments of DNA (often from different individuals or species) to form a new genetic combination called recombinant DNA. This is one of the techniques used in genetic engineering.

---

as physical abnormalities, cognitive impairments, and communication disorders. The reason for the severe anomalies is that impairment of chromosomal structure tends to affect a large number of genes. On the other hand, **genetic syndromes** often involve a single affected gene. The outward appearance of chromosomes may appear fine. It is a specific gene that is abnormal. The problems arising from a genetic syndrome can range from mild to severe, depending on the specific gene that is affected.

Chromosomal Syndromes

Approximately 7 out of every 1,000 births will be affected by a chromosomal disorder. These disorders account for approximately one half of all spontaneous abortions (i.e., miscarriages) that occur during the first trimester of pregnancy (Gerber, 1990). There are five basic abnormalities that can occur in chromosomal structure: (1) deletion of whole chromosomes, (2) deletion of parts of a chromosome, (3) addition of whole chromosomes, (4) addition of parts of chromosomes, and (5) restructuring (or rearranging) of chromosomes. Most people who have a chromosomal syndrome exhibit the chromosomal abnormality in every cell in the body. However, there are rare cases in which only a portion of the body's cells are affected. This condition is referred to as **mosaicism**. Individuals with mosaicism generally show less severe abnormalities than if all cells were affected. The chromosomal syndromes of: (1) Down syndrome, (2) Cri du Chat syndrome, and (3) Turner syndrome are profiled below.

Down Syndrome

Down syndrome is the most frequently occurring human chromosomal disorder. In this particular condition, the karyotype is characterized by a chromosomal addition to the 21st chromosome. The condition is referred to as trisomy 21, indicating the particular karyotype (Figure 11–9). The condition was named

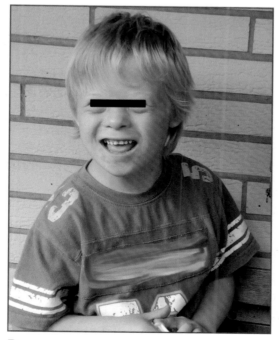

FIGURE 11–9. Down syndrome karyotype (**A**) and a photograph of a boy with Down syndrome (**B**). From Vanellus at Wikimedia Commons.

after **John Langdon Down** (1828–1896), an English physician who published *Observations of an Ethnic Classification of Idiots* in 1866. He identified a group of patients with similar features and called them mongoloid idiots. The term *idiot* was in common use at the time to describe intellectual impairment; *mongoloid* was in reference to the supposed similarity in appearance to people of east Asia. These days, neither term is socially acceptable. Although Down is credited with identifying the syndrome, the precise chromosomal structure of trisomy 21 was not identified until nearly 100 years later by **Jerome Lejeune** (1926–1994). Down syndrome is found to occur in approximately 1 out of every 800 births. Down syndrome is a chromosomal disorder caused by an error in cell division, and the likelihood of such an error increases with maternal age (Hook, Cross, & Schreinemachers, 1983), meaning that an older female is more prone to give birth to a child with Down syndrome. The occurrence dramatically increases to 1 out of every 25 births among women over the age of 45 years (Table 11–2). However, it is important to note that the combined effect of the father's age may also be a contributing factor. The average life expectancy of an individual with Down syndrome is 55 years of age.

The phenotype of Down syndrome is provided in Table 11–3. Included among these characteristics are heart anomalies, dry skin, fine soft hair, **hypotonia** (i.e., reduced muscle tone), brachycephaly (i.e., a widening of the skull with a flat back of head), Class III malocclusion, protruding tongue, and intellectual disability that is very rarely severe. Males with Down syndrome may also have hypogonadism—a defect of the reproductive system that results

Table 11–2. Approximate Occurrence of Down Syndrome Births According to the Mother's Age

Age of Mother (Years)	Frequency of Down Syndrome (Per Births)
15–19	1/1,250
20–24	1/1,400
25–29	1/1,100
30–32	1/875
33–35	1/500
36–38	1/225
39–41	1/100
42–44	1/50
45+	1/25

in lack of function of the gonads (i.e., sterility) in males. The communication disorder often found in Down syndrome is delayed onset of language. Although these children eventually will develop communication skills, the length of utterance and size of vocabulary is reduced and dependent primarily on the severity of intellectual disability. Children with Down syndrome also may show speech articulation difficulties resulting from reduced muscle tone in the oral cavity, combined with dentition irregularities. The hearing abilities of individuals with Down syndrome usually are normal, although children can experience higher than average bouts of otitis media.

Cri du Chat Syndrome

Jerome Lejeune (1926–1994) first described **Cri du Chat syndrome** in 1963.

Table 11–3. Phenotype of Some Chromosomal Syndromes

Chromosomal Syndrome	Phenotype
Down Syndrome	Hypotonia
	Protruding tongue
	Brachycephaly
	Heart anomaly
	Dry skin
	Fine soft hair
	Hypogonadism
	Obesity
	Short fifth finger
	Class III malocclusion
	Cognitive impairment
Cri du Chats Syndrome	High-pitched voice
	Hypotonia
	Microcephaly
	Orbital hypertelorisim
	Down-slanting eyes
	Ear tags
	Small stature
	Occasional cleft palate
	Severe cognitive impairment
Turner Syndrome	Short stature
	Short webbed neck
	Heart anomalies
	Renal anomalies
	Lack of sexual development
	Low-set ears
	Low hairline
	Shield-shaped chest
	Occasional cleft palate
	Puffy hands and feet
	Hearing loss

Legeune was a French pediatrician and geneticist who was also the first to identify the precise chromosomal structure of Down syndrome. Cri du Chat (meaning "cat's cry" in French) syndrome is named for the cat-like cry made by infants with this chromosomal disorder, which is caused by an abnormally small larynx. Cri du chat syndrome is also called 5p minus (5p–) syndrome because it is caused by a partial deletion of the short arm of chromosome 5 (Figure 11–10). The syndrome has been estimated to occur in 1 of every 50,000 live births. It accounts for 1 in every 500 cases of intellectual disability. Approxi-

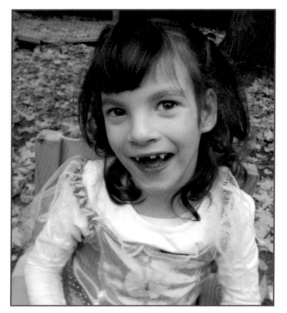

A

B

FIGURE 11–10. A. Karyotype of Cri du Chat syndrome. **B.** Photograph of Ariella at age six years. Photograph used with permission of the Cri du Chat Support Group of Australia.

mately 50 to 60 children are born with Cri du Chat syndrome in the United States each year. The syndrome is found to occur in all races and in both sexes. There is a slight female predominance with the ratio of occurrence estimated to be three girls to two boys. At birth, these children may show a failure to thrive because of feeding difficulties; however, those who do survive have a normal life expectancy. Individuals with Cri du Chat tend to be loving and highly social.

The phenotype of Cri du Chat syndrome is provided in Table 11–3. Individuals with this syndrome have unusual facial features such as down-slanting eyes, ear tags (i.e., small flap of skin on front of ear), small head size (i.e., **microcephaly**), small jaw size (i.e., **micrognathia**), and a large distance between the eyes (i.e., hypertelorism). The children also demonstrate hypotonia and may be born with a cleft palate. A severe intellectual impairment occurs because of the large deletion of genetic material from the chromosome. In addition to the classic feature of a cat-like cry or high-pitched voice, the voice also may have a nasal quality if the child was born with a cleft palate. As a result of the severe intellectual impairments, development of oral language can be a challenge. A small number of children never learn to speak; however, most are able to speak and make themselves understood to some degree, which they supplement with both formal and informal gestures. A conductive hearing loss may be present, resulting from persistent otitis media.

Turner Syndrome

Turner syndrome is named after the American physician **Henry Turner**

(1892–1970), who first described the condition in 1938. Turner syndrome affects only women and is caused by a total absence of one of the sex (23rd) chromosomes in some or all cells throughout the body (Figure 11–11). About 1% of all female conceptions have a missing X chromosome. Of these, the majority (99%) result in a miscarriage, usually during the first trimester of pregnancy. Turner syndrome affects around 1 out of every 2,500 live female births. Most women with Turner syndrome can live relatively normal lives. The prognosis for a person with Turner syndrome is dependent on other conditions that may be present. For example, there is a tendency toward heart or kidney defects, which may significantly impact the quality of life.

The phenotype of Turner syndrome is provided in Table 11–3. Individuals with this syndrome show short stature, a shield-like chest, stocky build, and puffy hands and feet. The neck is short and wide (web neck), and the ears are low-set. There is a lack of sexual development. Otitis media is common. There is no greater propensity to intellectual impairments than the general population. The phenotype of Turner syndrome is not easy to identify at birth. Many are identified around the time they enter school (due to their short stature) or around the time of puberty (due to a lack of sexual development). The primary communication disorder in Turner syndrome is hearing impairment. A sensorineural hearing loss has been found to occur in as many as 65% of all cases, and 10% of these individuals are deaf. Usually, language abilities are normal. Speech articulation difficulties may occur as a result of overcrowding of the teeth and a high arched palate.

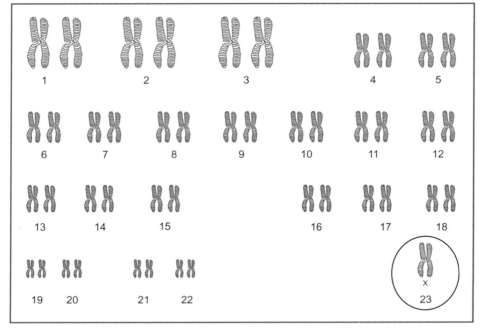

A

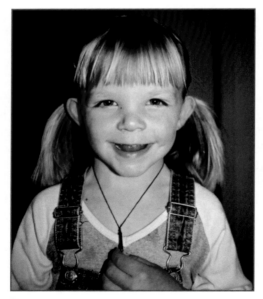

B

FIGURE 11–11. A. Turner syndrome karyotype. **B.** Photograph of Kasey at age four years. Photograph used with permission of the Turner Syndrome Support Group of New Zealand.

Genetic Syndromes

Although genetic syndromes are chromosome based, they are categorized separately. These are conditions that do not have a visible cellular abnormality. Most of these syndromes involve a problem with a single gene known as a **gene mutation**. There are three possible gene mutations: (1) deletion of a gene, (2) addition of a gene, and (3) rearrangement of genes. The human body consists of approximately 20,000 genes, so there are countless possibilities for gene mutations resulting in syndromes. There are close to 5,000 genetic disorders, and the list continues to grow (Shprintzen, 1997). The problems resulting from genetic syndromes range from mild to severe, depending on the specific gene and type of gene mutation. Some genetic syndromes are inherited and may have been present in past generations of the same family. Inherited genetic syndromes often involve mutation of a single gene. There are also genetic syndromes that fall under the class of **teratogenic** disorders. The term teratogen translates literally from its Greek roots meaning "monster maker" (*teratos* = monster, *gen* = life). Teratogenic disorders are polygenic, meaning more than one gene is likely to be mutated. Four genetic syndromes are covered below. Three of these syndromes are inherited: (1) Fragile X syndrome, (2) Prader-Willi syndrome, and (3) Crouzon syndrome. The fourth genetic syndrome is a teratogenic syndrome—fetal alcohol syndrome.

Fragile X Syndrome

Fragile X syndrome (also called Martin-Bell syndrome) is a genetic syndrome that affects a wide range of physical, intellectual, emotional, and behavioral features, which range from mild to severe in manifestation. The impairment is not readily identifiable at birth. Rather, the characteristic features begin to surface as the child develops. The condition was first reported by James Martin and Julia Bell in 1943. As the name of the syndrome suggests, this is a condition in which the 23rd ("X") chromosome is affected at the location of Xq27.3 (Figure 11–12). At this location,

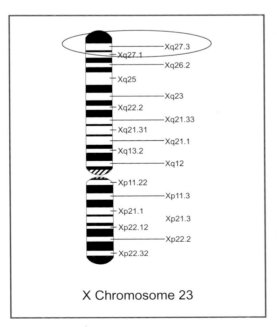

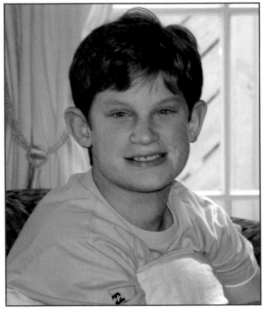

A

B

FIGURE 11–12. A. Fragile X syndrome karyotype. **B.** Photograph of Dominic at age 14 years. Photograph used with permission of the Fragile X Trust of New Zealand.

there is a mutation of a gene called FMR1. The FMR1 gene makes a protein that is needed for normal brain development. In this case, the gene is "turned off," so that no protein is made. Fragile X syndrome is the world's leading cause of inherited intellectual disability. This should not be confused with Down syndrome, which is the most common non-inherited cause of intellectual disability. The condition affects about 1 in 3,600 males and 1 in 5,000 females.

The phenotype of Fragile X syndrome is listed in Table 11–4. Some main physical features are: (1) a long face and prominent ears, especially in older males, (2) low muscle tone, (3) flat feet, (4) heart murmurs, and (5) frequent ear infections. The main behavioral features are: (1) hand biting and hand flapping, (2) poor eye contact, (3) sensory sensitivities such as aversion to touch and noise, (4) obsessive-compulsive disorder, and (5) socially engaging and

Table 11–4. Phenotype of Some Genetic Syndromes

Genetic Syndrome	Phenotype
Fragile X Syndrome	Mild-to-severe intellectual disability
	Autistic-like behaviors
	Pectus excavatum (sunken chest)
	Scoliosis
	Large, protruding ears
	Long, thin face
	Prominent forehead and jaw
	Dental overcrowding
	High-arched palate
Crouzon Syndrome	Premature fusion of cranial sutures
	Mid-face hypoplasia (underdeveloped)
	Beak-shaped nose
	Exorbitism (bulging eyes)
	Low-set ears
	Class III malocclusion
	Conductive hearing loss
	Possible otitis media
	Cognitive impairment is rare.
Prader-Willi Syndrome	Obesity
	Insatiable appetite
	Hypotonia
	Short stature
	Small hands and feet
	Hypogonadism
	Probable cognitive impairment

friendly. The main cognitive features are: (1) subtle learning difficulties to severe mental impairment, (2) delayed milestones such as walking and toileting, (3) attention deficit and hyperactivity, and (4) strong visual memory. The communication disorder in Fragile X syndrome includes speech sound articulation difficulties, disfluencies, and the presence of atypical speaking rate. Most males show moderate-to-severe delays in communication skills, whereas the communication skills of females are considerably less affected, depending on the severity of intellectual disability. There also is a high incidence of otitis media and intermittent hearing loss.

Crouzon Syndrome

Crouzon syndrome is a genetic disorder characterized by the premature fusion of certain skull bones (known as **craniosynostosis**). This early fusion prevents the skull from growing normally and affects the shape of the head and face. It is a type of a craniofacial syndrome (i.e., one that affects the developmental formation of the skull and face). Crouzon syndrome is caused by mutations in the FGFR2 gene, which is found on the long arm of chromosome 10 at the location of 10q25-10q26 (Figure 11–13). The gene is associated with growth factors of the face and skull. The condition was first identified in 1912 by **Louis Octave Crouzon** (1874–1938), a French neurosurgeon, through the case of a mother and child, both with Crouzon symptoms. People with Crouzon syndrome are of normal intelligence. The syndrome occurs in 1 out of every 60,000 live births and is the most prevalent form of craniosynostosis syndrome. The condition is readily identifiable at birth because of the observable craniofacial

abnormality. There is no difference in occurrence between females and males. Individuals with Crouzon syndrome have a normal life expectancy.

The phenotype of Crouzon syndrome is reflective of the premature fusion of the skull bones (see Table 11–4). Abnormal growth of these bones leads to wide-set, bulging eyes and vision problems caused by shallow eye sockets, a beaked nose, and an underdeveloped upper jaw. In addition, people with Crouzon syndrome may have dental problems. Surgery often is necessary to correct some of the craniofacial abnormalities. The skull abnormalities are corrected using a procedure known as a **craniectomy**, which involves surgical opening of the cranium to allow for more natural growth of the brain and skull. Facial reconstruction is performed to correct midface abnormalities. Individuals with Crouzon syndrome develop speech and language normally. If any communication disorders are apparent, they are a result of the physical problems related to the skull and face. For example, it is not unusual to observe speech articulation difficulties resulting from a Class III malocclusion. There may be a hyponasal voice quality due to a small nasal port. These children are also prone to chronic otitis media as a result of narrow ear canals.

Prader-Willi Syndrome

Prader-Willi syndrome is a complex genetic disorder that occurs in approximately 1 out of every 12,000 to 15,000 births. Prader-Willi syndrome was first described by Swiss doctors Andrea Prader, Alexis Labhart, and Heinrich Willi in 1956 based on the clinical characteristics of nine children they had examined. A primary feature of the

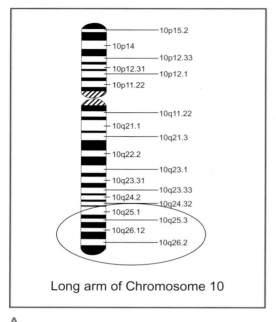

Long arm of Chromosome 10

A

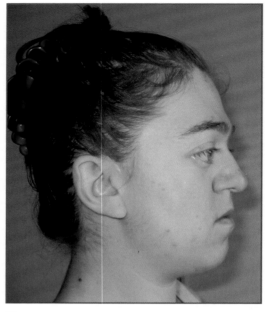

B

FIGURE 11–13. A. Crouzon syndrome karyotype. **B–C.** Photographs of Candar at age 24 years. Photographs used with permission.

C

syndrome is a chronic feeling of hunger that can lead to excessive eating and life-threatening obesity. Although Prader-Willi syndrome is considered a rare disorder, it is one of the conditions often encountered in genetics clinics and is the most common genetic cause of childhood obesity. Prader-Willi syndrome occurs as a result of a deletion of genetic material on the long arm of chromosome 15 at the location of 15q11-q13 (Figure 11–14). Prader-Willi syndrome is found in people of both sexes and all races and ethnicities. Currently, there is

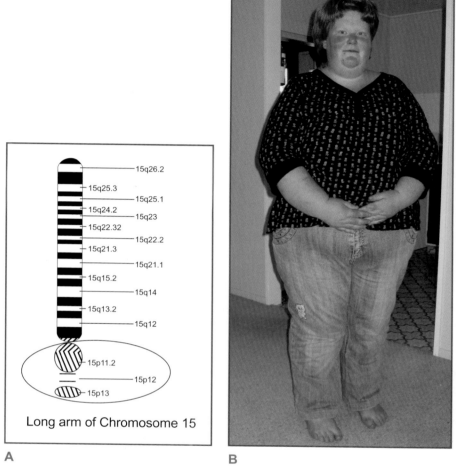

FIGURE 11–14. A. Prader-Willi syndrome karyotype. **B.** Photograph of young woman at age 24 years. Photograph used with permission.

no cure for Prader-Willi syndrome. For many individuals affected by the disorder, elimination of some of the most difficult aspects of the syndrome, such as the insatiable appetite and obesity, would constitute a cure. The implementation of growth hormone therapy has recently been explored as a treatment of Prader-Willi syndrome. Growth hormones serve to build muscle tone that allows better movement and thus more ability to burn calories. The life expec-

tancy for an individual with Prader-Willi syndrome is normal, and the prognosis is good, if weight gain is well controlled.

The phenotype of Prader-Willi syndrome includes small hands and feet, abnormal growth and body composition (obesity), low muscle tone, short stature, incomplete sexual development, and intellectual disabilities (see Table 11–4). There are two stages to Prader-Willi syndrome. During Stage 1, infants with Prader-Willi syndrome are of very low muscle tone and produce weak cries. They have difficulty sucking and are usually unable to breast-feed. As the children grow, they develop better muscle tone and strength. Motor milestones such as standing, walking, and running are achieved but delayed in comparison with same-age peers. Stage 2 of Prader-Willi syndrome occurs during the age range of two to six years. This stage is characterized by an insatiable appetite. During this time frame, children with Prader-Willi syndrome are likely to exhibit intellectual disabilities, with IQs ranging from low-normal to moderate mental impairment. Disordered speech and language often is observed among individuals with Prader-Willi syndrome that is associated with the child's overall level of cognitive functioning. The communication impairment found in Prader-Willi syndrome includes delayed speech and language development that parallels that found for achieving basic motor milestones. Children with Prader-Willi syndrome also may show hypernasal speech early in life that is linked to poor muscle tone. The hypernasality generally decreases as the child's strength and muscle tone improves.

Fetal Alcohol Syndrome

An infant born to a mother who drinks alcohol during her pregnancy, even in modest amounts, may be born with **fetal alcohol syndrome**. The condition of fetal alcohol syndrome results in growth retardation, unusual physical and facial features, and intellectual impairment. Children have suffered the consequences of their mothers' alcohol consumption since people began to drink alcohol. In 1973, the term fetal alcohol syndrome was coined by Kenneth Jones and David Smith, two pediatric dysmorphologists, who described the signs of alcohol exposure in infants at birth and early childhood. Fetal alcohol syndrome is a teratogenic disorder that causes gene mutation. On average, three out of five women drink alcohol. A woman's body metabolizes alcohol more quickly than a man's, and thus, they become intoxicated more easily. When pregnant women drink, the developing fetus receives a strong dose of alcohol. The internationally recognized rate of occurrence of fetal alcohol syndrome is 1 to 3 out of every 1,000 births. In 9 out of every 1,000 births, infants will show some (but not all) signs of alcohol exposure. This condition is referred to as alcohol-related neurodevelopmental disorder or fetal alcohol effects. It is estimated that 25 to 45% of women with chronic alcoholism will give birth to children with fetal alcohol syndrome if they drink heavily during pregnancy (Table 11–5).

It is difficult to pinpoint the exact gene (or genes) that are affected because

Table 11–5. Some Facts About Alcohol Consumption

- A "drink" is defined as a 12 oz. beer, a 1.5 oz. shot of 80-proof liquor, or a 4 oz. glass of table wine.
- In the United States, legally intoxicated is defined as a Blood Alcohol Level (BAL) of .08%.
- Permanent brain cell damage begins at a BAL of .07%.
- A 100-pound (45-kg) female consuming five standard drinks will reach a BAL of .25%, which is three times the legal BAL limit.
- BAL reduces .01% per hour.

the mutation is linked to: (1) the amount of alcohol consumed by the mother, (2) the time of pregnancy during which alcohol was consumed, and (3) the likely interaction of alcohol consumption with other drugs. The early months of fetal growth involve development of the face, limbs, heart, and brain. Therefore, mothers who drink during the first trimester of pregnancy give birth to children with the most severe problems because the alcohol abuse occurs during the period when many physical features of the child are developing. This is also a time when many women may not even realize they are pregnant. Women who abstain from alcohol in early pregnancy may feel comfortable drinking during the final months of the pregnancy. Yet it is during the last trimester of pregnancy that some of the most complex features of brain development take place. Even moderate alcohol intake, and especially periodic binge drinking, can seriously damage the developing nervous system of the fetus.

A list of the phenotype of fetal alcohol syndrome is provided in Figure 11–15.

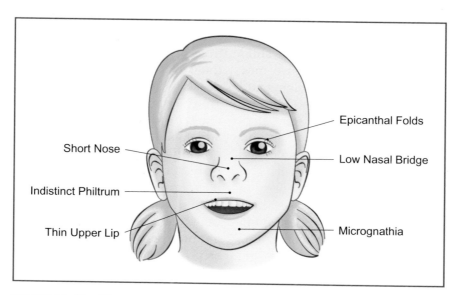

FIGURE 11–15. Phenotype of fetal alcohol syndrome.

FYI

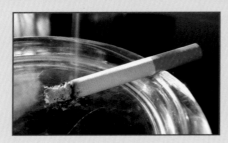

There is genetic evidence that suggests some people were "born to smoke." In 1999, researchers found that people who carry the gene *SLC6A3-9*, located on chromosome 5, were less likely to become addicted to cigarette smoking than those without the gene. The particular gene is found to be important for the transfer of the neurotransmitter dopamine, which is a natural stimulant created in the brain. Those without the gene may be more vulnerable to the addictive (i.e., stimulating) effects of tobacco.

The phenotype found in 50% (or more) of the cases of fetal alcohol syndrome include: (1) below average height and weight, (2) microcephaly, (3) micrognathia, (4) thin upper lip, (5) hyperactivity, and (6) intellectual impairment. Problems associated with fetal alcohol syndrome tend to intensify as children move into adulthood. These can include mental health problems, troubles with the law, and the inability to live independently. The communication problems found in fetal alcohol syndrome include a general overall delay in speech and language development. The child with fetal alcohol syndrome also may show speech articulation problems and swallowing problems due to poor motor coordination. If a child with fetal alcohol syndrome has an intellectual impairment, there is likely to be an associated language impairment, the severity of which is dependent on the severity of the intellectual disability. The condition of fetal alcohol syndrome, and all damage caused by prenatal alcohol exposure, is 100% preventable by simply choosing not to drink alcohol. Fetal alcohol syndrome cannot be cured, but the effects of the disabilities can be managed.

ASSESSMENT OF GENETICS AND SYNDROMES

We are continually learning more about the genetics of various diseases and syndromes and how these conditions run in families. Two forms of assessment are: (1) genetic counseling and (2) prenatal diagnosis. **Genetic counseling** is designed to help a person or family understand their risk for genetic conditions (such as Down syndrome), to educate the person or family about the condition, and to assess the risk of passing the condition on to children. Traditionally, a genetic counselor has a master's degree in genetic counseling and has studied genetic diseases and how they run in families. Table 11–6 provides a list of situations whereby a person may wish to seek genetic counseling. A recent trend in genetic counseling is for individuals to undergo **whole genome sequencing**. This is referred to as a form of "personalized" medicine, where a blood or saliva sample is collected and sent to a laboratory for analysis. The analysis provides the genome of

Table 11–6. Situations Where It Is Advisable to Seek Genetic Counseling

- Individuals who are concerned they might have an inherited disorder.
- Women who are pregnant or planning to be after the age of 35.
- Couples who already have a child with an inherited disorder.
- Women who have had three or more miscarriages.
- People concerned that their jobs, lifestyles, or medical history may pose a risk to the outcome of pregnancy. Common causes of concern include exposure to radiation, medications, illegal drugs, chemicals, or infections.
- Couples who would like testing or more information about genetic conditions that occur frequently in their ethnic group.
- Couples who are first cousins or other close blood relatives.
- Pregnant women whose ultrasound examinations or blood testing indicate that their pregnancy may be at increased risk for certain complications.

the individual, and this information is used to determine whether there are any specific genes (or mutations) that place the person at risk for various diseases. It is important to emphasize that being a carrier of a specific gene does not guarantee that the disease will occur.

As the term suggests, **prenatal diagnosis** involves assessing the fetus prior to birth. Two forms of prenatal testing used routinely for pregnant women are: (1) maternal blood sampling and (2) ultrasound scanning. Between 15 and 19 weeks of pregnancy, women are offered a blood test. A pregnancy blood test measures the exact amount of the pregnancy hormone called human chorionic gonadotropin in the bloodstream. This measurement can help give a rough estimate of the age of the fetus. It also can help determine if the pregnancy is progressing normally.

Ultrasound scans are performed on most pregnant women between 16 and 19 weeks of pregnancy. The process of fetal **ultrasound** testing was developed in the late 1960s and involves applying a clear, water-based conduction gel to the surface of the pregnant woman's abdomen that helps with the transmission of sound waves. A handheld probe called a transducer is then moved over

---

FYI

In the late 1920s, it was discovered that injecting a suspected mother's urine into a rabbit served as a form of pregnancy testing. The human chorionic gonadotropin pregnancy hormone found in the urine caused spontaneous ovulation among rabbits. Unfortunately, in order to determine if ovulation occurred in the rabbit, it needed to be dissected. Thus the euphemism, "the rabbit died" became associated with a positive test for pregnancy.

the area and delivers a series of sound waves that bounce off the curves and variations inside the body, including the fetus (Figure 11–16). These sound waves are translated into a pattern of light and dark areas that create an image of the fetus on a monitor. The procedure is noninvasive, safe, and painless for the mother and fetus. Generally, an obstetrician performs an ultrasound test to determine if a woman is pregnant and whether there is more than one fetus. An ultrasound test can be used to detect abnormalities in the development of the fetus such as growth retardation, heart and kidney defects, Down syndrome, and cleft palate. The test is also useful in identifying **neural tube defects** (i.e., abnormalities) of the brain and spinal cord. Two neural tube defects are spina bifida and anencephaly. In **spina bifida**, the fetal spinal column fails to close completely during the first month of pregnancy. There is usually nerve damage that causes at least some paralysis of the legs. In **anencephaly**, much of the brain does not develop. Babies with anencephaly are either stillborn or die shortly after birth.

For pregnancies where there is a risk of the fetus having a genetic abnormality, tissue for genetic testing can be obtained either by: (1) amniocentesis or (2) chorionic villus sampling. The **amniocentesis** procedure was developed in the early 1960s. The procedure involves withdrawing fluid from the amnion (the fluid-filled sack that contains the fetus). The fluid is taken from the woman's abdomen using a needle cannula (Figure 11–17). The cellular structure of the fluid is then analyzed to determine the karyotype of the fetus. Amniocentesis is performed during the

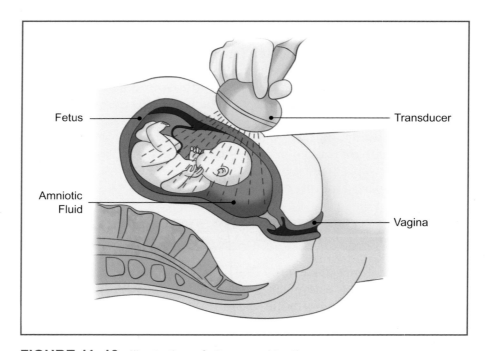

FIGURE 11–16. Illustration of ultrasound testing.

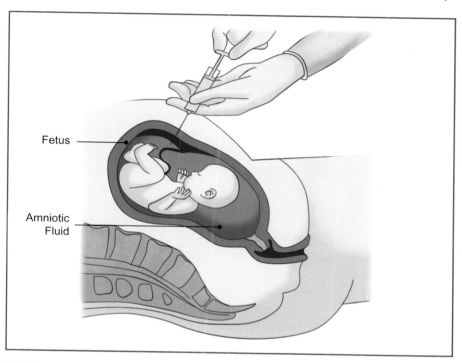

Fetus

Amniotic
Fluid

FIGURE 11–17. Illustration of amniocentesis in which amniotic fluid is withdrawn and later analyzed.

16th week of pregnancy, carries a low level of risk, and can be accomplished in an obstetrician's office.

Chorionic villus sampling was developed in 1975 by Chinese gynecologists as an aid to the early diagnosis of genetic disorders. In this approach, a catheter is inserted through the woman's cervix into the placenta. An abdominal ultrasound is also performed to determine the position of the uterus, the size of the gestational sac, and the position of the placenta within the uterus (Figure 11–18). A small piece of placenta tissue (i.e., chorionic villi) is removed from the uterus and examined microscopically for the existence of chromosomal abnormalities, as well as several hundred genetic disorders, such as cystic fibrosis and sickle cell disease. The main

advantage of chorionic villus sampling over amniocentesis is that the test can be performed earlier, generally between 11 and 12 weeks of pregnancy.

TREATMENT OF GENETIC CONDITIONS

Prophylactic Therapy

Prophylactic therapy involves the prevention of symptoms before they occur. One form of prophylactic therapy is the administration of vaccines to immunize against many diseases such as mumps, measles, and chicken pox. An example of prophylactic therapy involves treatment for a genetic condition known

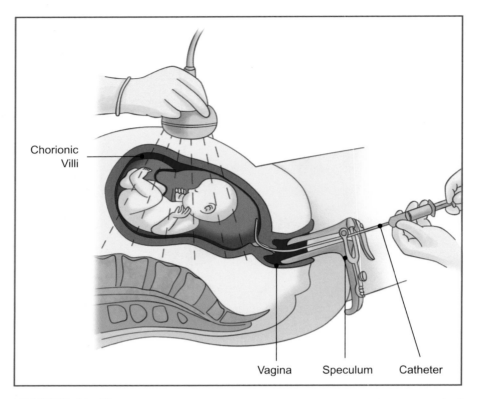

FIGURE 11–18. Illustration of chorionic villi sampling, involving removal of a small piece of placenta tissue (chorionic villi) from the uterus.

as phenylketonuria. Phenylketonuria is caused by mutations in the gene for phenylalanine hydroxylase, which is responsible for normal brain functioning. An infant's blood can be tested shortly after birth to determine whether phenylketonuria is present. If detected early, the baby's diet can be modified to ensure normal development and a normal life span.

Replacement Therapy

Replacement therapy involves replacing the gene product (i.e., protein) that is missing or defective in an affected person with a functioning gene product. For many years, such therapy has been available to individuals with conditions such as diabetes (where insulin is replaced) or growth hormone deficiency (where growth hormone is replaced). These disorders have been relatively easy to treat because the normal gene products are transported around the body in the bloodstream, and it is possible to inject the synthetic gene product intravenously. However, even for these disorders, the treatment has the disadvantage of having to be continually repeated.

Treatment of Symptoms

For most genetic disorders, the symptoms of the disorder are treated rather than the actual affected gene/chromosome. Such treatments include surgery, the administration of drugs, and control of a patient's environment. For example, it is not unusual for people with Down syndrome to be born with heart defects, which can be corrected surgically. For women with Turner syndrome, hormone-replacement therapy is given to prevent early-onset osteoporosis that occurs because of the absence of estrogen. The excessive eating and weight gain of patients with Prader-Willi syndrome has to be managed with strict diet control. Treatment of communication disorders among individuals with genetic abnormalities is directed toward underlying causes such as hearing loss or impaired speech motor control. In addition, young children may be placed in early intervention programs to provide optimal input for speech and language acquisition.

CULTURAL CONSIDERATIONS REGARDING GENETICS

It is often assumed that diseases found to occur within a family tree must be purely genetic. However, this family trend may reflect a common environment and lifestyle rather than a genetic influence. The term **ethnicity** is a complex construct that includes biology, history, cultural orientation and practice, language, religion, and lifestyle—all of these factors affect an individual's health (Pearce, Foliaki, Sporle, & Cunningham, 2004). For example, the Pellagra Commission was established in 1900 to investigate the problem of pellagra (a vitamin deficiency disease) in the southern United States. The commission concluded that pellagra was purely genetic because it occurred within the same families. Unfortunately, members of the commission failed to recognize that poverty and malnutrition also were major issues in the same families.

Even for classic genetic diseases, environmental factors usually have an important role. In fact, genetic studies can show the importance of environmental factors. A New Zealand study of alcoholism provides one example of a health-related genetic difference. Marshall et al. (1994) found that the ADH2-2 gene, which is believed to protect against alcoholism, was relatively common in the indigenous Maori people of New Zealand. This same gene is not found in New Zealand Europeans. Yet national statistics have revealed that alcohol-related health problems are more common in Maori, suggesting that the protective genetic factors are being outweighed by social, economic, cultural, and political factors. In summary, although some diseases are found to occur in some groups of people at a higher rate than others, the constant interaction between genes and the environment indicates that few diseases are purely hereditary.

CURRENT RESEARCH IN GENETICS

Junk DNA

Roughly 2% of the miles of DNA strings in our body contain genes that code proteins for specific functions. The remaining material is noncoded and was previously thought to be nonessential, thus giving rise to the phrase *junk DNA*. However, there is now emerg-

---
FYI

Cloning is the creation of an organism that is an exact genetic copy of another. This means that every piece of DNA is the same between the two organisms. Cloning is an asexual process because only one parent is required. Certain plants, such as types of grapes to make fine wines, have undergone cloning for hundreds of years. Only recently has the technology become available to clone animals, and the advent of this technology has sparked ethical debate.

---

ing research that shows this material may play an important role in the functioning of our bodies. For example, a group of scientists in England have recently discovered that at least one genetic malformation in a sequence of junk DNA can promote cancer growth (Cruickshanks, Vafadar-Isfahani, Dunican, & Tufarelli, 2013). A future area of genetics research lies in further understanding the nature of junk DNA proteins and how they work to create an individual person. This new and burgeoning scientific field is known as **proteomics**.

Genetics in Primary Communication Disorders

For years, communication disorders have been viewed as complex disorders that are caused by an interaction of many genes. Recently, the trend in genetics has been to study families with a history of specific communication disorders. This approach is designed to identify a gene sequence or regions on a chromosome that may be unique to the disorder. Language impairment, stuttering, speech sound disorders, hearing impairment, and dyslexia are all primary communication disorders that have a genetic component. Although not all instances of these disorders are a direct cause of genetic inheritance, the search is on for identifying the primary causal genes for primary communication disorders (Peter, 2012). This is quite possibly the most popular area of research currently taking place in the fields of audiology and speech-language pathology.

GENETICS AND SYNDROMES ON THE WORLD WIDE WEB

Listed below are websites that provide further information on the topics of genetics and syndromes. At the time of publication, each website was freely accessible.

Human Genome Project
http://video.pbs.org/video/2328723783

http://www.youtube.com/watch?v=4Gs9Cjwaxms

Human Genetics Disorders Video
http://video.pbs.org/video/2328386346

Information on Genetics
http://www.genetics.com

Inheritance of Genetic Disorders Video
http://www.teachersdomain
.org/resource/tdc02.sci.life.gen
.lp_disorder/

Down Syndrome Video
http://www.youtube.com/
watch?v=I13KxRYqoo0

Cri du Chat Syndrome Videos
http://www.youtube.com/
watch?v=--lx9c2EAwg

http://www.youtube.com/
watch?v=A47tRTi8YPw

Turner Syndrome Video
http://www.youtube.com/
watch?v=ldjb-FR-PKo

Crouzon Syndrome Video
http://www.youtube.com/
watch?v=X97fxLKjeUw

Fragile X Syndrome Video
http://livingwithfragilex.com/

Prader-Willi Syndrome Video
http://topdocumentaryfilms.com/
cant-stop-eating/

Fetal Alcohol Syndrome Video
http://fas.academicedge.com/fas_
media.html

STUDY QUESTIONS

1. List and define the basic terms related to genetics.
2. List and describe three chromosomal syndromes. What are the communication characteristics of each syndrome?
3. List and describe three genetic syndromes. What are the communication characteristics of each syndrome?
4. What are the various types of prenatal diagnosis?
5. What are the forms of treatment for genetic conditions?

REFERENCES

Cruickshanks, H. A., Vafadar-Isfahani, N., Dunican, D. S., & Tufarelli, C. (2013, May). Expression of a large LINE-1-driven antisense RNA is linked to epigenetic silencing of the metastasis suppressor gene TFPI-2 in cancer. *Nucleic Acids Research*, 1–13.

Gerber, A, (1990). *Prevention: The etiology of communicative disorders in children.* Englewood Cliffs, NJ: Prentice-Hall.

Hook, E. B., Cross, P. K., & Schreinemachers, D. M. (1983). Chromosomal abnormality rates at amniocentesis and in live-born infants. *Journal of the American Medical Association, 249,* 2034–2038.

Marshall, S. J., O'Brien, D., Wheeler, K., Hermans, I. F., Chambers, G. K., Robinson, G. M., & Stace, N. (1994). Genes and alcoholism: A preliminary report. *New Zealand Medical Journal, 107,* 106–107.

Pearce, N., Foliaki, S., Sporle, A., & Cunningham, C. (2004). Genetics, race, ethnicity and health. *British Medical Journal, 328,* 1070–1107.

Peter, B (2012, September 18). The future of genetics at our doorstep. *ASHA Leader,* 33–34.

Shprintzen, R. (1997). *Genetics, syndromes and communication disorders.* San Diego, CA: Singular.

SECTION 4
Audition

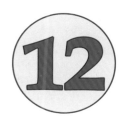

HEARING DISORDERS

OBJECTIVES

After reading this chapter, the student should be able to:

- Understand the concepts and terminology of the nature of sound.

- Understand basic audiology terminology.

- Describe various attributes of hearing loss including type, degree, and configuration of loss.

- Identify the primary types, causes, and characteristics of hearing disorders in children and adults.

- Describe common disorders of hearing associated with each part of the auditory system.

- Understand theory and practice of various audiological diagnostic tests.

- Describe the primary assessment of hearing disorders in children and adults.

INTRODUCTION

As noted in Chapters 1 and 2, communication involves the processes of encoding and decoding. Human communication is the exchange of a message between someone producing speech and someone listening to speech. A major portion of this book thus far has been dedicated to the wide range of communication disorders that result from a breakdown in the process of speech production. We now turn our attention to those communication disorders that stem from a disruption in hearing. There is perhaps no other health condition that can have as profound an effect on one's quality of life as a hearing disorder. Loss of hearing makes even routine communication difficult. This may result in frustration, withdrawal from social activities, depression, and even marital discord. People lose the ability to appreciate sounds of everyday living such as birds singing, children's voices, and even police sirens.

Hearing loss in adults is usually a condition that develops gradually over the years, and most people are not aware of the extent of their hearing loss until family or friends bring it to their attention. Even then, most adults will not seek help for their hearing until approximately seven years from the initial diagnosis of a hearing problem. A hearing loss that occurs early in childhood can have devastating consequences to a child's ability to learn. Such impairment also interferes with a child's psychological, emotional, and speech development. Even mild forms of hearing loss can cause great difficulties to people young and old. Loss of the ability to hear can be a serious problem, but in many cases, there is help available through medical or surgical treatment or with hearing aids. This chapter provides an introduction to the wide range of hearing disorders found in children and adults. Some disorders are more common than others, and there are unique ways of testing for various hearing disorders. Audiologists are professionals educated in the diagnosis and management of hearing disorders. For those interested in pursuing audiology as a career, this chapter should provide some insight into the complexities of the auditory system and the truly remarkable process of hearing.

TERMINOLOGY AND DEFINITIONS

The ear is one of the most amazing features of the human body, as well as the body of many living creatures. It is one of the smallest and most complex organs in the body and is capable of transforming airborne sound waves into a form the brain can understand. **Sound** results from a disturbance in air particles (i.e., molecules). Such disturbances are typically caused by the vibration of an elastic body such as a stereo speaker, bass drum, guitar string, or the vocal folds. Vibrations cause a disturbance of air particles. These particles bump into the particles close to them, which causes them to vibrate as well. The disturbance of particles move in a back and forth motion creating a **sound wave**. One complete back and forth motion of a particle is called a **cycle** of vibration. The **frequency** of a sound wave refers to how fast the particles vibrate and is measured by the number of complete vibrations that occur per unit of time. If a particle of air undergoes 1,000 vibrations in 1 second, then the frequency of the wave would be 1,000 cycles per second. The notation used to designate frequency is the **hertz** (Hz) **scale** (e.g., 1000 Hz). The hertz notation is used in honor of Heinrich Hertz (see later section). Low-frequency sounds are those that have a small number of vibrations per second. These vibrations are perceived as having a low-pitched sound. Alternatively, high-frequency sounds involve a large number of vibrations per second that we perceive as having a high-pitched quality. When a sound consists of only one frequency, it is referred to as a **pure tone**. A **complex sound** is one that contains more than one frequency. Sounds that have no consistent vibratory pattern are referred to as **noise**.

The back and forth motion of a pure tone can be represented graphi-cally as a **waveform** (Figure 12–1). On such a graph, the height of the sound wave is the point at which the particle is at its maximum point of disturbance. The terms used to describe the maximum disturbance of a sound wave are **amplitude** and **intensity**. The scale for measuring intensity is the **decibel scale** (dB). One decibel (1 dB) is considered the smallest difference in sound intensity that the human ear can discern. The decibel was named in honor of Alexander Graham Bell (see also Chapter 2). We perceive the intensity of a sound wave as its **loudness**. All sound waves can be described in regard to their frequency and intensity. For example, a sound wave may be produced with a single frequency of 2500 Hz and an intensity of 40 dB, or frequency components of 50 Hz and 70 Hz with an intensity of 100 dB. The variations in frequency and intensity for types of sound waves are

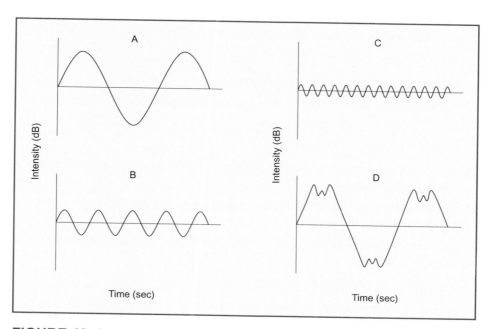

FIGURE 12–1. Examples of sound waves of varying frequency and intensity. **A.** The highest amplitude and lowest frequency, followed by **B** and **C**, respectively. **D.** A complex sound consisting of these same three sounds combined together.

endless. Illustrations of sound waves of varying frequency and intensity are shown in Figure 12–1.

Some facts and figures about hearing loss are provided in Table 12–1. It is estimated that approximately one in seven individuals has impaired hearing. This occurrence is found for countries throughout the world, including Europe, North America, and those in the southern hemisphere. Hearing impairment encompasses individuals who are deaf and hard of hearing. **Deafness** is defined as minimal hearing or complete loss of hearing. Deafness at birth is known as **congenital deafness**, whereas deafness that occurs after birth is called **adventitious deafness**. Some diseases that are known to cause adventitious deafness are meningitis, mumps, and chicken pox. Deafness that occurs prior to an individual learning to speak is called **prelingual deafness**, and **postlingual deafness** is hearing loss that happens after a period of language learning. **Hard of hearing** is defined as a hearing loss ranging from mild to severe for which a person usually receives some benefit from a **hearing aid**. Common causes of hearing loss are excessive noise exposure and aging. Not surprisingly, the occurrence of hearing loss is highest among the elderly. By the age of 65, one in every four individuals has a

---

Table 12–1.   Some Facts about Hearing Loss

- 22 million people in the United States have hearing loss.
- 9 million people in the United Kingdom have hearing loss.
- 3.5 million people in Australia have hearing loss.
- 4 million people in South Africa have hearing loss.
- 400,000 New Zealanders have hearing loss.
- Hearing loss is highly associated with aging.
- Approximately 60% of the hearing impaired are over the age of 65 years.
- Men are more likely than women to have hearing loss. Some 60% of people with hearing loss are men.
- Hearing loss is the third leading chronic disability, following arthritis and high blood pressure.
- The prevalence of hearing loss decreases as family income and education increase.
- People with hearing loss are generally less healthy than those with no hearing loss.
- Four out of five Americans with hearing loss do not use hearing aids.
- About 15% of university graduates have a level of hearing loss equal to or greater than their parents; a significant cause is listening to loud music.
- Minor decreases in hearing, especially of higher frequencies, are normal after the age of 18 years.

significant hearing loss. Hearing loss is the third most self-reported health problem of individuals 65 years of age or older, listed after arthritis and hypertension. It is estimated that untreated hearing impairments cost the United States economy $56 billion in lost productivity, special education, and medical care. The cost exceeds 200 billion euros across the European Union.

HISTORIC ASPECTS OF HEARING DISORDERS

Paleontologists who uncovered ancient skeletal remains have shown that hearing disorders such as middle ear infections (i.e., otitis media) occurred among early human populations. Skulls dating back to the Bronze Age (2000 BC) have shown evidence of temporal bone decay. Investigations of Egyptian mummies suggest that otitis media was present in Egyptian populations as far back as the 13th dynasty (1700 BC). Skulls uncovered from prehistoric Iran found evidence of otitis media among individuals from 1300 to 300 BC. Specific individuals who have either directly or indirectly contributed to our knowledge concerning hearing loss can be traced back approximately 200 years. Some of the more noteworthy contributors are mentioned below.

Prosper Ménière (1799–1862) was a French laryngologist (Figure 12–2), who at the age of 39, was appointed chief physician at the Institute for Deaf-Mutes in Paris, succeeding the renowned Gaspard Itard (noted for his work with the wild boy of Aveyron). Ménière was the first to describe the unusual ear disease that was later named in his honor. In 1861, he published a report entitled

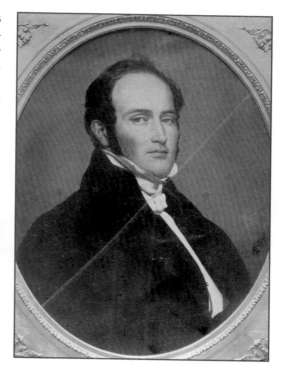

FIGURE 12–2. Prosper Ménière, French laryngologist who was the first to describe the unusual ear disease that was later named in his honor.

Lesions of the Inner Ear Giving Rise to Symptoms of Cerebral Congestion of Apoplectic Type. In this report, Ménière identified a condition in the inner ear that affected both hearing and balance. He concluded in this article that the auditory apparatus of the inner ear may be affected suddenly, causing ringing in the ear and loss of hearing. In addition, the balance structures of the inner ear could also be affected suddenly, resulting in attacks of dizziness and unsteady gait, which may be accompanied by nausea and vomiting. Ménière died in Paris of influenza pneumonia at the age of 63 years, the year after publication of his most famous work. Although Ménière's name is now known around the world, he did not receive the recognition due to him while he was alive.

Hermann von Helmholtz (1821–1894) was a German physicist who made outstanding contributions to the areas of human physiology, particularly in regard to the eye and ear (Figure 12–3). He invented the ophthalmoscope that was used for inspecting the interior of the eye and the ophthalmometer, a device used for measuring the eye's curvature. Helmholtz was also an authority on acoustics and hearing. In 1863, he published *On the Sensations of Tone as a Physiological Basis of the Theory of Music.* In this book, he described the placement of the higher frequency fibers at the basal end of the cochlea and the lower frequencies near the apex, which is now referred to as **tonotopic organization**.

Heinrich Hertz (1857–1894) was a German physicist who happened to be one of von Helmholtz's students (Figure 12–4). Hertz was the first to send and receive radio waves. He proved that electricity could be transmitted in

---

FYI

Gallaudet University, located in Washington, DC, was the first university in the world specifically designed to accommodate deaf and hard of hearing students. The university was established in 1864 during the presidency of Abraham Lincoln. The university is named after Thomas Hopkins Gallaudet who was the founder of the first school for deaf students in the United States. Hearing students are admitted to the graduate school, and degrees in audiology and speech-language pathology are offered.

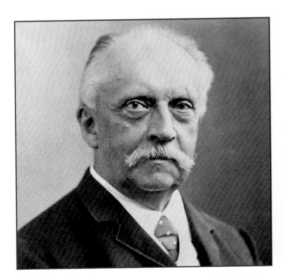

FIGURE 12–3. Hermann von Helmholtz, German physicist who made outstanding contributions to the areas of human physiology, particularly in regard to the eye and ear.

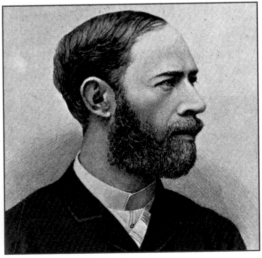

FIGURE 12–4. Heinrich Hertz, German physicist who was the first to send and receive electromagnetic radio waves.

electromagnetic waves, which travel at the speed of light. His experiments with electromagnetic waves eventually led to the development of the wireless telegraph and the radio. His name also became the term used for referring to the measure of frequency per unit of time, or the number of cycles per second (Hz). The hertz designation has been an official part of the international metric system since 1933. When we use the Hz notation to refer to a low-frequency or high-frequency hearing loss, we are acknowledging the pioneering work of Heinrich Hertz.

Hendrik Zwaardemaker (1857–1920) was both an otolaryngologist and a physiologist who was a professor at Utrecht University in the Netherlands (Figure 12–5). He was the first individual to describe the relationship between advanced aging and a high-frequency hearing loss, for which he coined the term **presbycusis**. Zwaardemaker studied various ways of assessing hearing and the use of whispered voice as a hearing test. He also worked on the physiology of speech production and examined acoustic properties of hearing aids. Since Zwaardemaker's initial description of presbycusis, extensive research has attempted to determine the precise physiological causes of presbycusis, which remain unknown.

Georg von Békésy (1899–1972) was a biophysicist born in Budapest, Hungary (Figure 12–6). His early research interest was focused on telecommunications and finding ways of improving the acoustic quality of long-distance telephone calls. However, he later turned his attention to the physics of sound and the physical processes involved in hearing. Békésy found that sound traveling

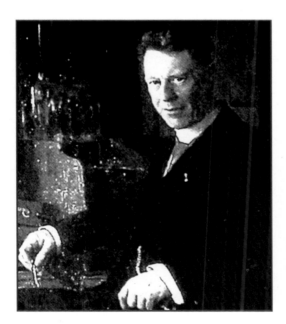

FIGURE 12–5. Hendrik Zwaardemaker, Dutch otolaryngologist who coined the term presbycusis.

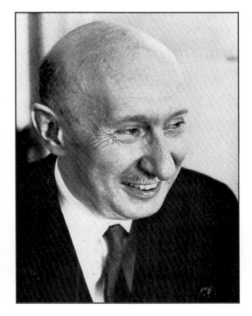

FIGURE 12–6. Georg von Békésy, Nobel Prize winner for his research on the functioning of the inner ear. From the University of Hawaii. Reprinted with permission.

through the cochlea flows as a series of waves. He demonstrated that these waves provide maximum stimulation of hair cells (i.e., auditory nerve receptors) at different places along the cochlea: low frequencies toward the apical end of the cochlea and high frequencies near its base. He discovered that the location of this maximum nerve receptor stimulation is the most important factor in determining the pitch and loudness of sounds. His work led to advances in ear surgery and the design of better hearing aids. In 1961, Békésy was awarded the Nobel Prize in Physiology and Medicine for his research on the function of the cochlea.

Rita Levi-Montalcini (1909–2012) was a Nobel Prize winning neurologist from Italy who discovered a protein that causes developing cells to grow by stimulating surrounding nerve tissue (Figure 12–7). She named this protein nerve growth factor. Since her initial discovery, nerve growth factor has been shown to play an important role in the growth of nerve fibers throughout the peripheral nervous system. The role of nerve growth factor in regenerating nerve fibers damaged in the cochlea of humans has yet to be proven; however, her initial discovery of this protein has opened an area of research that may someday lead to a cure for cochlea-based hearing loss.

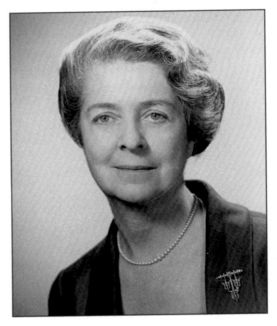

FIGURE 12–7. Rita Levi-Montalcini, Nobel Prize winning neurologist from Italy who discovered the protein called nerve growth factor.

(2) degree of hearing loss, (3) location of hearing loss, and (4) configuration of hearing loss.

Type of Hearing Loss

There are three types of hearing loss: (1) conductive, (2) sensorineural, and (3) mixed.

A **conductive hearing loss** is due to problems affecting sound transmission through the outer or middle ear. These problems disrupt the normal flow of sound entering the inner ear. People affected by a conductive hearing loss experience an overall reduction in the loudness of sounds and find it difficult to hear faint sounds. Most conductive losses are not permanent and can be treated medically or surgically.

TYPES OF HEARING DISORDERS

Hearing disorders can be described and categorized in a number of ways. For purposes of this introduction, they are presented below according to the categories of: (1) type of hearing loss,

However, if left untreated, conductive hearing losses can result in permanent impairment.

A **sensorineural hearing loss** occurs when there is damage to the inner ear or to the nerve pathways from the inner ear leading toward the brain. In addition to affecting loudness of hearing, a sensorineural loss can also affect the clarity of hearing. For example, normally we can hear sounds between the frequency range of 20 Hz to 20,000 Hz. In the case of a sensorineural hearing loss, a person may be unable to hear sounds higher than 2000 Hz, which can have a major impact on clearly understanding what is being said. Sensorineural hearing loss results in a permanent hearing disorder that cannot be corrected, although an individual's hearing can be improved by using some sort of hearing aid. A sensorineural hearing loss accounts for 90% of all types of hearing loss.

A **mixed hearing loss** is a combined conductive hearing loss and sensorineural hearing loss. The condition may result from a single pathology affecting both the middle ear and inner ear, or two separate independent pathologies. An example of mixed hearing would be a situation where a person may initially have a conductive hearing loss due to an ear infection and later develops a sensorineural hearing loss. Sometimes a mixed hearing loss is a temporary condition because the conductive component of the hearing loss can be successfully treated, leaving only the sensorineural hearing loss.

Degree of Hearing Loss

Degree of hearing loss refers to the **severity** of the loss. All types of hearing loss are defined by degrees. The severity of hearing loss can range from mild to profound, which represents the lowest or softest intensity level at which sound can be heard. A classification system for degree of hearing loss is listed in Table 12–2. Depending on the degree of hearing loss, various treatment options are suggested such as hearing aids, speech therapy, and counseling. The treatment approaches for working with hearing-impaired individuals are addressed in Chapter 13.

Location of Hearing Loss

A portion of Chapter 3 was dedicated to the anatomy of the auditory system. From this chapter, we learned that the entire auditory pathway can be neatly divided into two systems, peripheral and central auditory systems. Each of these systems provides an important contribution to the process of audition. Damage to any of the components composing the auditory system can result in

---

FYI

There is research indicating that the type of filling used to repair dental cavities might actually contribute to hearing loss. Use of amalgam fillings (an alloy of mercury) can have ototoxic effects and might be mistaken for presbycusis, especially among middle age and elderly adults who have had these fillings in their mouth over several years.

Table 12–2. Classification of Hearing Loss

Amount of Hearing Loss	Degree of Hearing Loss	Ability to Hear Speech
0–25 dB	None	No significant difficulty in hearing.
26–40 dB	Mild	Difficulty hearing soft speech and conversations, but can manage in quiet environments.
41–55 dB	Moderate	Difficulty understanding conversational speech, especially when there is background noise. Higher volume levels are required for listening to the television.
56–70 dB	Moderate-to-Severe	Speech clarity is significantly affected. Speech must be loud, and the person may have difficulty hearing in group conversations.
71–90 dB	Severe	Normal conversational speech cannot be heard. The person may also have difficulty with loud speech or only be able to understand shouted or amplified speech.
91+ dB	Profound	Unable to clearly understand even amplified speech.

different types and varying degrees of hearing loss. Disorders of hearing that occur at various locations throughout the auditory system are described below.

Disorders of the Outer Ear

When conditions occur that interfere or block the normal transmission of sound through the outer ear, a conductive hearing loss will occur. In most cases, this condition does not result in a severe hearing loss. Examples of outer ear disorders are: (1) atresia, (2) obstruction of the ear canal, and (3) otitis externa. The term **atresia** refers to an absence of a normal opening. Atresia can affect many structures in the body, and one of these structures is the ear canal. The absence of the external auditory canal is a congenital condition and almost always involves abnormalities of the

middle ear bones. A moderate conductive hearing loss typically is present in an atretic ear (Figure 12–8).

A common disorder of the outer ear involves an **obstruction** in the ear canal that prevents sound from normally entering the middle ear. The ear canal's natural secretion of ear wax, known as **cerumen** can become impacted to the point where normal hearing is affected (see Figure 12–8). Impacted cerumen is not unusual, with approximately 2 to 6% of the general population having this condition. A likely cause of impaction is through the misuse of cotton swabs, where the swab serves to push cerumen toward the tympanic membrane. As mentioned in Chapter 3, cerumen provides a beneficial function to the ear canal and normally does not need to be removed. Cerumen impaction is also prevalent among hearing

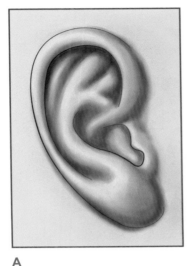
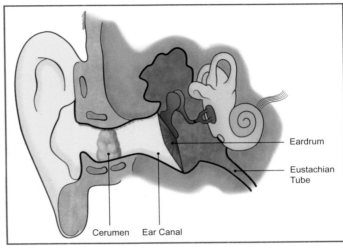

A   B

FIGURE 12–8. A. An illustration of atresia, where the ear canal fails to develop. **B.** An example of cerumen (earwax) impaction.

aid users. Problematic cerumen can be removed with dissolving drops, water jets ("irrigation"), or through the use of special instruments available to a qualified specialist.

Another disorder of the outer ear is **otitis externa**. The term otitis is Latin with *oto* referring to the ear, and *itis* meaning inflammation. So this particular condition is an infection of the outer (external) ear. The common term for otitis externa is swimmer's ear. In most cases, bacteria cause this infection in the thin layer of skin lining the canal. Our ear canals work best when they are dry, so if they are exposed to excess moisture, such as from frequent swimming, they are more likely to become infected. Swimmer's ear can be easily treated with antibiotic ear drops.

Disorders of the Middle Ear

Abnormalities of the middle ear will result in a conductive hearing loss. Examples of middle ear disorders are: (1) a perforated eardrum, (2) otitis media, and (3) otosclerosis. A hole or rupture in the tympanic membrane is called a **perforated eardrum**. This condition is accompanied by decreased hearing because the tympanic membrane ceases to work normally in the transmission of sound waves along the ossicular chain. The causes of a perforated eardrum are usually due to trauma or infection. Instances of trauma include a skull fracture or if a foreign object is pushed too far into the ear canal (Figure 12–9). A perforation can also result from a severe middle ear infection that causes the eardrum to rupture or tear. Most eardrum perforations heal on their own within weeks of the rupture, although some may take several months to heal. During the healing process, the ear must be protected from water to prevent further damage to the middle ear.

Otitis media refers to an inflammation of the middle ear cavity. Otitis media affects about two-thirds of children at least once before they reach their

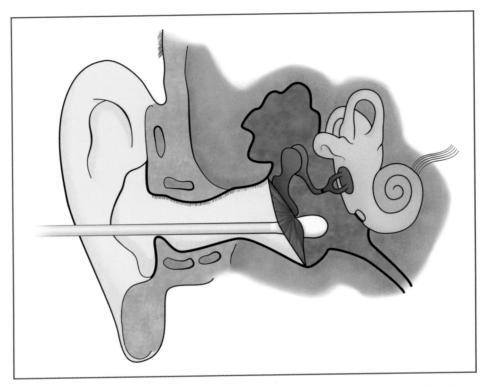

FIGURE 12–9. Example of a perforated tympanic membrane resulting from damage by a foreign object.

second birthday. The only childhood illness that occurs more often than otitis media is the common cold. An earache in children is often an indication of otitis media. The frequent occurrence of otitis media in young children is usually attributed to the small size, horizontal position, and immature functioning of their eustachian tube compared with adults, making it easier for infectious organisms in the mouth and nose to gain access to the middle ear (Figure 12–10). Otitis media can be further classified according to longevity and type of condition. Acute otitis media is an infection lasting less than three weeks. Subacute otitis media lasts between three weeks to three months, and chronic otitis media lasts longer than three months. **Otitis media with effusion** is a condition where a watery or mucus-like fluid fills the middle ear cavity. In some countries, the shorthand term used for otitis media with effusion is glue ear. Many times, the condition of otitis media can be diagnosed by examining the coloring of the tympanic membrane through the use of an **otoscope** (Figure 12–11). An otoscope is a standard piece of equipment found in most doctors' offices. Use of an otoscope allows for visualization of the outer ear, as well as a portion of the middle ear. Examination of the ear provides doctors with helpful information regarding a patient's overall health status.

Otosclerosis is the abnormal growth of spongy bone in the middle ear. This bone prevents the ossicular chain of

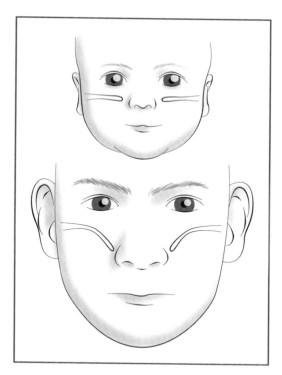

FIGURE 12–10. Depiction of infant and adult eustachian tubes. The horizontal angle of the tubes in infants makes them susceptible to ear infections.

the middle ear from working properly and causes hearing loss. The etiology of otosclerosis is not fully understood, although research has shown that otosclerosis tends to run in families so there may be a genetic component. On average, a person who has one parent with otosclerosis has a 25% chance of developing the disorder. Women are three times more likely to acquire the disease compared with men. There are also differences in regard to ethnicity with Caucasians more susceptible to the disease than Asians or Africans. One way of treating otosclerosis is to surgically repair the ossicular chain. Many times this involves **stapedectomy**, which is removal of all or a portion of the stapes and substitution of an artificial stapes.

Disorders of the Inner Ear

Damage to the inner ear will result in a sensorineural hearing loss. Problems of the inner ear represent the largest group of hearing disorders. These disorders can affect balance as well as hearing. Examples of inner ear disorders are: (1) prenatal causes, (2) meningitis, (3) ototoxic drugs, (4) Ménière disease, and (5) presbycusis. Prenatal causes are those that affect the mother and her developing fetus. The mother may acquire a virus during her pregnancy that has an adverse affect on the normal growth and development of the unborn child's cochlea. **Cytomegalovirus** is the most prevalent prenatal disease known to cause hearing loss. Cytomegalovirus is actually a very common viral illness. It belongs to the herpes virus family, which also includes viruses that are responsible for chicken pox, glandular fever, and cold sores. Between 50% and 85% of people in Australia, the United Kingdom, and the United States have had a cytomegalovirus infection by the time they are 40 years old. Cytomegalovirus infections are rarely serious in otherwise healthy children and adults. When symptoms do appear, they are similar to those seen in mononucleosis ("mono") and last a few weeks. Cytomegalovirus is only a risk when the mother develops a cytomegalovirus infection during pregnancy and passes this virus to the unborn baby before birth. The results can be severe with as many as 20% of these children failing to survive. The children who do survive may show intellectual disabilities, visual defects, and hearing loss. The severity of hearing loss can range from mild to profound.

Meningitis is an inflammation of the thin protective tissue that surrounds

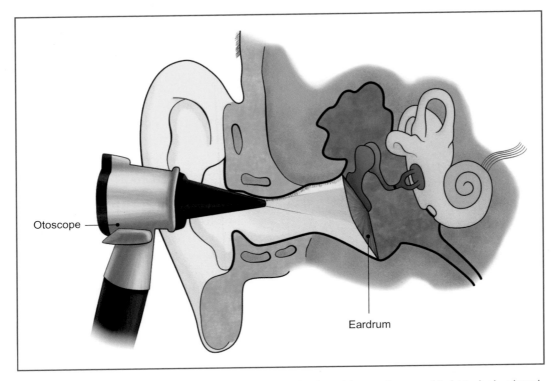

Otoscope

Eardrum

FIGURE 12–11. Example of an otoscope. The device shines a beam of light to help visualize and examine the condition of the ear canal and eardrum.

the brain and spinal cord, called the meninges. **Viral meningitis** usually does not cause serious illness, although in severe cases, it can cause prolonged fever and seizures. **Bacterial meningitis** is much rarer than viral meningitis but far more serious. Bacterial meningitis usually starts with bacteria that cause a cold-like infection. The infection can block blood vessels in the brain and lead to stroke and brain damage, as well as damage to other organs like the cochlea. Bacterial meningitis may lead to total deafness; however, early treatment with steroids can assist in reducing the severity of hearing loss.

An **ototoxic hearing loss** happens when someone takes or is given a drug that causes hearing loss as one of its side effects. There are roughly 200 prescription and over-the-counter drugs

recognized as ototoxic. Sometimes the drugs are needed to save lives, and hearing loss is the price paid for being able to live. Common medications that are known to be ototoxic include various antibiotics, chemotherapy medications, anesthetics, cardiac medications, steroids, mood altering drugs, and some vapors and solvents. Often an ototoxic hearing loss is reversible simply by discontinuation of the drug. People with an existing hearing loss need to be especially aware of the potential for ototoxic effects, as an ototoxic drug can worsen the hearing loss.

Ménière disease is an inner ear disorder caused by increased fluid pressure in the chambers of the inner ear. The disease affects both the balance and hearing systems of the inner ear, and usually just one ear is involved. There

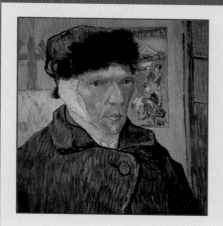
are various symptoms that are indicative of a person having Ménière disease. These symptoms include episodes of severe dizziness (i.e., vertigo), nausea, unilateral hearing loss, ringing in the ear (i.e., tinnitus), and a feeling of ear pressure or pain in the affected ear. The disease may be extremely debilitating. Episodes of dizziness can occur without warning and may last from minutes to several hours or even days. The cause of Ménière disease is unknown, although some feel it is a result of **endolymphatic hydrops**, which is the oversecretion of endolymph (i.e., the fluid contained within the cochlea). Surgery to drain excessive endolymph is found to help reduce the debilitating aspects of the disease. In extreme cases, the inner ear may be surgically destroyed to help alleviate vertigo and tinnitus, which results in permanent deafness of the affected ear.

Presbycusis is the gradual deterioration in hearing that happens as we grow older. It is likely the hearing mechanism begins to deteriorate shortly after birth, although most experts agree that by the age of 18 years, a natural reduction in the performance of our auditory system begins to occur. As we age, the

hair cells within the cochlea become damaged through normal wear and tear of use, particularly those that are found at the entrance (basal end) of the cochlea. This deterioration is synonymous with the entryway into a carpeted room. As years go by, the carpet fibers at the entryway of the room become flattened and damaged, whereas those at the back of the room retain their shape. As for the cochlea, this form of damage results in a high-frequency hearing loss that can start as early as middle age. The condition is to be expected in men by their early 60s and women by their late 60s. Presbycusis most often occurs in both ears. Because the process of loss is gradual, people who have presbycusis may not realize their hearing is diminishing. Between the ages of 65 to 75 years, about 35% of adults have a hearing loss. After the age of 75 years, hearing loss is found in almost 50% of all individuals.

Whereas presbycusis reflects a natural aging of the auditory system, **noise-induced hearing loss** is a form of impairment that mirrors that of presbycusis somewhat but can be found in people at a much younger age. This hearing loss is not a result of natural aging but rather damage due to exposure to excessive noise, whether at work or play. The National Foundation for the Deaf reports that one in four teenagers are likely to experience a hearing loss as a direct result of MP3 player listening habits. Among the elderly, it may be difficult to differentiate between presbycusis and noise-induced hearing loss simply because both pathologies affect hearing of high-frequency sounds. Noise-induced hearing loss is a preventable disorder that can be avoided by taking necessary precautions such as noise-reduction headphones or ear plugs.

Disorders of the Central Auditory System

Any damage to the auditory system running from the auditory nerve to the brain is called a **retrocochlear pathology** because the damage occurs beyond (or behind) the cochlea. One type of retrocochlear pathology is a tumor called an **acoustic neuroma** (Figure 12–12). An acoustic neuroma is a noncancerous (i.e., benign) brain tumor. All types of brain tumors are rare, and acoustic neuromas account for eight out of 100 primary brain tumors. An acoustic neuroma tends to grow very slowly and normally is not a life-threatening condition. In very rare cases, the tumor can grow large enough to press on the brain. However, most acoustic neuromas can be treated before they get to this stage. Typically, the tumor is only found on one side of the central auditory system. Approximately 50% of acoustic neuromas are treated by surgery where the tumor is removed. About 25% of neuro-

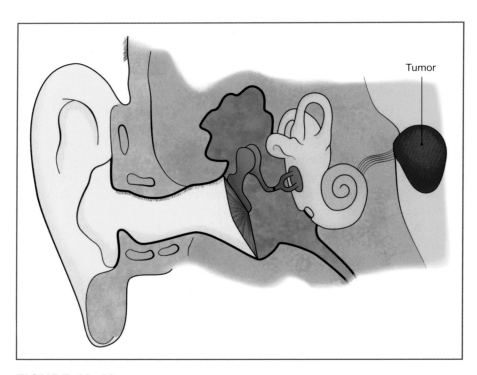

FIGURE 12–12. Illustration of an acoustic neuroma (tumor), resulting in a retrocochlear hearing loss.

mas are treated with radiation, and the remaining 25% are monitored (i.e., left untreated). Regardless of the treatment approach, an acoustic neuroma almost always results in total hearing loss in the affected ear. Each year in the United Kingdom and the United States approximately 13 people out of one million are diagnosed with an acoustic neuroma. Acoustic neuromas occur more often in women compared with men, although the reasons for this are not yet understood. People who are 30 to 60 years of age are usually affected.

Configuration of Hearing Loss

The configuration of a hearing loss refers to the extent of loss at various frequencies of hearing, ranging from low to high. The configuration of hearing loss gives an overall picture of a person's hearing acuity. For example, an individual who is unable to hear frequencies within the range of 2000 to 8000 Hz at a soft loudness level would show a **high-frequency hearing loss**. Some hearing loss configurations are flat, indicating the same amount of hearing loss for low-, middle-, and high-frequency sounds. Another aspect of hearing loss configuration is whether or not two ears are affected: A **unilateral hearing loss** means that only one ear is affected by the loss, and a **bilateral hearing loss** means both ears are affected. In addition, a hearing loss can be symmetrical or asymmetrical. A **symmetrical hearing loss** means the severity of loss and the frequencies affected are the same for both ears. An **asymmetrical hearing loss** means there is loss of hearing in both ears, but the severity of loss and frequencies affected are not identical. A final way of describing hearing loss

configuration relates to the change in hearing over time. A **progressive hearing loss** is one that becomes increasingly worse. This is found in conditions such as presbycusis. A **fluctuating hearing loss** is one whereby a person's hearing may improve or worsen from one day to next. This is often the case in conditions such as otitis media and Ménière disease.

Other Types of Hearing Disorders

There remain other types of hearing disorders that are less easy to classify according to a specific location along the auditory pathway. Two such types of disorder are tinnitus and auditory processing disorder. **Tinnitus** is the medical name used to describe a continuous noise in the ears. The term comes from the Latin word for *ringing*. Some people experience a mild ringing noise, whereas others are troubled by loud, high-pitched noises. Tinnitus can occur in one or both ears. Tinnitus is divided into two types: (1) objective and (2) subjective. Objective tinnitus is rare. In this condition, the faint noise generated in the ear can be heard (using special equipment) by somebody examining the patient. In such cases, the talents of an ENT surgeon are required to seek a surgical cure. Subjective tinnitus is by far the more frequently occurring form of the disorder. In this condition, the noise can only be heard by the patient. Subjective tinnitus is not a disease but a problem in the auditory pathway or in the central nervous system of the brain. There are many factors that have been associated with tinnitus including headaches, elevated blood pressure, emotional tension, exposure to loud noises, medications, allergies, and fatigue. Estimates from the United Kingdom, United States, Australia, and New Zealand indicate that tinnitus affects anywhere from 10 to 20% of the general population. Of these, about 1% experiences the condition to a disturbing degree.

Auditory processing refers to the way the brain makes sense out of the incoming signals from the auditory pathway. Auditory processing helps us to discriminate between different sounds, pick out sounds or speech from a noisy background, and understand speech when the sound quality is poor. The disorder known as an **auditory processing disorder** is a condition in which an individual demonstrates normal hearing and normal intelligence but may show a hearing problem in the sense that he or she is unable to process information normally. They can hear perfectly well but have trouble interpreting or understanding what is being said. Examples of the types of processing difficulties demonstrated by individuals with auditory processing disorder are shown in Table 12–3. The prevalence of auditory processing disorder in the general population has not been firmly established. Estimates indicate that auditory processing disorder occurs in approximately 3% of people, with a two-to-one ratio between males and females. Neurological disorders account for most instances of auditory processing disorder in adults. Among children,

Table 12–3. Types of Difficulties Shown by Individuals with an Auditory Processing Disorder

- Asks for things to be repeated
- Poor listening skills
- Mishears words
- Needs more time to process information
- Difficulty following multistep instructions given orally
- Difficulty hearing in background noise
- Distracted
- Low academic performance
- Language comprehension difficulty

a definitive neurological cause for auditory processing disorder is found in only 5% of diagnosed cases. The remaining occurrences have an unknown etiology. In these cases, auditory processing disorder has been called an invisible disability as there appears to be nothing physically wrong with the individual. The difficulties these individuals experience are often incorrectly assumed to be the result of an attention deficit or a lack of motivation. There are no established therapies for the treatment of individuals with auditory processing disorder. A general recommendation is to modify the environment by either minimizing background noise or increasing sound

FYI

Prolonged exposure to loud noise has resulted in many well-known musicians acquiring the condition of tinnitus. The list includes Jeff Beck, Bono, Bilinda Butcher, Cher, Eric Clapton, Phil Collins, Al Di Meola, Mick Fleetwood, Ted Nugent, Ozzy Osbourne, The Edge, Trent Reznor, Sting, Pete Townsend, and Neil Young.

amplification (such as in a classroom setting) to facilitate improved auditory processing.

ASSESSMENT OF HEARING DISORDERS

Audiometry is the quantitative measurement of hearing. Measurement of auditory function enables the audiologist to determine the type, degree, location, and configuration of hearing loss. Some of the tests performed to evaluate auditory function are: (1) pure-tone audiometry, (2) immittance testing, and (3) electrophysiologic testing.

Pure-Tone Audiometry

In **pure-tone audiometry**, a person's hearing acuity for each ear is measured for tones as low as 250 Hz and as high as 8000 Hz. Although our entire range of hearing extends from 20 Hz to 20,000 Hz, the 250 to 8000 Hz range is tested because this is the frequency range we use in order to clearly hear conversational speech. The device used to generate pure tones is called an **audiometer**. Pure-tone audiometry is usually completed while an individual is seated in a sound-isolated booth. During the test, the individual is asked to respond each time they hear the tone. Adult patients usually push a button when the tone is heard, and children will raise their hand (Figure 12–13). As part of the test, the audiologist determines the person's threshold for each of the tones. The **threshold** represents the loudness (dB) level at which tones are barely audible. Once determined, the threshold for each frequency is recorded on a graph known as an **audiogram**. The test frequencies (pure tones) are plotted on the horizontal axis of the audiogram, and the loudness threshold for each tone is indicated on the vertical axis. The symbols, "o" and "x" are used to indicate the thresholds of the right and left ear, respectively. A threshold value

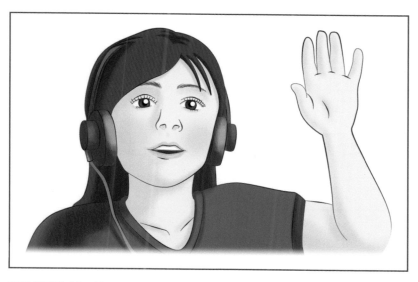

FIGURE 12–13. Example of pure-tone audiometry. A hand is raised in response to any sound that is heard.

of 0 to 20 dB is considered normal hearing acuity. It is possible to have scores less than 0, which indicate better than average hearing. A wide range of audiogram configurations are presented in Figure 12–14.

Two types of pure-tone testing are: (1) air conduction and (2) bone conduc-

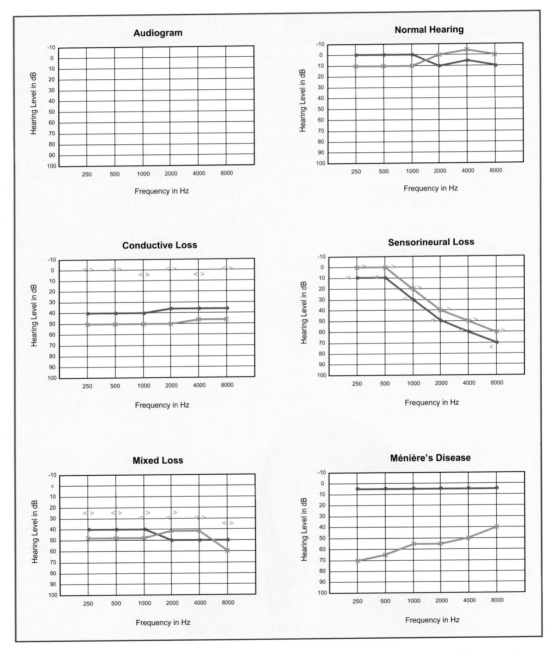

FIGURE 12–14. Audiograms depicting normal hearing and various types of hearing loss. The "x" symbol represents the left ear threshold, and the "o" symbol is the right ear. The "<" and ">" symbols represent bone conduction thresholds for the left and right ear, respectively.

tion. During **air conduction testing**, headphones are placed over the outer ear. Small foam insert-earphones are sometimes used in place of headphones. Insert-earphones are placed directly in the entrance to the ear canals. Air conduction testing is designed to examine a person's hearing of sounds as they travel through the air. The sound (pure tone) leaves the earphone and travels down the ear canal as an airborne acoustic signal. Air conduction testing allows the audiologist to examine a person's hearing as sound travels through the entire peripheral auditory system (Figure 12–15). It is not possible to determine the precise location of the impairment by air conduction testing alone. If the person's hearing thresholds for air conduction fall outside the normal range of hearing, it is necessary to perform a follow-up test known as **bone conduction testing**. In bone conduction testing, the pure tones are not presented as an airborne (acoustic) signal, but rather via a bone vibrator that is placed on the surface of the skull behind the ear (i.e., mastoid process of temporal bone). These tones are transmitted directly to the cochlea by vibrations in the skull, and toward the central auditory system (see Figure 12–15). Bone conduction testing bypasses the outer and middle ear systems because these parts of the auditory system are located outside of the skull. If a person was to show a hearing loss from air conduction testing but normal hearing from bone conduction testing, the hearing loss is likely to be an impairment of the outer or middle ear. This is called a conductive hearing loss (see Figure 12–14). A sensorineural hearing loss would be indicated if both air conduction and bone conduction hearing thresholds were higher than normal (see Figure 12–14). When both air and bone conduction thresholds are higher than normal but bone conduction was the higher of the two, a mixed hearing loss would be indicated.

Immittance Testing

The term immittance refers to ease or compliance of movement. In audiological testing, **immittance testing** is the ease with which sound travels from one medium to another, as from air to bone. These tests do not provide a direct measure of hearing loss, but rather yield information about the mobility of the tympanic membrane and functioning of the middle ear. Immittance tests are also considered **nonbehavioral tests** because the individual is not required to push a button or raise their hand for various tones. The response occurs naturally. Two types of immittance tests are: (1) tympanometry and (2) acoustic reflex.

Tympanometry is a testing methodology that gives useful information about the presence of fluid in the middle ear, mobility of the middle ear system, and ear canal volume. It provides a graphic representation of the relationship between air pressure in the

---

FYI

Sound can travel through any medium such as air, water, rock, and steel. Sound cannot travel through a vacuum because it is devoid of matter (i.e., particles). There is no sound in outer space.

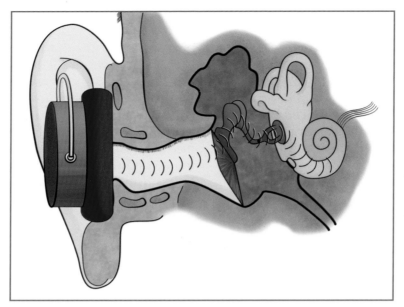

A

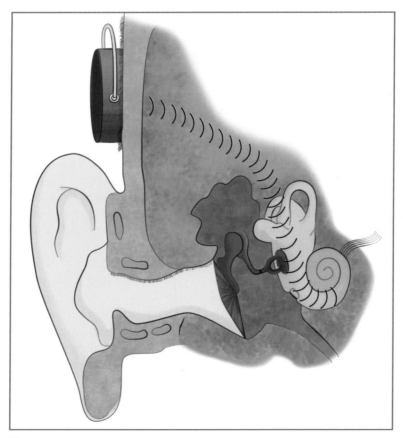

B

FIGURE 12–15. Example of air conduction (**A**) and bone conduction (**B**) pure-tone audiometric testing.

external ear canal compared with the movement of the tympanic membrane and middle ear ossicular chain. The test is noninvasive. A **tympanometer** instrument is used to perform the test. The instrument consists of a probe that is fitted snugly into the outer ear and slowly changes the pressure within the ear canal, at the same time transmitting a tone into the canal. The tone strikes the tympanic membrane, causing vibration of the middle ear. Some of this sound is reflected back and picked up by the tympanometer (Figure 12–16). The amount of sound that is reflected back from the eardrum as the pressure in the ear canal varies is quantified and plotted on a graph. These **tympanogram** plots are classified as type A (normal middle ear functioning), type B (flat, indicative of middle ear fluid or punctured eardrum), and type C (off-center, indicative of eustachian tube malfunction). Examples of tympanogram plots are shown in Figure 12–16.

The **acoustic reflex** is an involuntary contraction of the stapedius muscle located in the middle ear. The response is obtained by presenting high intensity sounds via a probe inserted into the ear canal. High-intensity sounds (e.g., 90 dB) are presented, and the probe detects the decibel level at which the stapedius muscle contracts. Acoustic reflex testing is completed with the same equipment used for tympanometry. Acoustic reflex testing is done in each ear following tympanometry. We all should show an acoustic reflex to loud sounds. The reflex is actually a protective response of the middle ear to prevent extremely loud sounds from entering (and subsequently damaging) the cochlea. If an acoustic reflex is not present, a middle ear or brainstem disorder would be suspected.

Electrophysiologic Testing

Electrophysiologic tests are nonbehavioral tests that are administered to difficult-to-assess individuals or to determine the specific site of an auditory lesion. **Otoacoustic emissions** and the **auditory brainstem response** are the most frequently performed electrophysiological tests. They are fast and easy to administer and do not require the individual to give a behavioral response (such as raising a hand). Otoacoustic emissions are faint acoustic sounds that are generated in the cochlea in response to sounds presented to the inner ear. They are considered to be epiphenomena (i.e., a secondary activity) and a byproduct of a normally functioning cochlea. A healthy cochlea creates internal vibrations whenever it processes sound. Impaired ears usually do not. These faint sound emissions travel back through the middle ear and into the ear canal where they can be measured with a tiny microphone. Emissions are thought to be generated by the hair cells within the cochlea. Because most forms of hearing involve the loss (i.e., death) of hair cells, the lack of otoacoustic emissions is a good predictor of cochlear hearing loss. Otoacoustic emissions are measured by a probe placed at the opening of the ear canal. An illustration of the otoacoustic emissions setup is shown in Figure 12–17.

In the **auditory brainstem response** technique, an **electroencephalograph** is used to measure brain wave activity associated with the reception of sound. Prior to the test, three electrodes are attached, one to the forehead and one on each ear. A series of acoustic clicks is then presented to one ear via an earphone. The electrodes pick up the brain's response to those clicks, which appears as a

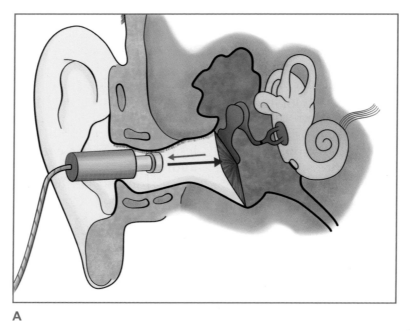

A

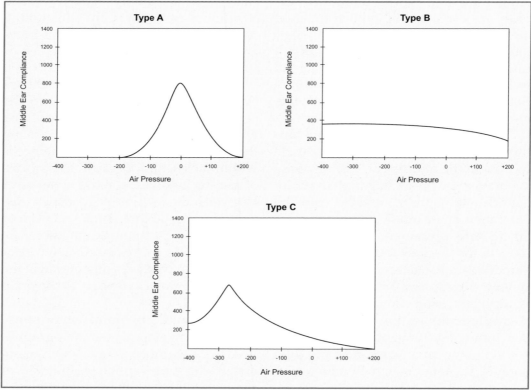

B

FIGURE 12–16. A. An illustration of tympanometry testing. A probe is inserted into the ear canal and delivers a tone to measure compliance of the tympanic membrane. Part of the probe tone is reflected backward, and some is admitted into the middle ear. **B.** Examples of three types of tympanograms.

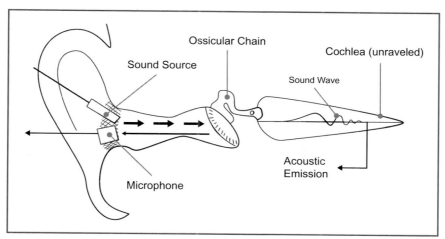

A

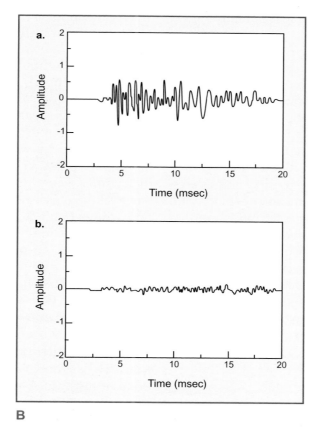

B

FIGURE 12–17. A. Depiction of the equipment setup for evoking and recording an otoacoustic emission. **B.** An example of normal otoacoustic emissions (*top panel*) and a low emission level (*bottom panel*), which may indicate cochlear dysfunction.

characteristic waveform with five peaks or waves that occur within the first 10 milliseconds of response. The waveform reflects the speed of electrical impulses traveling along the hearing pathway from the inner ear through the brainstem. The person being tested must remain very still during the test and may even be sleeping. An illustration of the auditory brainstem response setup is shown in Figure 12–18. If the auditory brainstem response waveform is missing one or more of the five peaks, or there is a time delay in the appearance of these peaks, the result is indicative of a significant hearing loss or neurological dysfunction.

Evaluating the hearing abilities of a newborn is a difficult task. Infants cannot respond with words or raise their hand to indicate what they hear and when. However, early detection of hearing problems is important. We have increasing evidence that difficulties in hearing during the infancy period may cause irreparable delays in a child's cognitive and communication development. Currently there is a worldwide emphasis for **universal newborn screening** of newborn hearing. Many countries (e.g., Canada, United Kingdom, United States, and New Zealand) have enacted mandatory screening of newborns shortly after birth. The otoacoustic emissions and auditory brainstem response tests are the primary instruments for evaluating a newborn's hearing.

CULTURAL CONSIDERATIONS AND HEARING DISORDERS

There are a wide range of cultural and ethnic variables in regard to hearing loss and specific types of hearing disorders. For example, the occurrence of otitis media among indigenous populations such as Hawaiians, New Zealand Maori, Australian Aboriginals, and Native Americans is unusually high. The high occurrence is attributed to the general social and physical environment, limited medical attention, allergies, and possibly also anatomical predispositions. For many nonindigenous children, especially those with good access to medical treatment, middle ear problems and associated hearing loss have been resolved by the time they arrive at school. For most indigenous children, the ramifications of chronic otitis media may disadvantage these children throughout the school years and into adulthood.

Epidemiological studies have consistently demonstrated that age-related hearing loss is most common in white men, followed by white women, black men, and black women, suggesting that whites are more vulnerable to the harmful effects of noise exposure than non-whites (Ishii & Talbott, 1998). It is interesting to note that tribal people in rural Africa do not seem to experience as much age-related hearing loss compared with adults with European backgrounds. One proposed explanation is that melanin-A pigment is found in higher levels among blacks compared with whites (Helzner et al., 2005). Research has shown that high concentrations of melanin-A within the cochlear hair cells may serve to protect hair cells from damage. In addition to race, gender has also been found to affect one's chances of developing an age-related hearing loss. Men are five times more likely than women to acquire a hearing loss at some point in their lifetime. This sex imbalance is attributed to likely

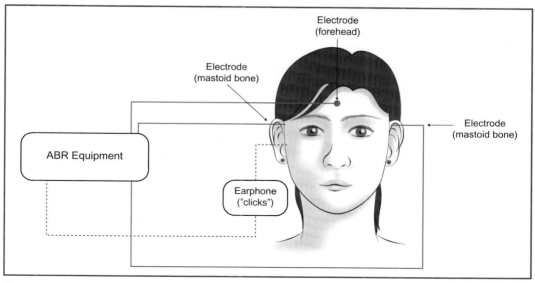

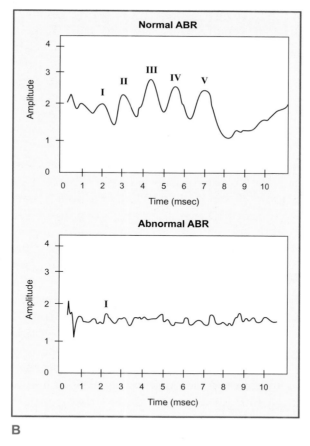

FIGURE 12–18. A. Depiction of the equipment setup for evoking and recording an auditory brainstem response. **B.** An example of normal auditory brainstem response with five distinct waveform peaks (*top panel*) and an abnormal auditory brainstem response indicative of a brainstem tumor (*lower panel*).

biological differences between men and women, as well as the tendency for men to work in occupations that may increase the chance of acquiring a noise-induced hearing loss.

Finally, hearing loss can affect one's culture in regard to participating in society at large. People with hearing loss are less likely to participate in social activities than people without hearing loss. For example, among people over the age of 65 years, those with a hearing loss are less likely to engage in community volunteer work compared with those without a hearing loss. Hearing loss can also affect an individual's emotional well-being. Among people age 70 and older, those with a hearing loss are more likely to experience bouts of depression compared with those without a hearing loss (Morgan-Jones, 2001).

CURRENT RESEARCH IN HEARING DISORDERS

Earbud Deafness

The baby boomer generation was the first to demonstrate that loud rock music was hazardous to hearing. The development of MP3 players is likely to significantly increase the occurrence of noise-induced hearing loss and tinnitus for Generation X and Y'ers. These devices use earbud earphones, rather than headphones, which are situated directly in the entrance of the ear canal. They efficiently funnel music down the ear canal and enable the user to turn up the volume without disrupting others. As a result, MP3 players easily desensitize the user to dangerously high sound levels. These devices are able to store thousands of songs that can be played continuously for hours without the need for recharging. Most MP3 players produce sound in excess of 100 dB. This situation sets the stage for prolonged exposure to high levels of loudness, aptly named Earbud Deafness Syndrome. Recent research has shown a jump in the prevalence of hearing loss in adolescents in the past 25 years, which is attributable to earbud use (Shargorodsky, Curhan, Curthan, & Eavey, 2010).

A recent survey at the University of Hong Kong examined the listening habits of 1,000 young adults who were MP3 users for more than one year (Hong Kong Society for the Deaf, 2007). The results found that 70% of users would turn up the volume of their music player in noisy surroundings. One third of the users perceived that their hearing sensitivity had worsened since they started using music players, and 20% experienced ringing in their ears within a short period of time after turning off their music players. Researchers have found that exposure to sounds in excess of 80 dB for only 90 minutes duration is sufficient to cause a hearing loss. Audi-

FYI

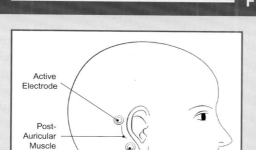

Researchers discovered that muscles located behind the ear could be deliberately activated (and measured) when sound was presented to the ears. The phenomenon has been referred to as the **postauricular muscle response**. This naturally occurring response has prompted a number of researchers to consider using the postauricular muscle response as a method of screening for hearing impairment, especially in the infant population (Purdy, Agung, Hartley, Patuzzi, & O'Beirne, 2005).

ologists recommend what is called the **60-60 rule**, which translates to a listening level of 60% (of the maximum volume) for no more than 60 minutes. The full impact of MP3 players on the occurrence of noise-induced hearing loss has yet to be determined. Early indications are that young people are putting themselves at risk for permanent hearing loss by exposing themselves to excessive noise.

Tinnitus

The American Tinnitus Association reports that approximately two million Americans suffer from severe tinnitus. The definitive cause of tinnitus has yet to be determined, and there is no magic pill for the treatment of tinnitus. We have known for some time that exposure to loud noise appears to be a factor that triggers the onset of tinnitus. Recent research indicates that tinnitus can either originate in the brain or cochlea. Imaging techniques such as functional magnetic resonance imaging and positron emission tomography have revealed that areas of the brain that process information from the ears are more active in tinnitus sufferers than in people without the condition. As a next stage, researchers are trying to stimulate these overactive areas of the brain to see whether they can reduce people's perceptions of tinnitus. There is also evidence that tinnitus may originate within the cellular structure of the cochlea. Scientists have discovered that a unique set of cells in the cochlea release a chemical called **adenosine triphosphate** (ATP), which causes the hearing system to generate brain activity in the absence of sound. By controlling the release of ATP, it may be possible to reduce or eliminate tinnitus (Tritsch, Yi, Gale, Glowatzki, & Bergles, 2007).

Some of the current treatment approaches for tinnitus include devices that look like hearing aids and produce sound that will mask or cover up tinnitus.

Cognitive behavioral therapy is a treatment administered by a psychotherapist that seeks to change people's attitudes and behavior. When used to treat tinnitus, it seems to improve patients' quality of life, even when the volume of noise from the tinnitus remains the same. Another new therapy is **neuromonics**, which was developed in Australia. This therapy involves the combined use of acoustic stimulation (namely music) with a structured program of counseling and support. The therapy approach is in need of independent assessment to demonstrate its benefits. Finally, research is underway exploring the use of a biomedical implant that stimulates the vagus nerve. The vagus nerve extends throughout the body with nerve connections to the ear. Stimulation of the vagus nerve serves to overexcite the auditory cortex, which may lead to a reduction in tinnitus symptoms (Porter et al., 2012).

Vestibular Prostheses

Neuroprosthetics is an area of considerable scientific and clinical interest. Since the introduction of the cardiac pacemaker in 1932, there have been developments in neuroprosthetic techniques for bladder and bowel control, deep brain stimulation for Parkinson disease (see Chapter 9), restoration of respiration for paralyzed individuals, and the development of cochlear implants to improve hearing (see Chapter 13). Individuals suffering from dizziness and balance disorders may also benefit from the progress made in neuroprosthetics. The inner ear's vestibular system provides information about self-motion and helps stabilize vision during movement. Damage to this system can result in dizziness, vertigo, nausea, blurred vision, and instability in walking. Medical, surgical, and rehabilitative approaches are all used to treat balance problems. Even though all of these approaches have greatly improved over time, they are still not 100% effective in all cases. Vestibular prostheses include a range of approaches to vestibular impairment. All approaches rely on motion detectors that measure head movement and send a signal back to the central nervous system to process these motion cues. Both implantable and nonimplantable prostheses are currently being developed. An implantable prosthesis delivers self-motion cues to the central nervous system via implanted stimulators directly within the vestibular nerve. A nonimplantable prosthesis is a less invasive means of providing some self-motion cues. They are sensory substitution devices that send motion and balance information to the central nervous system through sound, vision, tactile vibration, or electrostimulation of the tongue. Although not yet available clinically, vestibular prosthetics could provide another option for those with balance problems, as well as for those who are elderly and prone to falling (Wall, 2008).

HEARING DISORDERS ON THE WORLD WIDE WEB

Listed below are websites that provide further information on the topic of hearing disorders. At the time of publication, each website was freely accessible.

Child and Adult Hearing Test Video
http://www.youtube.com/user/ UniCanterburyCMDS/videos

The Wonderful Hearing and Sound Activity
http://www.wonderville.ca/asset/how-we-hear

Listen to Your Buds
http://www.asha.org/buds/

Pediatric Hearing Loss Video
http://www.infanthearing.org/videos/index.html

Sound Advice for Farmers
http://nasdonline.org/video/1/V000001/sound-advice-for-farming.html

Tinnitus Video
http://www.ata.org/about-ata/news-pubs/video

STUDY QUESTIONS

1. List and describe the various categories of deafness.
2. How do conductive and sensorineural hearing losses differ?
3. What are the major disorders of the outer, middle, and inner ear?
4. List and describe the tests used to evaluate auditory function.
5. What are some of the cultural and ethnic variables in regard to hearing loss?

REFERENCES

Helzner, E. P., Cauley, J. A., Pratt, S. R., Wisniewski, S. R., Zmuda, J. M., Talbott, E. O., . . . Newman, A. B. (2005). Race and sex differences in age-related hearing loss: The health, aging and body composition study. *Journal of the American Geriatric Society, 53*, 2119–2127.

Hong Kong Society for the Deaf. (2007). *A study on the impact of MP3 players on hearing amongst young people.* Retrieved from http://www.deaf.org.hk/documents/press_release/2005_7/mp3_press_030207_e.pdf

Ishii, E., & Talbott, E. (1998). Race/ethnicity differences in the prevalence of noise-induced hearing loss in a group of metal fabricating workers. *Journal of Occupational and Environmental Medicine, 40*, 661–666.

Morgan-Jones, R. A. (2001). *Hearing differently: The impact of hearing impairment on family life.* London, UK: Whurr.

Porter, B., Khodaparast, N., Fawaz, T., Cheung, R., Ahmed, S., Vrana, . . . & Kilgard, M. (2012). Repeatedly pairing vagus nerve stimulation with a movement reorganizes the cortex. *Cerebral Cortex, 22*, 2365–2374.

Purdy, S. C., Agung, K. B., Hartley, D., Patuzzi, R. B., & O'Beirne, G. A. (2005). The post-auricular muscle response: An objective electrophysiological method for evaluating hearing sensitivity. *International Journal of Audiology, 44*, 625–630.

Shargorodsky, J., Curhan, S., Curthan, G., & Eavey, R. (2010). Change in prevalence of hearing loss in U.S. adolescents. *Journal of the American Medical Association, 304*, 772–778.

Tritsch, N., Yi, E., Gale, J., Glowatzki, E., & Bergles, D. (2007). The origin of spontaneous activity in the developing auditory system. *Nature, 450*, 50–55.

Wall, C. (2008, July). Vestibular prostheses: Engineering and biomedical issues. *ASHA Leader, 13*(9), 14–17.

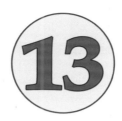

AUDITORY REHABILITATION

OBJECTIVES

After reading this chapter, the student should be able to:

■ Define aural rehabilitation and understand why the service is necessary for those who have hearing loss.

■ Describe the components of a hearing aid.

■ Understand the different types and styles of amplification or assistive listening devices plus the related advantages and disadvantages of each device.

■ Explain the nature and features of various auditory implants.

■ Describe the speech and language features that accompany a severe hearing impairment.

■ Describe the types of aural rehabilitation programs available to children and adults.

■ Discuss, compare, and contrast the different types of communication options, methods, training approaches, and philosophies (e.g., oral/aural, total communication, sign only, ASL/BSL).

■ Discuss issues pertaining to Deaf culture.

INTRODUCTION

Hearing loss is referred to as an invisible condition, yet its impact is anything but invisible (Tye-Murray, 2009). Whether the severity of hearing loss is mild or profound, it can have serious consequences on an individual's overall well-being. A number of devices to improve hearing and various forms of treatment have been developed to assist individuals with a diagnosed hearing loss. Decisions regarding the best approach are guided by factors such as the age of the person and the type of hearing problem they demonstrate, with the ultimate goal of improving an individual's communication and overall quality of life. The purpose of this chapter is to provide background on the tools and approaches used to help improve hearing and minimize the consequences of a hearing loss.

TERMINOLOGY AND DEFINITIONS

Aural rehabilitation involves techniques used with people who are hearing impaired to improve their ability to communicate, and this involves both listening and speaking. Presumably, these individuals once demonstrated normal hearing earlier in life. Since then, a hearing impairment has occurred, requiring assistance in improving their communication abilities in order to compensate for sounds of speech and daily living they no longer hear clearly. People who are hearing impaired at birth also require assistance in compensating for their hearing loss. For these individuals, the more appropriate term is **aural habilitation**. Aural rehabilita-

tion (including habilitation) is all about learning how to take advantage of what a person hears and sees in the environment. The particulars of a rehabilitation program are unique to each individual. A person's age, severity of hearing loss, and daily living environment are taken into consideration. For example, an individual who is **hard of hearing** shows a partial hearing impairment that may range from mild to severe. The individual's needs could be quite different from those of an individual with **deafness**, who has minimal or no hearing. Aural rehabilitation typically is provided by an audiologist, although speech-language pathologists and teachers of the deaf or hard of hearing may also make important contributions. There are various locations where aural rehabilitation occurs, including hospitals, nursing homes, community centers, as well as the classroom.

HISTORIC ASPECTS OF AURAL REHABILITATION

Origins of Aural Rehabilitation

The concept of aural rehabilitation was developed in the 1940s as a response to World War II. Prior to this time, there was no particular program for improving the quality of life for adults with postlingual hearing loss, despite schools for the deaf having been in existence since the late 1800s. Many individuals who served in the war developed severe cases of noise-induced hearing loss. These losses could not be treated using medical or surgical techniques. Military hospitals began to develop aural rehabilitation programs to assist these injured soldiers. Specialists in fields such as speech pathology, psychology, medicine, and deaf education were brought together to design aural rehabilitation programs. Lip reading was stressed as one of the major rehabilitation approaches. During the 1940s, wearable hearing aids were also available and, along with lip reading, became a significant component of rehabilitation.

The need for a specially qualified individual to assist with the needs of people with hearing loss eventually led to the creation of the profession of audiology. The establishment of audiology contributed to new techniques for diagnosing and managing hearing impairment for children and adults. However, the major focus of the audiology profession during the period of 1950 to 1980 was on the diagnosis of hearing loss, with far less attention placed on the rehabilitation of hearing loss. The lack of attention to rehabilitation was driven by the view that it was unethical for an audiologist to sell a hearing aid. Such an activity was left to salespeople who had little or no training in audiological care. Ironically, this created a situation in which the actual rehabilitation of indi-

viduals with hearing loss was performed by individuals far less qualified than audiologists. All of this changed in 1978 when the American Speech and Hearing Association permitted audiologists to dispense hearing aids. Today, audiologists are able to provide comprehensive diagnostic and rehabilitative services to individuals with hearing loss. This situation has led to enormous improvements in the provision of audiological care.

History of Hearing Devices

Dating back to the earliest hearing devices (or aids), their function has remained essentially unchanged: to increase the loudness of sound. Prior to the 20th century, the only way to provide amplification was to reduce the amount of outside, distracting noise. The primary way to accomplish this noise reduction was to filter out other noise by directing the desired sound straight into the ear with some kind of tube or trumpet (Figure 13–1). These

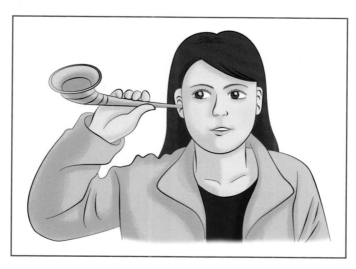

FIGURE 13–1. Early hearing aid, known as an ear trumpet. The instrument was designed to reduce the amount of distracting noise.

trumpets were large and awkward, although some models could be worn on the head and attached to a harness. Cupping your hand behind your ear gives a similar (but smaller) amplification effect.

Hearing aid technology has certainly come a long way in the past 100 years. Changes in hearing aids were linked to two important milestones in technology: (1) the advent of electricity and (2) Alexander Graham Bell's work on the telephone. Early electric hearing aids used the concept of a **microphone** that picks up sound, an **amplifier** which makes the sound louder, and a **speaker** that delivers the amplified sound to the ear. The first electric hearing aids were created around 1900 and were so large that they sat on a table. The cost of these was far beyond the means of most. In the early 1920s, hearing aid technology incorporated the use of vacuum tubes, which allowed a much more efficient method for amplifying sound. However, the early electric hearing aids were still unwieldy and could not be carried around easily. The miniaturization of batteries in the 1930s led to a significant decrease in the size of hearing aids. Hearing aids were made portable by allowing the user to wear a battery pack. By the early 1950s, vacuum tubes were replaced by transistors, and this resulted in a technological revolution in the design of hearing aids. Early transistor hearing aids were designed to fit within the frames of eyeglasses. Later, they were adapted to fit behind the ear. The 1990s saw a major shift in hearing aid technology from analog to digital circuitry, which led to major improvements in sound quality. In spite of the many changes in hearing aid design and technology over the past 100 years, they still rely on the concept of a microphone, amplifier, and speaker.

Deaf Education

Pedro Ponce de León (1520–1584), a Benedictine monk living in Spain, was the first teacher of the deaf in the modern era (Figure 13–2). His students were mostly children of aristocrats who had the financial means to provide their children with private tutoring. His work with these deaf children focused on helping them learn how to speak intelligibly. He also instructed the children in sign language. The monks observed daily periods of silence and had developed a series of hand gestures to help communicate during those times. Thus, it was natural for de León to apply this form of communication with his deaf students. The prevailing opinion among most Europeans in the 1500s was that people with deafness were incapable

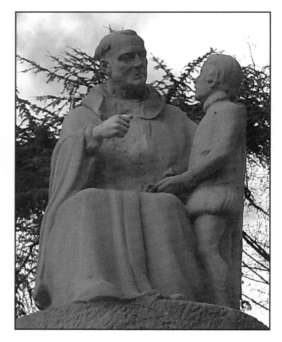

FIGURE 13–2. Monument of Pedro Ponce de León in Madrid, Spain who was the first teacher of the deaf circa 1550.

of being educated. Many even believed that the deaf were too intellectually disabled to be eligible for salvation under Christian doctrine. So de León's work with the deaf was considered quite bold and courageous. He was able to demonstrate that these children could not only learn to speak but could also learn to read and write.

Laurent Clerc (1785–1869) was born in a small village near Lyons, France (Figure 13–3A). Although he was French, Clerc is considered by many to be the "father of deaf education" in the United States. He was born hearing, but as an infant fell from his high chair, which resulted in a complete loss of hearing in both ears. He entered the Royal Institution for the Deaf in Paris where he excelled in his studies. His outstanding academic abilities, in spite of a profound hearing loss, caught the attention of a visiting American, **Thomas Hopkins Gallaudet** (1787–1851) (Figure 13–3B). Gallaudet invited Clerc to visit the United States, and the two eventually established the first school for the deaf in Hartford, Connecticut, now known as the American School for the Deaf. Clerc never returned to France and dedicated his life to educating deaf children. The American School for the Deaf remains the oldest existing school in the United States for the education of deaf students. Gallaudet University in Washington, DC, is named in honor of Thomas Gallaudet (see also Chapter 12).

Laura Bridgman (1829–1889) was born in Hanover, New Hampshire (Figure 13–4). At two years of age, she developed scarlet fever. The illness killed two of her older sisters and one of her brothers, but she survived, although without vision or hearing. A courageous individual, she was the first deaf-blind individual to be successfully educated in the modern era. She attended the Perkins School for the Blind in Massachusetts,

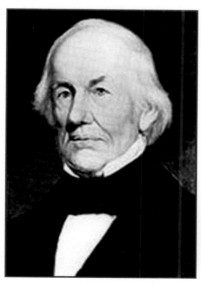
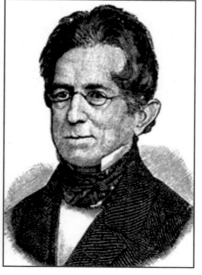

A   B

FIGURE 13–3. A. Laurent Clerc. **B.** Thomas Hopkins Gallaudet established the first school for the deaf in the United States.

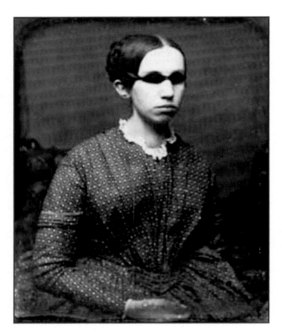

FIGURE 13–4. Laura Bridgman, the first person with deaf-blindness to be formally educated in the United States.

where she learned to read, write, and also sew. She eventually became a sewing teacher at the school and remained there until her death. Bridgman was famous for her accomplishments, which were described in newspapers and magazines worldwide. Her fame was later eclipsed by that of Helen Keller.

Helen Keller (1880–1968) was born in Tuscumbia, Alabama (Figure 13–5). Her birth history was quite similar to Laura Bridgman's—Helen had a normal birth but at the age of 19 months developed scarlet fever that left her deaf and blind. Her only companion until the age of six years was the family housekeeper, named Martha Washington. As Keller grew older, the family became increasingly frustrated in their attempts to communicate with their daughter. Helen's mother eventually read about the success of Laura Bridgman and later

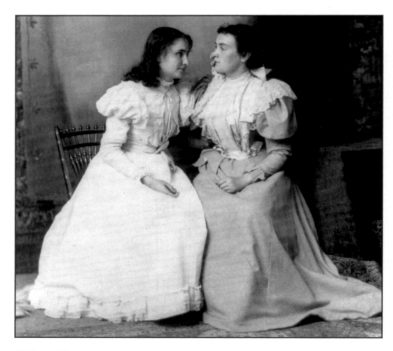

FIGURE 13–5. The student Helen Keller and her teacher Anne Sullivan.

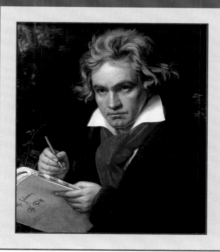

The life of German composer **Ludwig van Beethoven** (1770–1827) was affected by hearing problems. Beethoven did not become suddenly deaf—his loss of hearing was a slow process, spanning approximately 20 years. He was known to use a hearing trumpet. By the age of 50, he was totally deaf and could not hear music. In his years of total deafness, he completed his Ninth Symphony. It is said that after his first public performance of the symphony, he cried when he was turned around in order to see the audience's response to the music.

visited a local expert on the problems of deaf children. This expert was Alexander Graham Bell, and he recommended that the family take Helen to the Perkins School for the Blind. It was there that Helen met her teacher **Anne Sullivan** (1866–1936) who would become Helen's companion for the next 50 years. In 1904, Helen graduated from Radcliffe College, becoming the first deaf-blind person to earn a Bachelor of Arts degree. She and Anne went on a series of lecture tours around the world, speaking of her experiences. She became a major advocate for ensuring the rights of the deaf and blind. During her lifetime, she was introduced to every U.S. president from Grover Cleveland to Lyndon B. Johnson, and met many celebrities as well.

TREATMENT APPROACHES: HEARING REHABILITATION

One feature of aural rehabilitation is to directly treat the hearing loss. Three approaches to treating hearing loss are: (1) surgery, (2) hearing aid fitting, and (3) auditory implants.

Surgical Treatment

Two surgical procedures that address pathology of the tympanic membrane and middle ear are myringotomy and tympanoplasty. **Myringotomy** involves making a small incision in the eardrum to drain fluid that has accumulated in the middle ear space and serves to relieve pressure within the middle ear. The surgery is often performed on children who are prone to otitis media with effusion, although adults occasionally acquire similar problems requiring the myringotomy procedure. The buildup of fluid implies that the eustachian tube is not functioning and is unable to perform its normal role of keeping the middle ear dry and ventilated. The fluid buildup creates a conductive hearing loss, and once the fluid is drained, the child's hearing is essentially restored. As part of the surgery, a small **ventilation tube** (also called a **pressure equalization**

tube or **grommet**) is placed in the area of the incision. The tube serves to ventilate the middle ear and prevent fluid from accumulating (Figure 13–6). Most tubes are made of a synthetic plastic material, such as silicone or Teflon. They

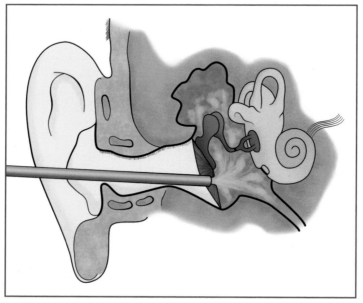

A

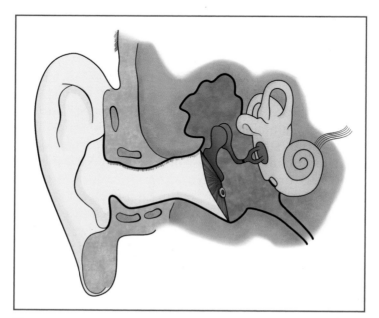

B

FIGURE 13–6. **A.** Myringotomy procedure. **B.** Insertion of a ventilation tube (i.e., grommet) in the tympanic membrane.

typically stay in place for around nine months before they are pushed out by the rapidly healing eardrum. A small scar usually forms in the eardrum, although the scarring does not impair hearing. The surgery is an outpatient procedure, meaning the patient returns home on the same day the surgery took place.

Tympanoplasty is a microsurgical procedure to repair a perforated tympanic membrane or reconstruct the small bones of the middle ear. The procedure can also help treat certain types of hearing loss and prevent infection of the middle ear. Three types of tympanoplasty are: (1) myringoplasty, which is a repair of a tear in the eardrum; (2) tympanoplasty with ossiculoplasty, which is a repair of a tear in the eardrum and correction of a defect in middle ear ossicles; and (3) tympanoplasty with mastoidectomy, which is a repair of an eardrum tear and removal of a bony infection in the area behind the ear. An illustration of tympanoplasty is shown in Figure 13–7.

Hearing Devices

The use of hearing aids to treat hearing loss typically is considered when no medical or surgical option is available to correct the loss. As mentioned earlier, a hearing aid consists of three major components: (1) the microphone, (2) amplifier, and (3) speaker. All components are housed in a plastic case that protects them and allows the hearing aid to be fitted on the ear (Figure 13–8). The microphone serves to transform the incoming acoustic sound into an electrical signal. The amplifier then increases the intensity of the electrical signal. A programmable filter is an additional feature of the amplifier. Filters have the ability to selectively modify sound, so only the sounds needed by the person with a hearing loss are amplified. The speaker converts the electrical signal that has been amplified back into an acoustic sound, which is transmitted down the ear canal. The hearing aid user can regulate loudness with a volume control.

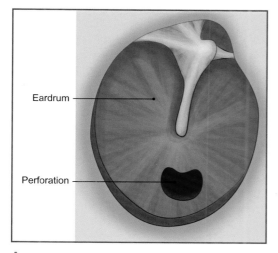

A

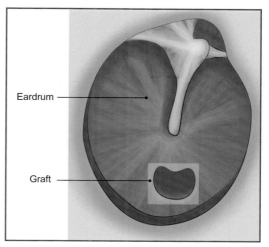

B

FIGURE 13–7. A. Example of a perforated (punctured) tympanic membrane. **B.** Tympanoplasty involving repair of the puncture.

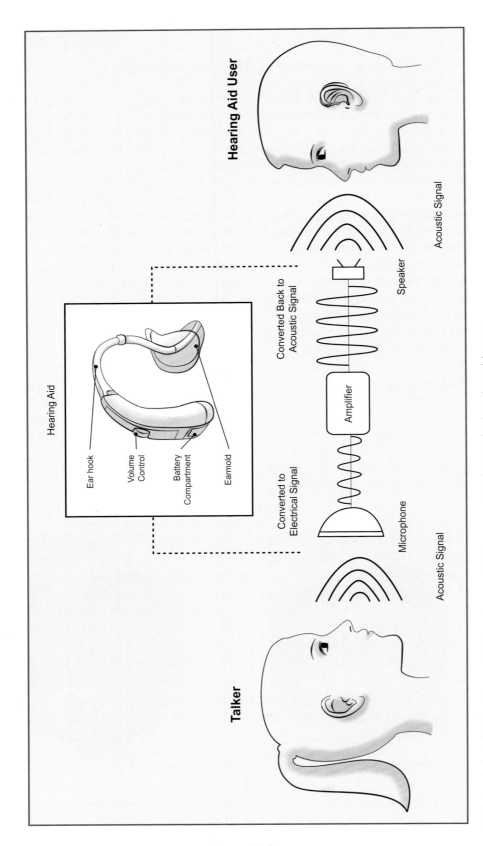

FIGURE 13–8. The transmission of sound between a speaker and a hearing aid user.

Some aids have other controls that can be used to make the signal clearer.

Hearing aids tend to be expensive, and the high cost is due to the manufacturing of miniaturized components. They are built to be durable, but like any electronic device, can be broken if dropped on a hard surface. Exposure to water also can lead to damage, so they must not be worn in the shower or when swimming. Hearing aids come in various sizes, generally corresponding to the amount of power (or amplification) that can be provided. Large hearing aids usually provide the most amplification and are prescribed for individuals with more severe hearing loss. A listing of the various types of hearing aids follows.

Behind-the-Ear Aids

A **behind-the-ear** (**BTE**) **aid** consists of two parts (Figure 13–9). One part is the actual hearing aid, and this is situated behind the ear; the other part is an acrylic/silicon earmold that fits in the outermost portion of the ear canal. The mold is connected to the hearing aid with a transparent tube that transmits the amplified sound from the hearing aid into the ear canal. People with a wide range of hearing losses, from mild to profound, can be fitted with BTE hearing aids. Because the components are housed outside of the ear, these aids tend to be the most durable. This durability makes them ideal for children, and the size of the hearing aid also provides a high level of amplification if needed. A popular modification to BTE aids is to fit the aid without a mold but with a small plastic tip on the end of the tubing (called an open-ear fitting). The soft silicone tip has holes so that the ear canal is not sealed off. The advantage of an open-fit BTE is the cosmetic appeal, as well as the open feeling in the ear canal.

In-the-Ear Aids

All components of an **in-the-ear** (**ITE**) **aid** are built into a custom-made mold

---

FYI

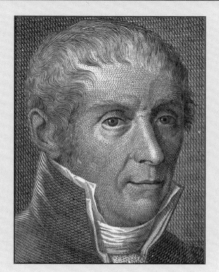

Count **Alessandro Volta** (1745–1827) was an Italian physicist born in Como, Italy. He is known for his pioneering work in electricity and inventing the voltaic pile, a forerunner of the electric battery, which produced a steady stream of electricity. The electrical unit known as the volt was named in his honor. Volta was also the first to note that the auditory system could be stimulated electrically. He inserted an electrical current into his ears via two metal rods. He reported a sensation that was like a "boom within the head" followed by a sound similar to that of "boiling of thick soup."

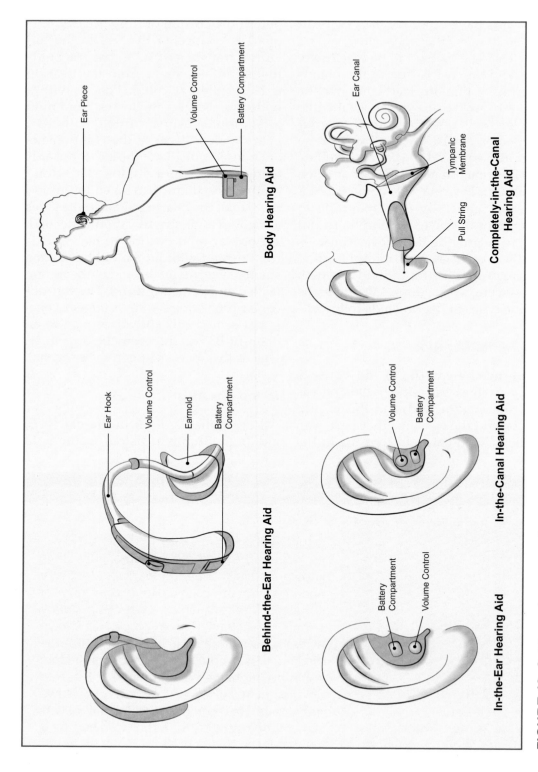

FIGURE 13–9. The various types of hearing aids currently available to individuals with varying degrees of hearing loss.

(see Figure 13–9) that fits snugly in the bowl of the outer ear. The mold is normally made to be similar to the color of one's skin. The ITE hearing aid can be used by people who have mild-to-severe hearing losses. This aid is not recommended for individuals who have a severe-to-profound hearing loss, or problems with finger or hand dexterity that make manipulating small controls difficult.

In-the-Canal Aids

The **in-the-canal (ITC) aid** is custom designed, smaller in size than the ITE aid, and fits partly in the ear canal (see Figure 13–9). It has a wide cosmetic appeal because it is less visible than ITE aids. Like the ITE, all components are housed within a single plastic shell. Because they are smaller in size, ITC aids are particularly good for management of mild-to-moderate hearing losses. People with this aid find it convenient for telephone and cell phone use.

Completely-in-the-Canal Aids

A **completely-in-the-canal (CIC)** aid is small and fits inside the ear canal and is barely visible (see Figure 13–9). This type of aid has the advantage of sitting very close to the eardrum, which improves sound quality and reduces wind noise and the "echo" sensation sometimes found in larger aids. The size of the CIC makes it very appealing from a cosmetic standpoint. The small size, however, also has some disadvantages, such as short battery life because the batteries are so small. Some people may not be good candidates for a CIC aid if they have unusually shaped ear canals or if they have a severe hearing loss. A slight variation on the CIC is

called the **invisible-in-the-canal (IIC)** aid and is placed deep in the ear canal. The IIC is designed for people with very active lives.

Body-Worn Aids

The earliest forms of modern hearing aids were body worn. This type of aid may seem outdated, but they are still in use today. These aids can be clearly distinguished from other hearing aids because they require a battery pack and amplifier that is worn in a harness on the body (or situated in a shirt pocket; see Figure 13–9). They are much less bulky than the older body aids and are more attractively designed. These days, **body aids** are used by individuals with a profound hearing loss because it is likely to provide the highest level of sound amplification. They also are prescribed for some individuals who do not have the manual dexterity to operate a BTE aid, as they are simple to operate with large controls and switches that are easy to handle. Finally, the cost of body aids tends to be substantially less than BTE-style aids.

Assistive Listening Devices

The hearing needs of some individuals cannot be successfully addressed with hearing aids alone. In these cases, devices have been created that are used to facilitate listening in various environments, especially those with excessive noise. Some **assistive listening devices** are designed to be used with hearing aids, whereas others are designed for independent use. Assistive listening devices can amplify a sound, but their primary purpose is to separate background (distracting) sounds from speech sounds. They improve what is known as the **signal-to-noise ratio**, which is the difference in level between the signal of interest and the background noise. Examples of assistive listening devices include: (1) a telecoil, (2) soundfield amplification, and (3) captioning. A helpful feature of most hearing aids is called the **telecoil**, or "t-switch." A telecoil is used when speaking and listening on a telephone. A hearing aid uses a microphone to pick up sound and send it into the ear canal. When the telecoil switch is activated, the hearing aid also can detect a magnetic signal transmitted through the actual telephone device. This magnetic signal serves to further enhance the signal-to-noise ratio allowing for better listening over the telephone. **Soundfield amplification** systems typically are found in classroom settings and are designed to amplify and broadcast the teacher's voice through loudspeakers. The system consists of a microphone/FM transmitter, amplifier, and one or more loudspeakers. **Captioning (closed)** is a form of assistive listening device, in which words that are said on a television show are embedded in the signal and become visible with a special decoder. The decoder lets a hearing-impaired individual see captions at the bottom of the screen that tell them what is being spoken in the television program. Most televisions have a built-in option to display closed captioning of broadcasts; however, this feature will only work if the specific television program has been captioned beforehand. These days, captioning can also be found on many 24-hour news channels, without the need of a decoder. These television stations provide a seemingly endless stream of text information in addition to what is being spoken.

Auditory Implants

An auditory implant provides a new mechanism for hearing when use of a traditional hearing aid alone is insufficient. An auditory implant is very different from a traditional hearing device. Hearing aids amplify sound, whereas auditory implants compensate for damaged or nonworking parts of the auditory system. There are four principal types of auditory implants: (1) bone-anchored hearing aid, (2) cochlear implant, (3) auditory brainstem implant, and (4) middle ear implant.

Bone-Anchored Hearing Aid

We typically think of hearing as a process of air conduction. That is, sound is transmitted through the air, which travels down the ear canal toward the eardrum, middle ear ossicles, and the inner ear. However, sound is also transmitted through bone conduction via the bones in the head that bypass the outer and middle ear going straight to the inner ear (see also Chapter 12). Conventional hearing aids sit in the ear canal and transmit sound via air conduction. Some people cannot use conventional hearing aids due to chronic outer or middle ear infection problems or lack of a functioning ear canal (e.g., atresia). A **bone-anchored hearing aid (BAHA)** is an auditory implant for people with hearing loss who cannot receive benefit from a normal hearing aid. The BAHA works **percutaneously** (i.e., through the skin) by vibrating the skull directly through a small titanium fixture that is implanted in the skull behind the ear (Figure 13–10). The device works by taking the sound from the outside and transmitting it to the inner ear through

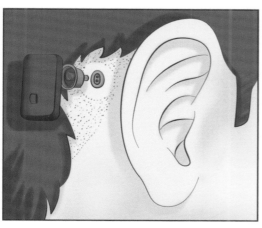
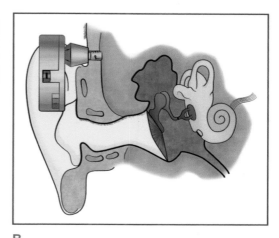

A

B

FIGURE 13–10. Illustration of a bone-anchored hearing aid (BAHA). **A.** The BAHA is attached to a small titanium implant behind the ear. **B.** The sound travels via the bones of the skull to the inner ear.

━━━━━ FYI ━━━━━

The early term used for a cochlear implant was a *bionic ear*. The prototype of current day cochlear implants was implanted in the first adult at the Royal Victorian Eye and Ear Hospital in Melbourne, Australia, in 1978.

---

the temporal bone. This bypasses the ear canal and the middle ear. The BAHA was first used in Europe in 1977 and has been approved for use in the United States since 1996 for conductive and mixed hearing losses.

Cochlear Implant

One of the most groundbreaking biomedical achievements in the last 30 years was the **cochlear implant**. Prior to 1975, the primary aural rehabilitation device for profoundly deaf or severely hearing-impaired children and adults was a BTE hearing aid. Anyone above 12 months of age, with severe-to-profound sensorineural hearing loss in both ears (70 dB or greater), who receives limited benefit from a hearing aid is a candidate for a cochlear implant. The major components of a cochlear implant are located outside, as well as inside the head. The components located outside the head are a microphone that picks up sounds in the environment, and a sound processor that arranges the sounds into an electrical signal that is transmitted through the skull. The transmitted signal sent through the skull is picked up by a receiver located inside the head. This receiver sends the electrical impulses to an array of 22 electrodes that stimulate different regions of the cochlea (Figure 13–11). A cochlear implant does not restore normal hearing. Instead, it can give a severely hearing-impaired person a useful representation

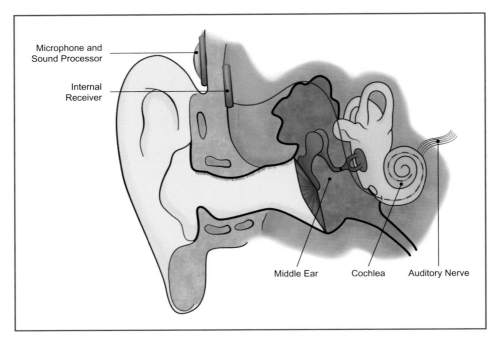

FIGURE 13–11. Illustration of a cochlear implant.

of sounds in the environment to assist with the understanding of speech. Although sound quality is sometimes described as mechanical, the cochlear implant provides users with the ability to sense sound that they could not otherwise hear. As of January 2011, the U.S. Department of Health reports that over 220,000 individuals in more than 120 countries have received a cochlear implant. In the United States, roughly 43,000 adults and 29,000 children have received a cochlear implant.

Auditory Brainstem Implant

An **auditory brainstem implant (ABI)** is the first device specifically designed to bypass the cochlea and the auditory nerve to transmit sound directly to the brainstem. Because it bypasses the auditory nerve, the device is most useful for people who have lost or will

lose their hearing in both ears following the removal of an auditory nerve tumor. Similar to a cochlear implant, the device involves components located outside and inside the head. The ABI device consists of a tiny microphone positioned by the ear, a sound processor, and an array of 21 electrodes implanted directly on a nerve center at the base of the brainstem called the cochlear nucleus. The microphone picks up sounds from the environment and transmits them to a receiver inside the skull. This receiver stimulates the brainstem electrodes, allowing for electrical impulses of sound to be transmitted to the brain (Figure 13–12). Most ABI recipients benefit from the device through increased sound awareness. Most patients are able to hear noises like a telephone ringing or horn honking, but the degree of hearing usefulness can vary greatly. At this point in time, few ABI recipients are able

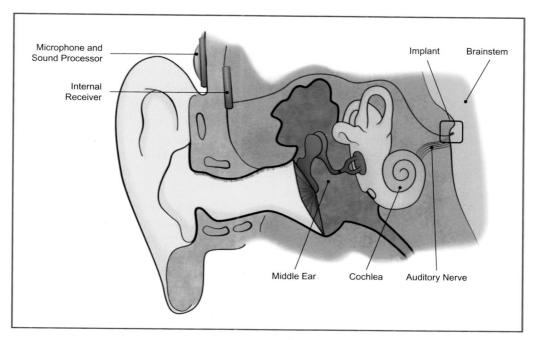

FIGURE 13–12. Illustration of an auditory brainstem implant.

to understand speech without lip reading, but this may improve in the future. However, the environmental and speech sounds that patients receive through the ABI help to significantly improve their communication and quality of life.

Middle Ear Implant

The newest type of implant to be developed is specific to the middle ear. This **middle ear implant** is not a hearing aid (i.e., the device does not amplify sounds). Instead, this implant is designed to convert sound into mechanical vibrations that are then delivered to the inner ear. Similar to a cochlear implant and ABI, a middle ear implant involves components located outside and inside the head. The external component receives sounds that are then delivered to a transducer implanted in the middle ear that causes the ossicles to vibrate.

A middle ear implant can be used to treat individuals with conductive, mixed, or sensorineural losses. The implant is ideal for individuals who cannot tolerate a traditional type of hearing aid that is inserted into the ear canal.

TREATMENT APPROACHES: SPEECH AND LANGUAGE REHABILITATION

Another aspect of aural rehabilitation concerns treatment of the speech and language abnormalities that may accompany a hearing impairment. Generally, the earlier the hearing loss occurs (e.g., congenital, prelingual) and the more severe the hearing loss (e.g., severe, profound), the greater its impact on speech and language. The presence of a severe hearing loss during the critical periods of speech and language development deprives a child of the opportunities to hear language and can thus affect a child's ability to develop the features of normal communication (i.e., form, content, and use). Some of the primary speech and language disorders that result from a severe hearing loss are provided in Table 13–1. A brief summary of these features is provided below followed by an assortment of treatment approaches.

Speech and Language Characteristics

Phonology

A child with a severe hearing loss is likely to show a speech sound disorder.

The child's ability to accurately produce consonants and vowels is influenced by two variables: (1) speech **sound visibility** and (2) **acoustic characteristics**. Some speech sounds are more easily perceived on the face of a speaker compared with others. For a severely hearing-impaired child, this visual information can assist in learning to produce speech sounds accurately. For example, the /f/ sound is highly visible compared with the /k/ sound. Not surprising, low visibility sounds such as /k/ are likely to be misarticulated more often than highly visible sounds.

All consonants and vowels have unique acoustic characteristics that are differentiated from one another in regard to duration (ms), loudness (dB),

Table 13–1. Characteristics of Speech and Language Found in Deaf and Severely Hard of Hearing Individuals	
Feature	*Characteristics*
Phonology	Consonant and vowel omissions, substitutions, and distortions.
	Less visible phonemes more likely to be misarticulated.
	Acoustic features of phonemes can influence perception and production.
Semantics	Vocabulary can range from normal to severely impaired.
Syntax	Short and simple sentences.
	Incorrect word order and sentence constructions.
Pragmatics	Limited understanding of figurative language, idioms, and metaphors.
	Restricted range of communicative intents such as conversational skills.
Voice	Quality is impaired, likely to be hypernasal.
	Pitch is likely to be high.
	Regulation of loudness may be impaired.
Suprasegmental Features	Slow speaking rate.
	Impaired speech intonation and phrasing.

and frequency (Hz). Depending on the configuration of a person's hearing loss, some sounds are less likely to be perceived clearly compared with others, and this can lead to inaccurate speech sound production. For example, assuming a child has a high-frequency hearing loss, sounds that are naturally produced with a high acoustic frequency (e.g., /s/, /sh/) are less likely to be perceived and produced clearly compared with sounds that have a low acoustic frequency (e.g., /m/, /z/). The general acoustic characteristics of speech sounds are shown in Figure 13–13. A hearing loss that falls outside the range of the acoustic char-

acteristics for various speech sounds would presumably be problematic for a hearing-impaired individual to perceive. In turn, the same sounds may be difficult to produce accurately.

Voice

Voice disorders are often found in the severely hard of hearing and deaf populations. Foremost among these voice problems is the production of **hypernasal speech**. This excessive nasality is thought to occur due to a lack of auditory feedback during speaking. We tend to take for granted that we produce

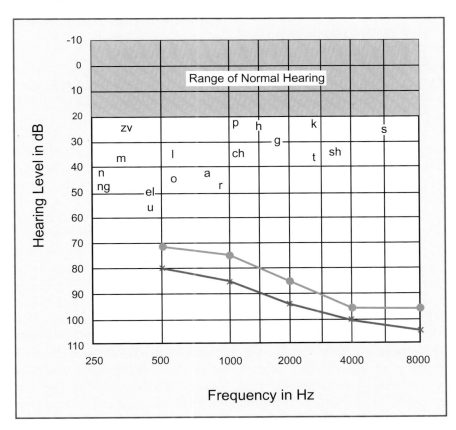

FIGURE 13–13. Depiction of the acoustic features of various consonants and vowels overlaid on an audiogram. In the case of an individual with a severe bilateral hearing loss, it is unlikely these sounds would be audible.

most speech sound by closing off the nasal cavity. Without auditory feedback, a deaf speaker may not learn the motor routines needed to separate the oral and nasal cavities, resulting in inadequate velopharyngeal closure and subsequent speech nasality. A second feature of voice found to be impaired is voice pitch, particularly among individuals with deafness. Attempts to produce voice, without being able to hear one's voice, tend to result in excessive tension in the region of the larynx. This results in abnormally tense vocal fold vibration that leads to the production of a high-pitched voice.

Language

Deaf children acquire language in the same developmental stages as a child with normal hearing; however, deaf children generally develop language at a slower pace. The primary deficit area is in the area of language **syntax** and includes problems with grammatical markers, articles, and word endings. The deficit likely results from a combination of factors. The syntactic structure of English is both complex and subtle with a number of inconsistencies. For example, consider these three sentences: (1) "I am going home," (2) "I am going to school," and (3) "I am going to the store." It is not surprising to find an individual with hearing impairment unable to grasp the subtleties of these differences and say something like, "I am going to home" or "I am going school" (Schow & Nerbonne, 2007). Another factor influencing an individual's correct use of syntax may stem from the mismatch between the language systems used by deaf and hearing individuals. For example, the language structure of American Sign Language is quite different from Standard English. For a deaf child who first learned American Sign Language, the later acquisition of Standard English may prove challenging.

Speaking Rate

There is considerable research confirming that hearing-impaired individuals speak more slowly than normally hearing speakers. Prelingually deaf children speak at one-fourth the rate of normally hearing children and adults. And even after practice, the deaf child's speaking rate is still one half that of normally hearing children and adults (Dwyer, Robb, O'Beirne, & Gilbert, 2009).

Rehabilitation Approaches

Speech Reading

For people with deafness, use of their eyes rather than ears provides the critical link with the world. One way of taking advantage of this visual link for communication is the act of speech reading. **Speech reading**, sometimes called lip reading, involves the decoding of language spoken by an individual by paying close attention to the speaker's mouth. The speech reader will also use the speaker's facial expressions, gestures, and hand movements as visual cues. All of this decoding is performed without being able to hear the speaker's voice. Even under optimal conditions, speech reading involves a great deal of guesswork. When we speak English, only 30% of the consonants and vowels are clearly visible on the mouth. For example, compare the highly visible "f" and "th" sounds with the nearly invisible "t" and "k" sounds (Figure 13–14). The speech reader needs to become adept at filling-in the gaps between vis-

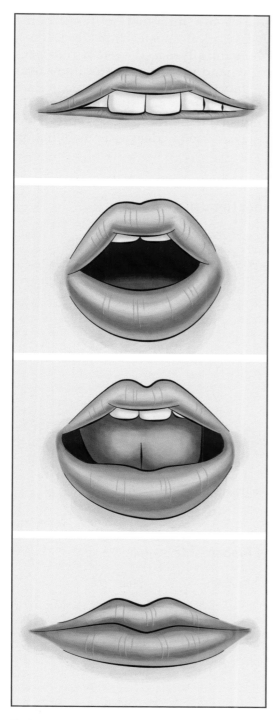

FIGURE 13–14. Various mouth shapes that can be seen during speech reading. Can you identify the sounds being produced by this speaker?

ible and invisible sounds to read words and phrases. People with deafness who are experienced speech readers can decode approximately 40% of single words. Speech reading is not normally used as the sole means of aural rehabilitation. Speech reading is a strategy that is used in combination with other assistive listening devices to communicate effectively.

Cued Speech

Cued speech was created as a means of helping to solve the decoding problems related to speech reading. Some speech sounds are not readily visible (e.g., "t," "k"), and some speech sounds look almost identical. Consider the differences between the sounds "m," "b," and "p." All of these sounds are produced with the lips closed and could easily be confused by the speech reader when trying to distinguish the words "my," "buy," or "pie." Cued speech is a supplement to spoken language in which the speaker uses a set of sound-related hand shapes while talking to a severely hard of hearing individual. These hand shapes are intended to remove the guesswork from speech reading. It is a phonemically based system that uses eight hand shapes in four locations near the face. A total of 36 different cues are used to clarify 44 different sounds in English (Figure 13–15). Cued speech has not been used widely as a rehabilitation

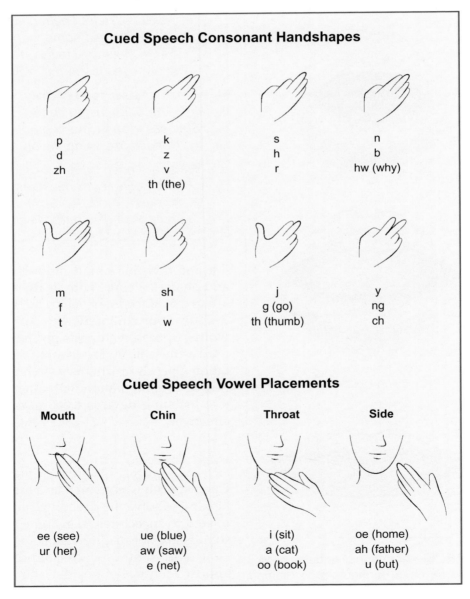

FIGURE 13–15. The hand symbols used for cued speech.

technique. The major limitation is that the system is not applicable to every-day communication situations. Both the speaker and the speech reader need to be familiar with the cued speech system of communication.

Oral/Aural Approach

The terms **oral** and **aural** refer to the mouth and ear, respectively. Thus, the oral/aural approach to speech and language rehabilitation focuses on improving both speech and hearing abilities. This method stresses the use of speech articulation, hearing aids, and speech reading skills. A primary objective is to develop clear spoken language abilities to enable the person to function in a hearing society. People using this method are discouraged from relying exclusively on visual cues (such as sign language). Use of various biofeedback devices can be helpful in the development of oral skills. For example, the **nasometer** (see Chapter 7) is designed to measure both oral and nasal airflow during speech. The device provides a visual display of both types of flow that can be used by the speaker as a form of feedback to subsequently modify excessive nasality. An instrument known as a **Visi-Pitch** can be useful in helping to reduce a high-pitched voice. The device provides a visual display of fundamental frequency (i.e., pitch) during speak-ing activities. The severely hearing impaired individual learns to associate the visual display with the feeling of tension in the throat linked to loudness and pitch of voice. This has been referred to as *muscle memory.*

Manual Approach

Manual communication is often thought of as **sign language**. The language involves movement of the hands, body, face, and head as the primary mode of communication. Advocates of the manual communication approach believe that knowledge and understanding of language is more important than the ability to speak clearly. Because deaf and severely hard of hearing individuals use the visual mode more readily, communicating through the visual mode is a natural form of expression. Two examples of manual communication are **finger spelling** and sign language. Finger spelling is the process of creating words using a finger alphabet and is generally used alongside sign language to spell out names, places, and unusual words that do not have their own, distinct sign. The finger alphabet used in Canada and the United States is based on hand shapes formed using one hand. The finger alphabet used in the United Kingdom, Australia, and New Zealand uses two hands (Figure 13–16). Sign language is the process of forming

---

FYI

In April 2006, the New Zealand government officially declared New Zealand sign language as one of three official languages in the country. The two other official languages of the country are English and Maori. Other countries that have made a similar declaration concerning sign language include Sweden, Denmark, Finland, Norway, Switzerland, Ireland, Portugal, and Greece.

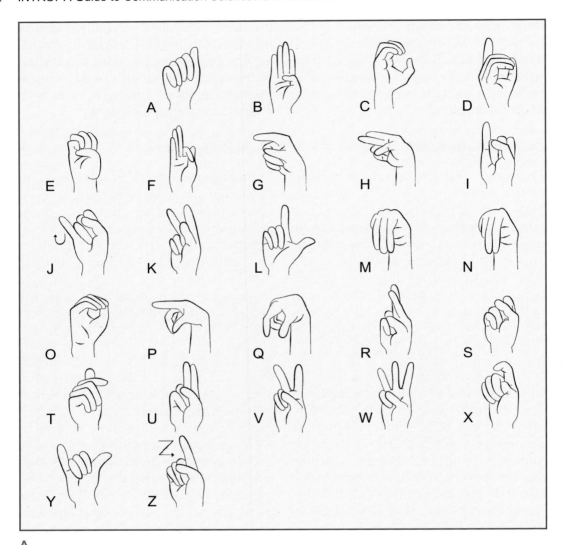

A

FIGURE 13–16. A. Manual finger spelling alphabet used in America. *continues*

sentences using various hand shapes that reflect specific words. American Sign Language is the visual/gestural language used by many people in the Deaf community in the United States, Canada, and parts of Mexico, although it originated in Europe. It is considered a distinct language and not just a visual representation of English. American Sign Language has its own grammar and syntax and does not follow the word order we would normal use when speaking English. British Sign Language is the sign language used in the United Kingdom and is quite distinct from American Sign Language in the hand shapes for various words, as well as grammar and syntax. The Australian sign language and New Zealand sign language systems have evolved from British Sign Language.

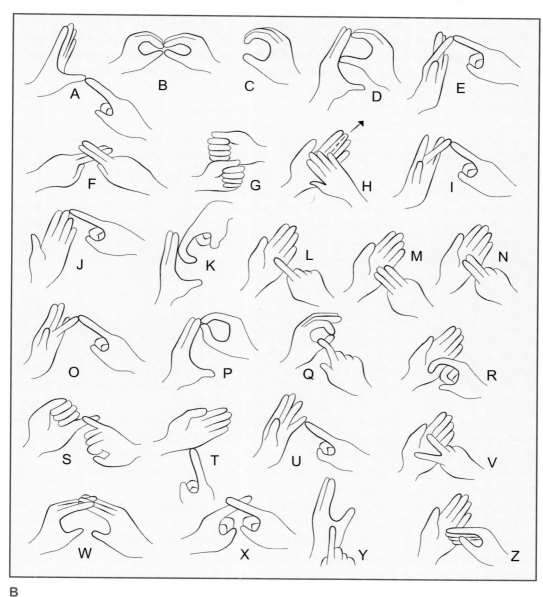

B

FIGURE 13–16. *continued* **B.** Manual finger spelling alphabet used in the United Kingdom.

Simultaneous Communication Approach

Simultaneous communication (Sim-Com) is an aural rehabilitation approach that encourages all possible modes of communication to help a hearing-impaired individual communicate effectively. The various modes of communication include using a combination of spoken language, sign language, finger spelling, speech reading, amplification, writing, and gestures. SimCom is a common form of communication used in educational settings for deaf children. Advocates of this approach believe that individuals can learn and use language in a way best suited to their needs, while developing communication skills to function in the hearing world.

The Deaf and Blind Person

A critical feature of most aural rehabilitation programs is to capitalize on an individual's existing communication skills. This includes sound amplification and utilizing visual cues such as speech, reading, and sign language. Alternatively, an individual with blindness relies primarily on auditory cues to communicate effectively. In the case of an individual who has lost vision and hearing, aural rehabilitation is particularly challenging. **Deaf-blindness** is defined as a combination of both auditory and visual disabilities that can contribute to severe disorders of development, learning, and communication. The prevalence of deaf-blindness is approximately 1 per 10,000 individuals. For the profoundly deaf and blind individual, the primary means by which he or she experiences the outside world is through touch. The National Foundation of the Blind lists a number of methods of communication that are available to the deaf-blind person. These include (1) manual alphabet, (2) print-in-palm, (3) Braille, and (4) the Tadoma method.

Manual Alphabet

The use of a manual alphabet involves the speaker (encoder) to produce a series of hand motions that depict letters of the alphabet. The deaf-blind person than decodes these symbols into words by placing his or her hand over the hand of the person making the letters. The manual alphabet can be one of the quickest and most versatile communication methods for a deaf-blind person.

Print-in-Palm

The basics of **print-in-palm** are similar to the manual alphabet. In this case, the speaker communicates with the deaf-blind person by tracing the shapes of block (capital) letters on the palm of their hand with an index finger. Using this system does not involve learning a unique manual alphabet, simply the letters making the standard alphabet.

Braille

Braille is a tactile reading and writing system that was developed by the Frenchman, **Louis Braille** (1809–1852) who also happened to be blind. Based on a system of six raised dots that occur in different patterns, an entire alphabet, including punctuation, can be coded. The user learns to sequence the patterns and translate them into words and language.

Tadoma Method

The **Tadoma method** was developed in Sweden in the 1920s and named after two children (Tad and Oma) who were deaf and blind. The deaf-blind individual places a thumb on a speaker's lips and spreads their remaining fingers along the speaker's face and neck (Figure 13–17). Communication is transmitted through vibrations, motions of the jaw, and facial expressions of the speaker. Although the Tadoma method is very difficult and time consuming to learn, it has proven successful, allowing fluent Tadoma users the ability to comprehend as well as produce spoken language.

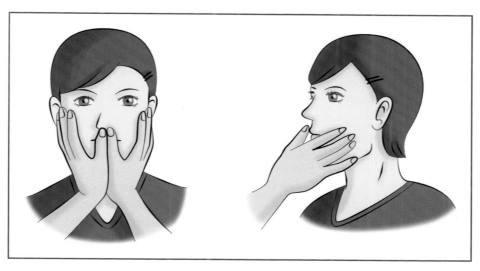

FIGURE 13–17. Illustration of the Tadoma method used by individuals with deaf-blindness to comprehend spoken language.

CULTURAL CONSIDERATIONS AND AURAL REHABILITATION

Culture is defined as a system of values, attitudes, beliefs, and learned behaviors shared by a population. Culture is shaped by factors such as geographic location, education, age, and sex. A person's hearing abilities can also be a defining feature of one's culture. This is especially the case among those with a profound hearing loss. Sociologists have identified two opposing perspectives on culture and deafness, which are referred to as the medical model and cultural model. In the **medical model**, deafness is viewed as an illness and disability. Indeed the term *hearing impaired* can be construed as reflective of the medical model. The disability can be treated by surgery and/or prosthetic devices like a cochlear implant or hearing aid. The condition can also be treated by allied health professionals including audiolo-

gists and speech-language pathologists. The medical model discourages separatism from the hearing world; instead, emphasis is placed on encouraging deaf people to acquire oral language skills. The use of sign language is discouraged. In the **cultural model**, deaf people are seen as nondefective persons, who are members of a minority culture. Deafness is not an illness or impairment but a difference, so there is no need for surgical intervention. Deaf and hard of hearing people are disabled only by barriers created by other people trying to make them fit into the hearing world. The cultural model sees the Deaf community as having its own unique culture. Evidence of Deaf culture is found in a number of ways. Deaf and hard of hearing people produce plays, books, artwork, magazines, and movies targeted at deaf and hard of hearing audiences. Socialization in the Deaf community takes many forms. A particularly popular means of socialization is meeting at a restaurant, which has come to be known as a *signing*

FYI

There is a bit of debate as to whether chronic snoring actually can cause a noise-induced hearing loss. The noise generated by a person snoring can sometimes exceed 70 dB (comparable with the loudness of a vacuum cleaner), so it is no wonder its relationship to hearing loss is being explored.

---

supper or American Sign Language dinner. Another popular social vehicle is the *Deaf coffee*, a meeting at a local café to chat. The Deaf community also has its own online dating sites.

There are also cultural assumptions in regard to the manner in which the word deaf is written. The term *deaf,* as written with a lower case "d," is used to refer to people who are profoundly hearing impaired and choose to use oral communication as their first language of communication. The term *Deaf,* as written with a capital "D," is used to describe people who are profoundly hearing impaired and use sign language as their major mode of communication. Capital "D" deafness denotes the social, political, and cultural strands of members belonging to the Deaf community.

CURRENT RESEARCH IN AURAL REHABILITATION

Smart Phones

As mobile phones become more advanced so too are the applications available to individuals with a hearing impairment. Apple reports that iPhones may soon be able to detect and warn a user with severe hearing loss of immediate environmental sounds such as door bells or smoke alarms. Apple also plans to create phones that can remotely adjust hearing aid settings. Recent changes imposed by the U.S. Federal Communications Commission has required that individuals with disabilities, such as hearing loss, be allowed access to modern devices such as smart phones. So it seems that these communication devices will soon be designed to directly interact with hearing aid and cochlear implant users (Cutter, 2013).

Hearing Aid Frequency Transposition

People with severe-to-profound, high-frequency hearing loss face challenges to hearing because they are not able to clearly hear the entire range of speech sounds (250–8,000 Hz). One approach to helping these individuals is to design a hearing aid that delivers high-frequency speech sounds to the lower frequency region. This is referred to as **frequency transposition** (McDermott, 2011). There have been many attempts to do this, going back more than 30 years. However, previous attempts to transpose frequencies ended up obscuring the overall quality of the sound delivered to the ear. Modern day hearing aids use a digital processing technology that allows for improved transposition of frequencies and ultimately may help individuals with a high-frequency hearing loss (Kuk, Keenan, Auriemmo, & Korhonen, 2009).

Online Hearing Measurement

It is now possible to complete a hearing test online. Several hearing aid companies (e.g., Phonak, Starkey), as well as universities, provide these tests to individuals at no charge. This allows an individual who may be unsure of their hearing abilities the opportunity to seek information in the privacy and comfort of their home. This option is also particularly attractive to individuals who many not have insurance or cannot afford a visit to the doctor unless it is absolutely necessary. These tests provide a rough indication of a person's hearing ability. Online tests are not designed to replace a hearing evaluation performed by an audiologist but serve as a first step in the process of seeking help for their hearing loss.

Neuroimaging and Cochlear Implants

The study of congenitally deaf individuals provides a unique opportunity to understand the organization and potential for reorganization of regions in the brain following cochlear implantation. Cochlear implants provide auditory sensation to parts of the brain that had previously received no sensation. A current line of research is to use neuroimaging techniques such as magnetic resonance imaging and positron emission tomography scans to examine the structural organization of various regions of the brain. In the past, the effectiveness of a cochlear implant typically was evaluated by a subjective appraisal of the individual's speech recognition and speech production abilities. However, these assessments do not provide information regarding sites in the brain that are responsible for good (or poor) results. The use of neuroimaging techniques allows researchers to examine the cortical areas that are used by a cochlear implant user and to evalu-

ate the consequences of electrical stimulation by the cochlear implant (Sevy et al., 2010).

AURAL REHABILITATION ON THE WORLD WIDE WEB

Listed below are websites that provide further information on the topic of aural rehabilitation. At the time of publication, each website was freely accessible.

Better Hearing Institute Video
http://www.betterhearing.org/video/pbs/spotlight.cfm

Hearnet.Com Public Service Announcements
http://www.hearnet.com/features/feature_PSA.shtml

Oral Deaf Education Video
http://www.oraldeafed.org/

Hearing Aid and Implant Video
http://www.medel.com/int/index/

Deaf-Blind Resource
http://nfb.org/deaf-blind-resources

Hellen Keller Videos
http://www.youtube.com/watch?v=Gv1uLfF35Uw

http://www.youtube.com/watch?v=8ch_H8pt9M8

STUDY QUESTIONS

1. What are the various types of hearing aids that are currently available?
2. What are the four principal types of auditory implants?

3. What are the possible communication characteristics of a profoundly hearing-impaired person?
4. What are the types of rehabilitation approaches to working with a profoundly hearing-impaired person?
5. What are the various forms of communication available to the deaf-blind person?

REFERENCES

Cleys, G. (1997). *A lipreaders poem.* Retrieved from http://www.geocities.com/Heartland/Park/7180/lippoem.html

Cutter, M. (2013, January 1). Smarter phones for hearing impairment. *ASHA Leader,* 17.

Dwyer, C., Robb, M., O'Beirne, G., & Gilbert, H. (2009). The influence of speaking rate on nasality in the speech of hearing impaired individuals. *Journal of Speech, Language, and Hearing Research, 52,* 1321–1333.

Kuk, F., Keenan, D., Auriemmo, J., & Korhonen, P. (2009, January). Re-evaluating the efficacy of frequency transposition. *ASHA Leader, 4*(1), 14–17.

McDermott, H. (2011). A technical comparison of digital frequency-lowering algorithms available in two current hearing aids. *PLoS ONE, 6*(7).

Schow, R., & Nerbonne, M. (2007). *Introduction to audiologic rehabilitation* (5th ed.). Boston, MA: Pearson Education.

Sevy, A., Bortfeld, H., Huppert, T., Beauchamp, M., Tonini, R., & Oghalai, J. (2010). Neuroimaging with near-infrared spectroscopy demonstrates speech-evoked activity in the auditory cortex of deaf children following cochlear implantation. *Hearing Research, 270,* 39–47.

Tye-Murray, N. (2009). *Foundations of aural rehabilitation: Children, adults, and their family members* (3rd ed.). Clifton Park, NY: Delmar Cengage Learning.

GLOSSARY

60-60 rule: Hearing prevention rule which translates to a listening level of 60% of the maximum volume for no more than 60 minutes.

abducted: To move away from the midline position. Vocal fold opening is a form of abduction.

abductor type spasmodic dsyphonia: Severe voice disorder resulting from an inability to normally open the vocal folds to create a speaking voice.

accent: A characteristic of speech pronunciation as determined by regional or social background.

acid reflux: Regurgitation of stomach acid into the esophagus.

acoustic characteristics: Features of speech sounds that are described according to the domains of amplitude, frequency and time.

acoustic neuroma: A benign tumor located on the eighth cranial nerve that may affect hearing and balance.

acoustic reflex: An involuntary muscle contraction that occurs in the middle year as a result of sudden loudness in sound.

acquired disorder: A communication impairment that results after a period of normal communication. A traumatic brain injury is a form of acquired disorder.

acrocentric chromosome: A chromosome with its centromere located near the end of the chromosome.

active muscular process: The contraction of muscles for a specified movement. Breath inhalation involves an active muscular process.

acute care hospital: A hospital that provides short-term and highly specialized, patient care.

addition: Type of speech sound misarticulation in which one or more consonants or vowels are included in the target word production.

adducted: To move toward the midline position. Vocal fold closing is a form of adduction.

adductor type spasmodic dsyphonia: Severe voice disorder resulting from an inability to normally close the vocal folds to create a speaking voice.

adenoids: Pairs of lymphoid tissue located in the various regions in the back of the pharynx that serve to filter out debris from inhaled air. A related term is tonsils.

adenosine triphosphate (ATP): An adrenaline nucleotide that is used during muscle contraction. ATP is thought to provide natural protection from acquiring a noise-induced hearing loss.

adult-centered therapy: Form of speech and language therapy in which the adult plays a dominant and directive role in a child's therapy session.

adventitious deafness: Form of acquired communication disorder, where a hearing loss occurred after a period of normal hearing. An acoustic neuroma could result in an adventitious hearing loss.

affricates: A category of consonants classified according to the manner in which they are articulated in the vocal tract. The consonant /ch/ is an example of an affricate.

age of mastery: An approach to determining a child's acquisition of speech sounds. Each sound is expected to be acquired (mastered) by a particular age.

age of suppression: An approach to determining a child's suppression of phonological processes. Each process (e.g., final consonant deletion) is expected to disappear by a particular age.

air conduction testing: Form of hearing test where sounds are presented through earphones directly into the ear canal.

alaryngeal speech: A unique form of speaking in the absence of a larynx. Removal of the larynx is often a result of cancer.

alphabet: A standard set of letters used to display spoken language. Each symbol generally assumes a sound (phoneme) of the language.

altered auditory feedback: Collective term for masking, delayed auditory feedback, and frequency altered feedback. These forms of feedback are used in the treatment of stuttering.

alternative or augmentative communication: A unique form of communication to assist people with severe expressive communication difficulties.

alveolar ridge: The gum ridge of the upper jaw (maxilla) located directly behind the teeth.

alveoli: The final branches of the respiratory tree in the lungs that function to exchange gas between the lungs and the bloodstream.

Alzheimer, Alois: German psychiatrist who was the first to identify the unique brain disease related to cell death.

Alzheimer disease: Most common form of dementia characterized by progressive memory loss and intellectual abilities.

amniocentesis: Medical procedure used in the prenatal diagnosis of chromosomal and fetal abnormalities.

amplifier: A key feature of a hearing aid, designed to boost the loudness level of incoming sound before entering the ear canal.

amplitude: The height of a sound wave. Related terms are intensity and loudness.

amyotrophic lateral sclerosis: A progressive and fatal neurodegenerative disease—also known as motor neuron disease or Lou Gehrig disease.

anatomy: The science concerning the structure of the body.

anencephaly: Condition present at birth that affects the formation of the brain and the skull bones that surround the head.

ankyloglossia: Condition caused by an abnormally short lingual frenulum. The condition is commonly referred to as "tongue tie."

anomic aphasia: An expressive language disorder characterized by a severe problem with recalling words.

anthropometry: The science that relates to the measurement of body dimensions.

aphasia: A disorder that results from damage to the regions of the brain that are responsible for language. A similar term is dysphasia.

aphonia: Medical term used to describe a condition in which a person is unable to speak, or has lost their voice.

apical: Relating to the tip or apex.

app: Abbreviated term for application; which is a software program for use on the Internet, computer, phone or other electronic device.

approximates: A classification of consonant sounds that have articulatory and acoustic qualities that fall somewhere between true consonants and vowels. Examples include /w/ and /r/.

apraxia: Neurological disorder that is characterized by an inability to perform purposeful movements on command. Apraxia of speech is a unique form of speech sound disorder.

Aristotle: Greek philosopher who contributed important writings in the areas of logic, art, psychology, and nature.

articulation: The location at which two structures make contact. Speech articulation concerns the manner in which various anatomical structures work together to create speech sounds.

articulation approach: Treatment for speech sound disorders that focuses on the motoric aspects of speech production.

articulation disorder: Mispronunciation of speech sounds.

articulatory system: The anatomical structures used for creating the sounds of speech, which include cavities, muscles, and bone.

arytenoid cartilages: A pair of triangular shaped cartilages within the larynx that serve as points of attachment for the vocal folds.

Asperger, Hans: Austrian pediatrician and child psychiatrist who was the first to describe "autistic psychopathology," which was later named Asperger syndrome.

aspiration: Inhalation of foreign material such as food or fluids in the lungs.

aspiration pneumonia: The entrance of food or fluids into the trachea that leads to the eventual development of harmful bacteria that forms in the lungs ore bronchial tubes.

assistive listening device: Any type of device that helps an individual to function better in their daily communication. Closed captioning on a television is a form of an assistive listening device.

asymmetrical hearing loss: A hearing loss in both ears; however, the degree and configuration of hearing loss is not identical.

atresia: Absence or incomplete development of the of the ear canal.

audiogram: A graph used to depict an individual's hearing.

audiologist: Professional who specializes in the diagnosis and management of disorders of the auditory and vestibular portions of the ear.

audiology: Branch of science that is concerned with balance, hearing, and related disorders.

audiometer: Machine (typically a computer) that is used for measuring hearing sensitivity.

audition: The act of hearing.

auditory communication: Use and perception of sound that forms the basis of communication.

auditory brainstem implant: Device designed to bypass the cochlea and the auditory nerve to transmit sound directly to the brainstem.

auditory brainstem response: An electrical signal evoked from the brainstem in response to an auditory signal. This response is often used as a test of hearing in infants.

auditory cortex: Region of the brain responsible for the processing of auditory (sound) information—also called Heschl's gyrus, which is located in the temporal lobes.

auditory nerve: The nerve that caries auditory and balance information from the inner ear to the brainstem —also known as the cochlear nerve or the eighth cranial nerve.

auditory processing disorder: Broad term used to describe a variety of problems with the brain that can interfere with the understanding of auditory information.

aural: Relating to the ear or to the sense of hearing.

aural habilitation: The management of hearing loss for an individual born with a hearing impairment.

aural rehabilitation: The management of hearing loss for an individual who originally had normal hearing

auricle: The outer ear—also known as the pinna.

autism spectrum disorders: Group of autistic conditions with similar features that may vary in symptoms and severity.

babbling: The repeated production of the same or nearly similar syllable strings. A common type of vocalization produced by children during the period of 4 to 10 months of age.

bacterial meningitis: Inflammation of the meninges due to bacterial infection.

badge: A visual display to communicate status or accomplishment.

barium: Soft metallic element that is silvery white in its purest form. If swallowed, the substance is clearly visible during x-ray examination.

basal: Relating to, or forming, the base.

basilar membrane: Located within the cochlea and separates the cochlear duct from the scala tympani.

behaviorist theory: Theory based on the assumption that a child's speech and language developed is shaped by individuals and events in the child's environment.

behind-the-ear aid (BTE): A type of hearing aid where the primary components of the aid are situated and fit behind the ear.

Bell, Alexander Graham: Inventor of the telephone.

Bell, Alexander Melville: Scientist with interests in speech and deafness. Father of Alexander Graham Bell.

beneficence: The act of doing good or being charitable.

Berners-Lee, Timothy: Known as the inventor of the World Wide Web.

between-word disfluencies: Speech disfluencies that occur across words, such as a phrase repetition or an interjection.

bilabial: A class of consonants categorized according to the place of articulation in the vocal tract. Examples of bilabial consonants are /b/ and /m/.

bilateral cleft lip: A cleft that involves separation of the lip on both sides of the mouth, often shown as a large open gap.

bilateral hearing loss: An impairment of hearing that occurs in both ears.

bilingualism: The ability to communicate in two languages, which may include, speaking, listening, reading, and writing.

biofeedback: Teaching a client to control various functions of the body through relaxation, visualization, and cognitive control processes.

birth defect: An abnormality of structure, function, or body chemistry usually present at birth that can result in physical or intellectual disability.

Blackwell, Elizabeth: First woman in the United States to graduate from medical school and practice medicine.

blocks: A type of speech disfluency characterized by a complete, momentary stoppage in the forward flow of speech.

blogging: Contraction of the terms Web and log. A website usually maintained by an individual that contains regular entries and personal commentaries.

Bloom, Lois: Professor of speech-language pathology who developed the framework of form-content-use to define communicative competency.

bodily movements: Features of stuttering whereby certain body parts, such as the head and eyes move during moments of stuttering.

body aid: Type of hearing aid that involves a battery pack and amplifier worn in a harness that delivers sound to the ears. A very powerful hearing aid.

body language: A form of nonverbal communication that involves use of various parts of the body.

bolus: Food that has been chewed and mixed in the mouth with saliva.

bone conduction testing: Test of hearing that bypasses the outer and middle ear by sending sound vibrations through the skull bones toward the cochlea.

bone-anchored hearing aid (BAHA): A surgical implant for the treatment of hearing loss that works through bone conduction.

bound morphemes: A morpheme that cannot stand alone as an independent word while carrying lexical meaning when attached to another morpheme.

brachycephaly: Condition in which the head is disproportionately wide (or flattened).

bradykinesia: An abnormal slowness in the execution of movement.

braille: Tactile reading and writing system bade on a series of raised dots.

Braille, Louis: Frenchman who developed a reading and writing system based on a series of six raised dots that occur in varying patterns.

brainstem nuclei: A cluster of sensory or motor nuclei located in the brainstem.

breathy voice: Quality of voice production where excessive air accompanies the voice.

Bridgman, Laura: First deaf-blind child in the United States to gain a formal education.

Broca, Paul: French neurosurgeon responsible for naming the region in the left frontal lobe responsible for speech production (Broca's area).

Broca's aphasia: Expressive language disorder where a person is able to comprehend language but has difficulty executing the motor movements to produce words. A form of nonfluent aphasia.

Broca's area: Region of the left cerebral temporal lobe that plays a role in the expression of speech and language.

Brodmann's areas: A series of 52 distinct regions of the cerebral cortex that are identified according to cellular structure and function.

Brodmann, Korbinian: German neurologist who mapped the cerebral cortex into 52 distinct functional areas.

Brodnitz, Friedrich: Well-known medical specialist in the treatment of vocal disorders, particularly those associated with singing.

bronchial tubes: Series of subdivided tubes that carry air to and from the mouth and the lungs. The smallest of these tubes are called bronchioles.

bronchioles The smallest air passageways comprising the lungs.

Brown, Hallie Quinn: The daughter of former slaves who was a black civil rights leader, teacher, and elocutionist.

Brown, Roger: American psychologist who developed the mean length of utterance measure to chart morphological development.

Bryngelson, Bryng: Pioneer in the speech-language pathology profession in the United States. He had a particular interest in the area of stuttering.

Butler, Margaret F.: A pioneer in the area of otolaryngology.

Campbell-Swinton, Alan Archibald: Engineer who was the first to envision the development of a television signal.

captioning (closed): An assistive listening device that provides a visual display of text on a television.

Carhart, Raymond: The "Father of Modern-day Audiology in the United States."

Carter, Henry Vandyke: Individual responsible for drawing all of the anatomical illustrations in the famous textbook, *Gray's Anatomy.*

case history: A detailed account of facts gathered about an individual or family that have analytical value for medical, educational, or psychological conditions.

Casserius, Julio: Italian anatomist who made an important contribution to the study of voice.

castrato: An adult male with a singing voice equivalent to a soprano that occurs as a result of castration or an endocrine disorder.

cell: The basic unit of life.

cellular anatomy and physiology: The microscopic study of cells and tissues—also called histology.

central auditory system: Portion of the auditory system consisting of the auditory nerve, brainstem, and brain.

central nervous system Portion of the nervous system consisting of the brain, brainstem, and spinal cord.

centromere: Region of a chromosome where the arms of a chromosome intersect.

cerebral palsy A nonprogressive disorder that affects muscle tone, movement, and motor skills.

cerebrovascular accident: A condition where the blood supply to the brain is disturbed in some way resulting in brain cell death—also called stroke.

cerebrum: The largest portion of the brain divided into two hemispheres.

Certificate of Clinical Competency: A qualification granted by the American Speech, Language, and Hearing Association to audiologists and speech-language pathologists who meet the educational and clinical criteria for independent practice.

cerumen: A normally extruded product of the ear canal—also known as earwax.

cervical (neck) auscultation: Use of a stethoscope placed on the neck to listen to sounds produced during swallowing.

chemical communication: Form of communication where an animal species produces a chemical that is interpreted by other members of the same species.

child-centered therapy: Approach to working with a communicatively impaired child where the therapist provides treatment to the child that is geared around the child's naturally occurring play activity.

childhood apraxia of speech: A type of speech sound production disorder characterized by inconsistent mis-articulations patterns. Considered to be a rare and poorly understood disorder.

Chomsky, Noam: American linguist who proposed the nativist theory of early language acquisition.

chorionic villus sampling: A medical procedure used in the prenatal diagnosis of chromosomal and fetal abnormalities.

chromosomes: A threadlike strand of DNA and proteins that are found in every cell nucleus of a living organism.

chromosomal syndrome: A birth defect resulting from visible changes in the chromosomal structure of the individual.

circumlocutions: A roundabout manner of talking rather than using specific, direct language.

Class I malocclusion: Normal alignment of the upper and lower jaw, with the exception of some minor dental abnormalities.

Class II malocclusion: Abnormal alignment of the upper and lower jaw, indicative of a severe overbite.

Class III malocclusion: Abnormal alignment of the upper and lower jaw, indicative of a severe underbite.

cleft lip or palate: The lack of fusion of the lip and/or palate during embryonic development.

cleft palate team: A team of specialists in various aspects of medical, health, and educational care who work together to assist individuals with a cleft lip/palate.

Clerc, Laurent: The "Father of Deaf Education in the United States."

cliché level: A form of communication between individuals that involves a low-level of intimacy.

clinical assessment: A common approach to the initial screening of dysphagia that occurs in a clinic setting.

cloning: The process of producing a genetically identical organism.

cluttering: A fluency disorder characterized by excessively fast speaking rate and word formulation difficulties.

cochlea: Snail-shell-shaped structure that serves as the hearing organ of the inner ear.

cochlear implant: Surgically implanted device in the cochlea that provides individuals with a sense of sound.

cochlear nucleus: The location in the central auditory system where the auditory nerve inserts to the base of the brainstem.

code of ethics: A series of broad statements created by a professional body to guide members of the association in their ethical decision making.

cognitive behavioral therapy: A psychotherapy approach that focuses on

cytomegalovirus: A form of the herpes virus that rarely causes serious illness in healthy adults. However, the disease can have devastating effects on a newborn.

Darwin, Charles: English naturalist who laid the foundations of the theory of evolution.

de León, Pedro Ponce: Spanish monk who is often credited as being the first teacher of the deaf.

deaf-blindness: A condition in which both sound and sight are profoundly impaired.

deafness: Minimal hearing or complete loss of hearing.

debate: Form of communication that involves engagement in argument by discussing opposing points of view.

decibel scale (dB): The unit of measure for loudness.

decode: To extract the underlying meaning of a signal.

deep brain stimulation: Surgical treatment involving the implantation of a brain pacemaker that sends electrical signals to specific parts of the brain. Used as an approach to the treatment of Parkinson disease.

deglutition: The medical term for swallowing.

Déjerine-Klumpke, Augusta: Pioneering neurologist known for her contributions to neurology and neuroanatomy.

demands and capacities theory: A theory of stuttering that views moments of disfluency as resulting when a child's capacities for fluency are not equal to speech performance demands.

dementia: A progressive decline in cognitive function due to damage or disease in the body.

denotative: A word that has distinct meaning.

dentition: The type, number, and alignment of a set of teeth.

deoxyribonucleic acid (DNA): The genetic material found in the cells of all living organisms.

description: A language therapy technique involving labeling by the therapist to call attention to the child about the labels and descriptions of objects and activities.

developmental disorder: A condition that is assumed to have been present at birth; however, in some cases the manifestation of the disorder is not visible until the child matures.

dialect: A variety of language that is spoken among a particular group. A dialect is rule-governed and has distinct linguistic features.

dialogue: A form of communication that involves a conversation between two or more people.

diaphragm: A dome-shaped muscle that sits below the lungs. The muscle is most active during the process of inspiration.

Dieffenbach, Johann Friedrich: German surgeon who performed pioneering surgery for maxillofacial disorders.

direct laryngoscopy: Procedure in which an otolaryngologist uses an instrument such as a flexible scope to examine the vocal folds.

discourse: A type of communication that involves a verbal exchange.

discussion: A formal discourse on a topic.

disfluency: A disruption in the forward flow of speech.

disfluency cluster: The occurrence of two or more disfluencies on the same word and/or adjacent words.

displays: Form of visual communication used by animals to attract or warn-off a predator.

dissection: The process of disassembling and observing an anatomical structure to determine its internal structure.

distortion: Type of speech sound misarticulations in which a consonant or vowel is misarticulated to such an extent that the sound produced is unrecognizable.

Down, John Langdon: English physician who is best known for his description of what is now called Down syndrome.

Down syndrome: Chromosomal disorder caused by the presence of an extra 21st chromosome—also known as trisomy 21.

drug therapy: An approach to the treatment of disease by the administration of drugs, chemicals, and antibiotics.

DuMont, Allen B.: Inventor of the picture tube that allowed for mass production of television sets.

Dutrochet, Henri: French physiologist who is credited with identifying the cell.

dysarthria: A motor speech disorder characterized by poor speech sound articulation.

dysphagia: Medical term for the symptom of difficulty in swallowing.

dysphonation: An unusual form of voice production, often characterized by moments of chaotic vocal fold vibration.

echolalia: The repetition of words or phrases made by another individual. A feature of speaking often associated with autism. The manner of echolalia can be either immediate or delayed.

echolocation: A sensory system used by animals such as dolphins and bats using high-pitched sounds to determine the direction and distance of objects—also called biosonar.

edema: Medical condition in which abnormally large volumes of fluid enter muscle tissue.

effortful swallowing: A dysphagia treatment technique that involves the deliberate and forceful act of swallowing.

elective therapy: Form of speech-language therapy that is based on helping an individual improve their communication abilities, although there is no diagnosed communication disorder. A person who speaks English as a Second Language may see elective therapy to help reduce their accent.

electroencephalography: The recording of electrical activity along the scalp produced by the firing of neurons within the brain.

electrolarynx: Device that is intended to reproduce the role of the vocal folds in patients who have had their larynx removed. A handheld device that produces audible vibrations is placed against the neck and the person mouths speech sounds.

electromyography: A technique for testing and recording the electrical activity of muscles.

electronic devices: A category of instruments used to help diminish moments of stuttering.

electropalatograph: Device that records the timing and location of tongue contact with the hard palate during speaking activities—also called a palatometer.

Elocutionary Movement: Approach to speaking in the 18th century concerned with the skill of communication in public settings, such as poetry readings, speeches, or plays.

embolism: An obstruction in a blood vessel due to a blot clot.

embryo: An organism in its early stages of development, especially before it reaches a recognizable form.

embryology: Branch of biology that deals with the formation and early development of living organisms.

Empedocles: Greek philosopher who speculated on the origins of life and human development.

encode: The process of creating a message into code.

endolymph: Thick fluid that fills the cochlear duct of the inner ear.

endolymphatic hydrops: An overaccumulation of endolymph in the inner ear. Often found to be a cause of Ménière disease.

English as a second language (ESL): A person who first acquired a language other than English.

enteral tubes: A tube used for the delivery of nutrition that bypasses normal ingestion of food through the mouth.

epidemiology: Branch of medicine that deals with the causes, distribution, and control of disease within a population.

epiglottis: A leaf-shaped flap of cartilage that covers the trachea during moments of swallowing.

esophageal dysphagia: A disorder of swallowing that is due to abnormal function in the esophagus.

esophageal speech: An alternative approach to producing speech without using the vocal folds. A form of speaking used by people having undergone a laryngectomy.

esophageal stage: The third and final stage in the process of swallowing.

esophagitis: Inflammation of the lining of the esophagus.

esophagus: The muscular tube that connects the throat to the stomach. Commonly known as the gullet.

ethical behavior: Behavior that conforms to accepted professional standards of conduct.

ethnicity: Term that represents social groups with a shared sense of identity, geography, culture, and history.

ethology: The study of animal behavior with special interest in genetically programmed behaviors known as instincts.

etiology: The study of causation.

Eustachi, Bartolomeo: Italian anatomist who described structures of the human body including the eustachian tube of the ear.

eustachian tube: Hollow structure of bone and cartilage extending from the middle ear to the rear of the throat (pharynx).

evidence-based practice: A decision-making process that is based on considering the best available research. In medicine, it is used to help make informed, clinical decisions for patient care.

exhalation phase: The outward flow of air composing one phase of the breathing cycle.

external auditory meatus: A cartilaginous and bony tube that runs from the outer ear to the tympanic membrane—also called the ear canal.

fact level: Form of communication between individuals that involves a low level of intimacy, such as the simple exchange of factual information.

Fairbanks, Grant: Professor in the field of communication disorders who made major contributions to the area of treatment of speech sound disorders.

falsetto: Voice register of males that is above (higher than) the normal speaking range.

fast mapping: A mental process whereby a new concept can be learned based on a single exposure to the concept.

feedback loops: Information about the result of an event or action is sent back to the original input of the system. In the case of communication, the speaker obtains feedback from the listener regarding the original message uttered.

feeding tube: Medical device used to provide nutrition to a person who is unable to obtain nutrition through swallowing.

feelings level: Form of communication between individuals that involves a high level of intimacy between speakers.

Ferrein, Antoine: French anatomist known for his work concerning the physiology of the voice. He is credited with coining the term, vocal cords.

Fetal alcohol syndrome: Birth defect that affects physical and cognitive development resulting from mothers who consumed alcohol during pregnancy.

fetus: Unborn child, spanning the period from eight weeks following conception to the moment of birth.

fiberoptic endoscopic evaluation of swallowing: Procedure for evaluating the oral stage of swallowing based on examination of the oral/pharyngeal cavity with the use of a fiberoptic endoscope.

finger spelling: The representation of letters and numbers of a writing system with the use of one or two hands. A system of communication commonly used by individuals with severe and profound hearing loss.

fissure: A long narrow opening. Fissures along the cerebral cortex provide points of demarcation for the various lobes of the brain.

fistula: A narrow opening or passageway caused by disease or injury.

fixed articulators: Speech articulators that have no moveable action. Examples of fixed articulators include the teeth and hard palate.

fluctuating hearing loss: Condition in which a person's hearing may improve or worsen from one day to the next.

fluency: The effortless flow of speech that includes proper use of rhythm, rate, pausing, and language formulation.

fluency disorder: A disruption in the forward flow of speech.

fluency shaping: A comprehensive therapy for the treatment of stuttering that focuses on changing all speaking behavior, not just moments of stuttering.

fluent aphasia: Language disorder in which a person has difficulty comprehending spoken and written language, although their ability to speak seems to remain relatively intact.

form: The shape or structure of an item that provides distinctive character.

formal communication: Style of communication that follows a specific code for particular settings.

FOXP2: Gene located on chromosome 7 that has been implicated in the development of normal speech and language skills.

Fragile X syndrome: Most common form of inherited intellectual disability that results in a mutation of a gene located on the X chromosome.

Franco, Pierre: Sixteenth-century Swiss surgeon known as the "Father of Cleft Palate Surgery."

free morpheme: The smallest unit of language that can occur by itself.

frequency: The number of vibrations that occur per second.

frequency transposition: Technique used in the programming of hearing aids that extends the audibility of higher frequency sounds for people who cannot receive this information from a conventional hearing aid.

Freud, Sigmund: Austrian neurologist who is considered the founding father of psychoanalysis.

fricatives: A category of consonants sounds classified according to the manner in which they are articulated in the vocal tract. The /s/ and /f/ consonants are examples of fricatives.

front-back confusion: Impairment in the ability to perceive the origin (direction) of a sound source.

frontal lobes: The front of the cerebral cortex, primarily involved in the execution of motor movement as well as mental reasoning.

functional disorder Any disorder that results in the absence of a known anatomical, physiological, or neurological cause.

functional dysphagia: Form of dysphagia that has no identifiable, organic cause.

fundamental frequency: The lowest frequency component of a complex sound.

Gage, Phineas: One of the earliest documented cases of a severe brain injury and its impact on mental function following recovery.

Galen, Claudius: Second-century physiologist who is often considered the founder of laryngology and voice science.

Gall, Franz Joseph: German anatomist and pioneer in the study of brain functions who developed a system for studying the brain by noting the shape of the skull called phrenology.

Gallaudet, Thomas Hopkins: American educator and founder of the first American school for the deaf.

García, Manuel: Spaniard who developed the laryngeal mirror.

gastroesophageal reflux disease: A chronic condition in which stomach acid is regurgitated resulting in heartburn and indigestion.

gastronomy tube: Feeding tube used in situations when a person is unable to swallow normally. The tube is placed directly into the stomach and is used to deliver nutrition to the body—also called a percutaneous endoscopic gastrostomy (PEG) tube.

gaze-coupling: An early form of communicative exchange between a young infant and parent where the infant turns toward the speaker and gains eye contact.

gene mutation: A permanent change in the DNA that makes up a gene.

gene splicing: Form of genetic engineering where specific genes are inserted into the genome of a different organism.

genes: Hereditary unit that occupies a specific location on a chromosome and determines a particular characteristic in an organism.

genetic: Relating to genes or heredity.

genetic counseling: A service that is designed to help families who may be at risk for an inherited disease or abnormal pregnancy outcome, and to discuss the chances of having children who are affected.

genetic syndromes: A disorder caused by abnormalities in one or more genes.

genetics: Branch of biology that deals with hereditary and the transmission of characteristics among organisms.

genome: The total DNA sequence that characterizes a species, including humans.

genotype: The genetic makeup of an organism.

geographic dialects: Variations in the style of speaking according to geographic region. A New England dialect is an example of a geographic dialect.

geographic region: Demarcated areas of the world. Some disease conditions vary in regard to geographic region.

Glasgow Coma Scale: Scoring system used to describe the level of consciousness in a person following a traumatic brain injury.

glides A category of consonants sounds classified according to the manner in which they are articulated in the vocal tract. The /w/ is an example of a glide.

globus: The sensation of a lump in the throat.

glossectomy: Surgical removal of the tongue.

glottal: Location in the vocal tract that is just above the vocal folds (glottis).

glottal stop /ʔ/: A speech sound produced by a momentary complete closure of the glottis followed by an explosive release.

glottis: The space between the open vocal folds.

Goodall, Jane: Renowned English primatologist and ethologist—one of the world's foremost authorities on the behavior of chimpanzees.

graphic cuing: Language treatment technique for individuals with brain injury that involves providing familiar photographs to facilitate communication.

Gray, Henry: Nineteenth-century English anatomist whose classic publication regarding human anatomy is still used today.

grommet: See pressure-equalization tube.

gross anatomy: Study of organs, parts, and structures of a body that are visible to the naked eye.

group communication: The interactive exchange of information that occurs among more than 3 people, and usually no more than 20 people.

Gutenberg, Johann: Inventor of the printing press in the 15th century.

Gutzmann, Hermann: German physician who studied speech disorders from a medical point of view.

gyri: A bump or ridge like those found along the surface of the cerebral cortex.

habitual pitch: The speaking voice that is most commonly used.

hair cells: Sensory receptors that are found in the inner ear (cochlea and vestibular apparatus).

hard of hearing: A person who has any level of hearing impairment other than deafness.

hard palate: Bony roof of the mouth that separates the nasal cavity from the oral cavity.

Hawk, Sara Stinchfield: First individual in the United States to obtain a PhD in speech-language pathology.

hearing aid: Device that can amplify sound waves in order to help a hard-of-hearing person perceive sounds more clearly.

helicotrema: An opening at the apical end of the cochlea that connects the scala vestibuli canal with the scala typani canal.

helix: The cartilaginous rim of the outer ear.

hemiparesis: Body weakness or paralysis occurring on one side of the body only.

hemispheres: The two halves of a circle. The cerebrum (brain) is divided into a left and right hemisphere.

hemorrhage: Excessive loss of blood from blood vessels.

Henry, Joseph: American scientist of the 18th century whose early work in electromagnetism eventually led to the development of the telegraph.

heredity: The genetic transmission of characteristics from parent to offspring.

Hertz, Heinrich: German physicist who was the first to send and receive radio waves.

hertz (Hz) scale: Notation used to refer to frequency, or the number of vibrations per second. Developed in honor of Heinrich Hertz.

hieratic: A cursive form of Egyptian hieroglyphics.

hieroglyphics: System of writing using pictorial symbols to represent sounds or meanings.

high-frequency hearing loss: A configuration of hearing loss where a person is unable to clearly perceive sounds that are in excess of 1000 to 2000 Hz.

Hippocrates: Greek physician who described the importance of the lungs, trachea, lips, and tongue in phonation in the early fifth century BC.

hoarse voice: A description of voice quality, involving an unusually low-pitched voice.

holism theory: Theory that views brain functioning as a single, non-localized, organ.

Hooke, Robert: English philosopher who coined the term *cell* to refer to the basic unit of life.

Human Genome Project: An international scientific undertaking to determine the complete structure of the human genetic material known as DNA.

Husson, Raoul: Developed one of the earliest modern theories of normal voice production known as the neurochronaxic theory.

hyoid bone A horseshoe-shaped bone that is located high in the neck. The most superior portion of the laryngeal framework.

hyperfunctional voice: Speaking with excessive muscular effort and force resulting in a tense, high-pitched voice. A form of spasmodic dysphonia.

hypernasal speech: Abnormal speech characterized by the excess flow of sound through the nasal cavity.

hypnotherapy: Approach to the treatment of a variety of health conditions by hypnotism or by inducing prolonged sleep.

hypofunctional voice: Refers to inadequate muscle tone of the laryngeal mechanism during the production of voice often resulting in weak, low-pitched voice that may also sound breathy. Found in some conditions associated with muscle weakness such as amyotrophic lateral sclerosis.

hypotonia: Decrease of normal muscle tone or tension.

idioglossia: Term used to describe a unique, specialized language thought to be indicative of the early speech spoken by twins.

idioms: Words or phrases that cannot be taken literally.

idiopathic: A condition that is of unknown origin.

immittance testing: Form of audiological testing that provides information regarding eardrum mobility and eardrum function—often called tympanometry.

informal communication: Specific code of communication that allows for a varied manner of speaking.

in-the-canal aid (ITC): Type of hearing aid where all components of the aid are situated directly within the ear canal.

in-the-ear aid (ITE): Type of hearing aid where all components of the aid are situated within the entrance of the ear canal.

incidence: The number of new cases that occur during a particular period of time.

incomplete cleft lip: A cleft that does not penetrate the nostrils.

incomplete cleft palate: A cleft that does not encompass the entire hard and soft palate structure, only a portion is affected.

incus: The middle bone of the three small bones (ossicles) of the middle ear, also known as the anvil to reflect its unique shape.

indirect laryngoscopy: Procedure in which an otolaryngologist uses an instrument, such as a mirror, to examine the vocal folds.

infant: A child under the age of 12 months. Derived from the Latin word meaning "without speech."

infant mortality: The death of a child less than one year of age. Often used as a barometer of the social well being of a country.

ingestion: The consumption of food or drink by an organism.

inhalation phase: The inward flow of air composing one phase of a breathing cycle.

inhibiting: The inability to suppress emotions. Some individuals with brain injury may show difficulty with inhibiting.

initial assessment: The first phase in the diagnosis of aphasia where the speech-language pathologist meets with the patient while still in the hospital.

instant messaging: Form of real-time communication between two or more people based on typed text over the Internet.

intelligence quotient (IQ): A measure used to estimate intellect, usually calculated by examining the ratio of a person's mental age compared with their chronological age.

intelligibility: Term used to describe the clarity of a person's speech sound productions.

International Classification of Functioning (ICF) Framework developed by the World Health Organization that classifies health according to a number of domains.

intensity: The maximum disturbance of a sound wave. Also referred to as amplitude.

interactionist theory: A theory of language development whereby children acquire their language through a combination of behavioral and nativist processes.

International Phonetic Alphabet (IPA): System of phonetic notation developed by the International Phonetic Association that can be used to represent the sounds of any language.

Internet: An interconnected system of networks that connects computers around the world.

interpersonal communication: Form of communication that occurs between two or more people.

invisible-in-the-canal aid (IIC): Miniature hearing aid that sits deep in the ear canal.

Iowa Scale for Rating the Severity of Stuttering: Scale used for determining the severity of speech disfluency based on noting the number and type of speech disfluencies occurring within a conversational speech sample.

Itard, Jean-Marc Gaspard: French physician known for his work with deaf and intellectually impaired individuals, particularly Victor, the wild boy of Aveyron.

itinerant speech-language pathologist: A speech-language pathologist who works in a number of settings. Speech-language pathologists who work for a school system tend to work in more than one school setting.

Janssen, Zaccharias: Dutch spectacle-maker who is believed to be the inventor of the microscope.

Jean, Andre: French physiologist who has studied the role of the brainstem in the process of swallowing.

Jefferson, Thomas: Third President of the United States and a follower of the Elocutionary Movement.

Johnson, Wendell: American speech-language pathologist known for his work in stuttering.

Kanner, Leo: Austrian psychiatrist known for his work in autism.

karyotype: The arrangement of chromosomes within a cell.

Keller, Helen: The first deaf-blind person to achieve a university education, who later became an advocate for individuals with disabilities.

King Louis II: King of France during the period of 843 to 879 who was also known to stutter.

L1: Abbreviation used to designate the first or dominant language.

L2: Abbreviation used to designate the second or less dominant language.

labio-dental: A class of consonants that are categorized according to their place of articulation within the vocal tract. The /f/ and /v/ are examples of labio-dental consonants.

laceration: A wound or cut to that involves direct tearing of tissue.

Lahey, Margaret: Developed a framework for describing the various strands of language, according to form, content, and use.

Lashley, Karl: First individual to define autism, based on examination of 11 self-absorbed children who had autistic disturbances of affect contact.

language: The expression of human communication through which information can be experienced, explained, and shared.

language acquisition device: Proposed by Noam Chomsky as a special biological brain mechanism that humans are born with that enables them to learn language.

language content: Aspect of language that concerns meanings of individual words and words in combination. Another name for language content is semantics.

language delay: A language disorder indicating that the child's language system is similar to younger, nondisordered children.

language deviance: A language disorder whereby the child is exhibiting a linguistic system that is unlike that of younger nondisordered children.

language difference Situation in which the language features of a community differ from the majority. The rules are normal for the smaller community.

language expansions: Language therapy approach in which the therapist restates the child's utterance using a fuller and grammatically correct language model.

language form: Aspect of language that concerns the features of phonology, morphology, and syntax.

language sampling: Feature of a language assessment in which a representative sample of the child's typical expressive language behavior is collected and later analyzed.

language use: Aspect of language in a social context. Another name for language use is pragmatics.

Larsen, George L.: American speech-language pathologist who was one of the first individuals to develop specific treatment techniques for individuals with dysphagia.

laryngeal system: The anatomical structures that comprise the larynx, which include cartilages, muscles, and bone.

laryngectomy: Partial or complete removal of the larynx, including the vocal folds. The most common form of surgery to treat laryngeal cancer.

laryngitis: Inflammation of the vocal folds, associated with symptoms of sore throat and swallowing difficulty.

larynx: Structure that consists of a number of muscles and cartilages that work cooperatively to produce voice.

late talker: A term used to describe children between the ages of 16 to 30 months who are slow in acquiring their first 50 words.

Lee Silverman Voice Treatment (LSVT): A structured programmatic approach to voice therapy. The premise of the approach is to encourage a full, loud speaking voice to improve overall voice quality as well as speech clarity.

left neglect: Situation in which a person who experiences a right hemisphere stroke no longer acknowledges the left side of their body.

Lejeune, Jerome: French geneticist who discovered the chromosome abnormalies in humans that causes Down syndrome, as well as Cri du Chat syndrome.

Levi-Montalcine, Rita: Italian neurologist who discovered a protein that causes developing cells to grow. Her research has implications for helping to restore hearing.

Lidcombe Program: Stuttering treatment program developed in Australia for children younger than six years of age.

limbic system: A region deep within the cerebrum that includes part of or most of the other lobes (i.e., frontal, parietal, and temporal). The limbic system is involved in affective behaviors such as emotion and motivation.

lingua-alveolar: A class of consonants categorized according to their place of articulation within the vocal tract. Examples of lingua-alveolar consonants are /t/ and /s/.

linguadental: A class of consonants categorized according to their place of articulation within the vocal tract. An example of a linguadental consonant is /th/.

lingual frenulum: Tendon that extends from the floor of the mouth to the underside of the tongue.

linguapalatal: A class of consonants categorized according to their place of articulation within the vocal tract. An example of a linguapalatal consonant is /sh/.

linguavelar: A class of consonants categorized according to their place of articulation within the vocal tract. Examples of linguavelar consonants are /k/ and /g/.

lips: Two bands of muscular tissue.

liquids: A class of consonant sounds organized according to the manner in which they are articulated in the vocal tract. The consonants /r/ and /l/ are examples of liquids.

lobule: An anatomical extension such as that found at the base of the outer ear.

localism theory: A theory of brain functioning that assigns specific functions of the brain to specific regions of the brain.

Logemann, Jeri A.: American speech-language pathologist who is a pioneer in the assessment and treatment of dysphagia.

logopedics: Commonly used term in Europe to refer to the study and treatment of communication disorders.

loudness: The psychological perception of the intensity of an acoustic signal.

lower respiratory tract: The cavities of the body that include the trachea, bronchial tubes, and lungs.

lungs: Two spongy organs that function to remove carbon dioxide from the body and provide it with oxygen.

magnetic resonance imaging (MRI): Test that uses a magnetic field and pulses of radio wave energy to make a picture of organs and structures inside the body.

maintenance: The type of swallow used to remove natural build-up of saliva in the oral cavity.

malingerer: Someone who intentionally fakes or exaggerates a psychological or physical condition for personal gain.

malleus: Outermost of the three small bones (ossicles) of the middle ear, also known as the hammer to reflect its unique shape.

malocclusion: An uneven alignment between the upper and lower teeth.

mandible: Anatomical name for the lower jaw.

manner of articulation: Classification of consonant sounds in regard to how they are articulated in the vocal tract.

manual communication: Use of hand gestures to transfer information between individuals.

Marconi, Gugliemo: Italian inventor who is generally credited with creating the radio.

mass communication: Exchange of information to a large public audience through some sort of medium, such as radio, television, or the Internet.

mastication: The act of chewing.

maximal contrast approach: Treatment approach for phonological disorders that is designed to enact widespread change. Rather than targeting early developing sounds, later developing sounds are the focus of therapy.

mean length of utterance (MLU): A measure that examines a child's increasing ability to combine words and produce complex utterances by noting the average length of utterances according to grammatical morphemes.

medical model: Approach to the identification of disorders on the basis of an identifiable physical cause.

memory: A person's ability to remember things.

Mendel, Gregor: Austrian botanist who is known as the "Father of Modern Genetics," based on his work with pea plants.

Ménière disease: Disorder of the inner ear that can affect balance and hearing.

Ménière, Prosper: French otolaryngologist who was the first to describe a form of vertigo (dizziness) that is now known as Ménière disease.

meningitis: Infection of the fluid that surrounds the brain and spinal cord. The condition is caused by either viral or bacterial infection.

metacentric chromosome: A chromosome with a centrally placed centromere that divides the chromosome into two arms having approximately equal length.

metalinguistic awareness: The ability to reflect consciously on the nature and properties of language.

microblogging: The act of posting short messages on a social network website.

microcephaly: Abnormal smallness of the head.

microform cleft: Rare anomaly that can appear as a small scar on the lip.

micrognathia: A condition of abnormal smallness of the upper and lower jaws, usually the mandible.

microphone: A transducer that is designed to transform acoustic energy into an equivalent electrical representation.

middle ear implant: A surgical procedure designed to stimulate movement of the ossicles of the middle ear to incoming sound, as a means of improving hearing.

minimal pair: Refers to a situation where two words differ in pronunciation by only one sound, and the change in sound results in a change in word meaning. The words "dear" and "gear" are examples of minimal pairs.

misarticulation: Any deviation, great or small, in the pronunciation of consonant or vowel phonemes.

mixed (or global) aphasia: Communication disorder that involves impairment in both comprehension and production of language—generally considered the most severe form of aphasia.

mixed dysarthria: A non-pure form of dysarthria involving a combination of two or more types.

mixed hearing loss: Simultaneous occurrence of both a conductive hearing loss and sensorineural hearing loss.

mobile phone: A wireless telephone. The term was originally confined to telephones that were found in automobiles.

modal register: The middle register of one's speaking voice.

model: Academic term used to refer to an abstract idea.

modified barium swallow: Radiological imaging procedure that is used for the evaluation and treatment of swallowing disorders.

Montessori-based intervention: Language treatment technique using structured activities that take place in the context of social interaction.

monotonic voice: Lack of natural melodic voice inflection. A condition associated with the speaking voice of individuals with Parkinson disease.

Morgan, Thomas Hunt: Pioneer in the area of genetics. Received the Nobel Prize for his work on hereditary traits of fruit flies.

morphology: The smallest meaningful units of language.

Morse code: Alphabetic system for the telegraph that uses a combination of short and long clicks to create words.

Morse, Samuel: American creator of the telegraph in the 19th century.

mosaicism: Condition in which the cells composing an organism are not identical, having differing genotypes.

motor speech disorders: Impaired speech sound production ability resulting from motor pathway damage affecting the muscles responsible for producing speech.

mouth breathing: Process of inhalation and exhalation through the oral cavity rather than the nasal cavity.

movable articulators: Anatomical structures involved in speech production that are capable of moving. Examples of movable articulators include the lips, tongue, and soft palate.

multifactorial: The cause of a communication disorder attributed to more than one variable.

multilingualism: Individual who has knowledge of two or more languages. This knowledge may include the ability to speak, understand, read, or write more then one language.

multiple sclerosis: Disease in which the nerves of the central nervous system degenerate causing an impairment of movement, sensation, and body functions.

Mutual Recognition of Credentials Agreement: Pact signed by various speech-language pathology professional organizations worldwide that provides a framework for professionals from one country to practice as therapists in another country.

myelin sheath: The insulating envelope that surrounds the core of a nerve fiber (axon) to facilitate the transmission of nerve impulses.

myoelastic aerodynamic theory of phonation: Well-accepted theory of voice production that involves coordination of muscle tension and breath pressure.

myringotomy: Surgical incision into the tympanic membrane (eardrum) that is usually performed to relieve pressure or fluid buildup in the middle ear.

nares: The external openings of the nose—also called nostrils.

nasal cavity: The cavity lying between the floor of the cranium and the roof of the mouth and extending from the nostrils to the pharynx.

nasals: A class of consonant sounds categorized according to the manner in which they are articulated in the vocal tract. The consonants /m/ and /n/ are examples of nasal consonants.

nasogastric tube (NG tube): Type of feeding tube used on a short-term basis and involves passing a tube through the nose, pharynx, and esophagus directly into the stomach.

nasometer: Commercially available instrument designed to measure both oral and nasal airflow emitted during speech production.

nativist theory: A theory of normal language acquisition proposed by Noam Chomsky, which suggests that humans are born with the biological makeup to learn language.

natural theory: A theory of phonological development proposed by David Stampe based on the natural occurrence and suppression of phonological patterns (or processes).

needs level: The level of communication that occurs between two people who know one another intimately. They seem to know intuitively what the other person thinks.

Negus, Sir Victor: British laryngologist who was a pioneer in detailing the anatomy of the human and animal larynx.

neural plasticity: Refers to the ability of the brain and/or certain parts of the nervous system to change in order to adapt to new conditions, such as an injury.

neural tube defects: Congenital abnormality of the brain and spinal cord resulting from incomplete closing of the neural tube during embryonic development. Spina bifida is an example of a neural tube defect.

neurochronaxic theory: A theory proposed in 1950 that viewed the frequency of vocal fold vibration as being dependent on excitation of nerve cells from the laryngeal nerve.

neurogenic: Refers to having its origin or starting with the nervous system.

neurogenic stuttering: Form of stuttering characterized by a high number of involuntary repetitions or prolongations of speech that do not seem to be a result of poor (hesitant) language formulation difficulties or as a result of psychiatric problems. A condition sometimes found in Parkinson disease.

neurological: Relating to nerves and the nervous system.

neuromonics: Treatment for tinnitus that combines the use of a novel approach to acoustic stimulation with a structured program of counseling and support by a clinician.

neuromuscular electrical stimulation (E-Stim): An electrical current is used to stimulate the same electrical impulses that are activated during normal exercise. By passively activating the muscle, the body responds in much the same way as during normal exercise.

neuroplasticity: The brain's ability to reorganize itself by forming new neural connections throughout life

neuroprosthetics: The design and manufacture of neural prosthetics that can serve as a substitute for a motor or sensory modality that may have been damaged. A cochlear implant is a form of a neuroprosthetic device.

neuropsycholinguistic theory: A theory of stuttering based on the assumption that producing fluent speech involves sophisticated timing between the formulation of language and the actual motor execution of speech movement. Stuttering results in a situation where there is a disruption in the timing (integration) of linguistic formulation and speech movement.

noise: Acoustic sound wave that has random variations in amplitude and frequency. A lack of periodicity (back and forth vibration).

noise-induced hearing loss: Hearing impairment that results from exposure to excessively loud sounds.

nonbehavioral tests: Form of audiology testing that does not require the person to push a button or raise their hand in response to sounds. Rather, the tests are designed to measure natural physiological responses to sounds. The auditory brainstem response is a nonbehavioral test.

nonfluent aphasia: Language disorder in which an individual has difficulty expressing himself when speaking or writing, although their ability to understand language seems to remain relatively intact.

nonmaleficence: Ethical principle in health sciences and public health practice in which the professional strives to do no harm to the patient.

nonstandardized testing: Form of assessment in which there is no consistent or standardized manner to perform the assessment. This form of assessment generally provides the examiner with more flexibility. The collection and subsequent analysis of a language sample is a common form of nonstandardized testing.

nonverbal communication: Form of communication in which the exchange of information occurs without the use of spoken words. The use of eye contact is a form of nonverbal communication.

norms: A standard, model, or pattern regarded as typical. Norms are often used to assess individuals who are suspected of having a communication disorder.

nucleus: The central part of a cell that contains hereditary material.

objective assessment: Approach to evaluating a communication disorder using commercially available test instruments.

obstruction: An obstacle or blockage that impedes progress. A common disorder of the outer ear involves an obstruction of the ear canal.

obturator: A prosthetic device serving to close an opening in the body, such as a cleft palate.

occipital lobes: The posterior lobe of each cerebral hemisphere that contain the visual centers of the brain.

occlusion: The fitting together of the upper and lower teeth.

odynophagia: Pain associated with the act of swallowing.

omission: Pattern of speech misarticulations whereby the intended speech sound is deleted.

onomatopoeia: Use of sounds to signify a word based on the sound associated with the particular word. For example, beep-beep would be a form onomatopoeia to signify the word car.

onset: To start or begin. The onset of stuttering typically occurs at three years of age.

Operation Smile: International charity program for treating facial deformities such as cleft lip and palate.

opinion level: The level of communication that occurs between two people on somewhat of a personal level and includes comments, concerns, expectations, and personal goals.

optimality theory: A theoretical approach to describing the structure of grammar in a given language.

optimum pitch The level at which we can produce our strongest voice.

oral: The mouth.

oral cavity: The space inside the mouth that runs from the inside of the lips to the back of the throat.

ora-facial examination: A routine assessment of the structure and function of the mouth and face in regard to their influence on speech sound production.

oral stage: The first stage in the three-stage process of swallowing.

organ of Corti: Specialized structure located within the scala media of the cochlea. The organ contains hair cells that assist in the transfer of sound through the auditory system.

organic disorder: Medical or health condition with a known physical cause.

organizational communication: Type of communication that occurs in environments such as workplace offices and corporations.

oropharyngeal dysphagia: Most common form of dysphagia that reflects an impairment in the transfer of liquid or food from the mouth and pharynx to the opening of the esophagus.

orthognathic surgery: Procedure that is designed to correct conditions of the jaws and face related to structure and growth.

orthographic transcription: A type of annotation system used for detailing a sample of spoken language. The standard alphabet is used to write every word that is spoken.

Orton, Samuel: American physician who was interested in the area of learning disabilities, particularly those associated with reading.

ossicular chain: The three tiny bones that compose the middle ear, consisting of the malleus, incus, and stapes.

other disfluencies: Class of speech disfluencies that are found to occur in people who do not stutter, as well as those who do stutter. An example of an OD is a phrase repetition.

otitis externa: Infection of the ear canal, often associated with persistent exposure to water. Also called swimmer's ear.

otitis media: Infection of the middle ear space behind the eardrum. The duration of a bout of otitis media can range from acute to subacute, or chronic.

otitis media with effusion: Form of otitis media characterized by buildup of fluid in the middle ear space—also called glue ear.

otoacoustic emissions: Tiny sounds that emerge from the inner ear either spontaneously or shortly after the ear is exposed to an external sound. A screening test for newborn hearing.

otolaryngologist: Surgeon who specializes in the diagnosis and treatment of disorders of the ear, nose, or throat (also called an ENT).

otosclerosis: Hereditary disorder that results in abnormal growth in the middle ear that causes hearing loss.

otoscope: Instrument consisting of a light and magnifying lens that is used for examining the external auditory meatus (ear canal) and tympanic membrane (eardrum).

ototoxic hearing loss: A hearing impairment (both temporary and permanent) that can result from high doses of certain drugs.

overt behavior: Openly visible behavior.

Pagoclone: Antianxiety drug that is currently being evaluated as a treatment for stuttering.

papilloma: Benign wartlike tumors that form over muscle tissue. Papillomas have been found to form on the vocal folds.

papyrus: Thick, paperlike material produced from the papyrus plant. Used by ancient Egyptians as an early form of paper.

paralanguage: The nonverbal features that accompany speech and help convey meaning.

parallel talk: Language therapy approach in which the therapist describes out loud what the child is seeing, hearing, or thinking during the play activity.

Pare, Ambroise: French surgeon in the 16th century.

parent-directed therapy: Feature of speech and language therapy in which parents are an active and integral part of the child's therapy program.

parenteral tube: Feeding tube in which nutrition is delivered to the body intravenously—also called an IV tube.

parietal lobes: The lobes located at the top of the cerebral cortex that are largely responsible for sensation.

Parkinson disease: Degenerative neurological syndrome of the central nervous system that is characterized by rhythmical muscular tremors.

particulate theories: Early theories of genetics that posited that information from each part of the parent had to be communicated to create the corresponding body part in the offspring.

Passavant, Philip Gustav: German surgeon who was one of the first to propose a series of surgical solutions to help reduce hypernasal speech in cleft lip and palate.

passive muscular process: The relaxation of muscles for a specified movement. Breath exhalation involves a passive muscular process.

pediatric dysphagia: A swallowing disorder in children.

Penfield, Wilder: Famous brain surgeon who made contributions in mapping brain function.

percentage of consonants correct: Measure used to determine the severity of an individual's speech sound disorder. The percentage is calculated by examining the total number of consonants composing a speech sample in comparison with the number of consonants produced accurately by the speaker.

percutaneously: Effected or passed through the skin.

perforated eardrum: Puncture in the tympanic membrane.

perilymph: Fluid that is scala vestibuli and scala media ducts of the cochlea.

peripheral auditory system: Portion of the hearing anatomy that consists of the outer, middle, and inner ear structures.

peripheral nervous system: Portion of the nervous system that lies outside the brain and spinal cord.

peristalsis: Rippling, wavelike muscle contractions, which occur when food is digested.

per oral: Through or by way of the mouth.

personality and emotional adjustment theory: A theory that considers an individual's personality and subsequent behavioral patterns in the development of a voice disorder.

pervasive developmental disorder: Group of disorders characterized by delays in development of social, language, motor, and/or cognitive skills.

pharyngeal cavity: See definition for pharynx.

pharyngeal flap: Surgical procedure designed to reduce hypernasality. A flap of skin creates a bridge between the back of the throat and the soft palate.

pharyngeal fricative /ʃ/: A unique consonant that is articulated with the root of the tongue against the pharynx.

pharyngeal stage: The second stage in the three-stage process of normal swallowing, where the tongue transports material toward the back of the throat.

pharyngoplasty: Form of surgery to reduce nasality in speech by narrowing the pharynx.

pharynx: Hollow muscular tube that runs from the back of the nose to the top of the trachea (windpipe) and esophagus (food tube)—also called the throat.

phenotype: The observable physical characteristics of an organism.

phenylketonuria: Genetic disorder that is characterized by an inability of the body to utilize the amino acid, phenylalanine, which is essential for delivering protein to the body.

pheromones: Chemical secreted by the body that triggers a natural behavioral response in another member of the same species.

philtrum: Shallow groove or depression running down the center of the outer surface of the upper lip.

phonation: Sound made by the vibration of the vocal folds and modified by the resonance of the vocal tract.

phonatory disorder: An abnormality in the ability to produce one's voice.

phonemes: The consonant and vowel sounds spoken in a language.

phonetic inventory: A list of speech sounds that a person is able to accurately articulate.

phonetic-motoric disorder: A theory of speech apraxia where the disorder is attributed to difficulty with the linguistic/phonetic organization and motoric execution of speech.

phoniatrics: The medical research and treatment of organs involved in speech production.

phonomicrosurgery: Surgical treatment of voice pathology using a microscope and microinstruments.

phonological approach: Form of treating phonological disorders based on a linguistic (as opposed to motoric) approach.

phonological awareness: An understanding of the sounds of words and word parts, including the ability to identify and manipulate larger

parts of the spoken language such as words, syllables, and rhyme.

phonological difference: Pattern of speaking found in bilingual speakers where the individual's dominant language affects the pronunciation of the less dominant language. The patterns are predictable based on the phonological features of the dominant language, and therefore not considered to reflect a phonological disorder.

phonological disorder: Impairment in the accurate production of speech sounds.

phonological interference: Pattern of speech sound production found in bilingual speakers, where the phonological patterns of one language affect (interfere with) the pronunciation patterns in another language.

phonological processes: Systematic pattern of speech sound production that affects an entire class of speech sounds. Stopping of fricatives is an example of a phonological process.

phonology: The study of the speech sounds of a language.

phonosurgery: Medical operation designed to repair damage to the vocal folds.

phonotrauma: Any form of abuse to the vocal folds.

phrenology: The study of the shape of the skull that was thought to reveal a person's character and mental capacity.

physical appearance: A form of communication that is transmitted based on physical features of the individual.

physiology: The biological study of the function of living organisms and their parts.

Piaget, Jean: Swiss psychologist known for his study of the intellectual growth of children.

picture-naming task: Common method of sampling a person's speech sound production skills in which a person is asked to name a picture containing specific consonant and vowels sounds.

pinna: Most visible portion of the outer ear—also known as the auricle.

pipe speech: Manner of speaking where the upper and lower jaws are immobilized. This effect can be achieved by biting the end of a pipe and speaking at the same time.

pitch: Perceptual impression of the vocal fundamental frequency of an individual's speaking voice.

place of articulation: Description of consonant sounds in regard to the location in the vocal tract where the sound was articulated.

Plato: Ancient Greek philosopher.

positron emission tomography (PET) scan: Method of body scanning in which a small amount of radio-labeled compound is injected or inhaled in the tissue to be studied.

postauricular muscle response: Electrophysiological method of testing hearing sensitivity based on detecting muscular activity located behind the outer ear in response to sound.

postlingual deafness: Profound hearing loss that occurred after a person learned to talk.

Prader-Willi syndrome: Disorder caused by a genetic deletion of portions of chromosome 15.

pragmatics: The study of language as it is used in a social context.

prelingual deafness: Profound hearing loss that was present before a child learned to talk.

prelinguistic: Refers to the vocal behaviors a child demonstrates prior to producing first-words (language). The production of babbling is a prelinguistic vocal behavior.

premorbid state: An individual's health status before the occurrence of a physical disease or emotional illness.

prenatal diagnosis: The process of assessing the health status of a fetus prior to birth.

presbycusis: Type of hearing loss that gradually occurs as people grow older.

pressure equalization tube: Small tube that is inserted through the tympanic membrane (eardrum) to provide ventilation to the middle ear, also known as a grommet.

prevalence: Total number of cases of a disease in a given population at a specific time.

primary assessment: The full assessment of language expression and comprehension in an individual with suspected aphasia.

primary auditory center: Region in the temporal lobe of the brain that is responsible for the sensation of sound, also called Heschl's gyrus.

primary characteristics: The core features. The primary characteristics of stuttering are the moments of stuttering that occur while speaking.

print-in-palm: Approach used to communicate with a deaf-blind person by tracing the shapes of block letters on the palm of their hand with an index finger.

product: Something produced by mechanical or human effort or by a natural process.

progressive hearing loss A hearing loss that gets worse over time. Persistent exposure to loud noise can result in a progressive hearing loss.

proteomics: Branch of genetics that studies the proteins expressed by the genome of an organism.

proxemics: The study of cultural, behavioral, and sociological aspects of spatial distance between individuals.

psychogenic disorder: A disorder that stems from mental or emotional problems as opposed to having a known physiological cause.

psychogenic stuttering: Type of stuttering that is thought to be caused by emotional trauma or problems with thought or reasoning.

psychological disturbance: A disorder of the mind involving thoughts, behaviors, and emotions that cause either self or others significant distress.

psychosocial behavior: The mental and physical reactions that occur when an individual is placed in an environmental setting

puberphonia: Unusually high-pitched speaking voice that persists beyond puberty.

public communication: Form of communication that is used to promote ideas and social causes.

pulse register: Lowest range of speaking voice—also known as vocal fry register.

pure tone: A sound composed of a single frequency.

pure-tone audiometry: Use of single-frequency sounds (tones) in the evaluation of a person's hearing sensitivity.

qualitative: An evaluation based on description of attributes, characteristics, and properties without the use of numbers.

quantitative: An evaluation based on numeric description of attributes, characteristics and properties.

race: Group of people classified on the basis of common history, nationality, geographic distribution, or genetically transmitted physical characteristics.

radio: The wireless transmission of electromagnetic waves that are decoded into audible sounds.

range of motion: Description of movement in regard to maximal and minimal movement.

rate of movement: Description of movement in regard to the speed at which the movement is performed.

reciprocity: Mutual agreement or dependence. Professional reciprocity refers to an agreement between associations regarding the qualifications to practice as an audiologist or speech-language pathologist in another state or country.

reflux: A flowing back of fluid, often associated with the human digestive system and the reflux of gastric juices.

register of voice: The range of voice produced by humans including low-, medium-, and high-pitched sounds.

rehabilitation hospital: A hospital that is devoted to providing rehabilitation care to patients with various neurological or orthopedic conditions on an inpatient basis.

residual errors: Pattern of speech sound misarticulations that involve either a fricative or liquid consonant.

respiratory cycle: One complete breath, including an inspiratory and expiratory phase.

respiratory training: Treatment approach to improving voice quality that involves focus on proper breathing techniques.

retrocochlear pathology: Abnormality of the auditory system that occurs beyond the cochlea, most often seen as tumor of the auditory nerve or brainstem.

reverse swallow: See definition for tongue thrust.

rhetoric: The art or study of using language persuasively and effectively.

rib cage: Twelve sets of bones that encloses the lungs and heart.

right hemisphere theory of recovery: Theory related to left hemisphere brain damage where the right hemisphere takes over all functions that would have normally occurred in the left hemisphere.

Rustin, Lena: British speech-language pathologist who was an expert clinician in the area of stuttering management.

S * T = P: Abbreviation for the source-filter theory of phonation.

SALT (systematic analysis of language transcripts): Computer software program designed to provide a detailed grammatical analysis of a sample of spoken (and transcribed) English.

savant: A scholar or learned person.

scala media: The middle chamber of the cochlea located between the scala tympani and scala media. The chamber is filled with endolymph. Also called the cochlear duct.

scala tympani: The lower chamber of the cochlea that is filled with perilymph.

scala vestibuli: The upper chamber of the cochlea that is filled with perilymph.

schisis: Medical term for opening, which is used to describe an orofacial cleft.

Schuell, Hildred: American speech-language pathologist who devoted her career to the evaluation and treatment of aphasia.

Schulthess, Rudolf: Swiss scientist who theorized that stuttering was due to spasms of the larynx.

Scripture, Edward Wheeler: One of the first Americans trained in the field of psychology who developed skills in hearing measurement such as threshold testing and magnitude estimation. He was interested in various aspects of disordered speech production.

Seashore, Carl: American psychologist interested in music, voice, and hearing. He built the first audiometer.

secondary characteristics: Features that are not part of the primary form.

secondary characteristics of stuttering: Those behaviors that occur in addition to the primary (moment) of stuttering.

self-talk: The internal dialogue we use to view the world, explain situations, and communicate to ourselves.

semantics: The study or science of meaning in language.

semicircular canals: Three tiny circular tubes of the inner ear that are positioned at right angles to each other. They serve as the body's balance organ.

semiotics: The theory and study of signs and symbols, especially as they relate to communication.

sensorineural hearing loss: Most common type of hearing loss resulting from damage to the inner ear, or regions of the central auditory system.

severity: Term used to describe degrees of hearing loss ranging from mild to profound.

severity scale: An approach to estimate the severity of communication using a fixed numeric scale, such as

1 to 9, with 1 = low severity and 10 = high severity.

sign language: A language that uses a system of manual, facial, and other body movements as a means of communication.

signal-to-noise ratio: A measure of signal strength relative to background noise. The ratio is usually measured in decibels (dB).

simultaneous bilingualism: An individual who has acquired two or more languages with equal skill in both.

simultaneous communication (SimCom): Combined use of sign language and speech to communicate.

single words: Earliest identifiable language productions produced by children, usually by the age of 12 months.

Skinner, Burrhus Frederic (B. F.): American psychologist who published significant scientific works in the analysis of behavior.

Smile Train: International charity that provides cleft lip and palate surgery to children in need, as well as providing medical training to doctors.

social media: A network of friends, colleagues, and other personal contacts.

socioeconomic dialect: A manner of speaking that is associated with an individual's financial and/or social status.

socioeconomic status: A measure based on financial and social indicators.

SODA: An acronym that describes the notation of disorderd speech patterns, s = substittion, o = omission, d = distortion, a = addition.

soft palate: The soft tissue that composes the back of the roof of the mouth, also known as the velum.

sound: Vibrations that are transmitted through a medium. Sound can be described according to its duration, amplitude, and frequency of vibration.

sound sequencing: Therapy approach for speech apraxia where the sounds of a word are first produced individually before producing the word in its entirety.

sound visibility: Notion that some speech sounds are more readily visible on a talker's face compared with others. For example, the /f/ sound is high visibility, whereas the /h/ sound has low visibility.

sound wave: A pressure wave that is propagated through air (or other media) that is generally audible to the human ear.

soundfield amplification: System often used in classrooms for hearing-impaired children, whereby the teacher's voice is transmitted through a microphone and loudspeaker.

sound-to-symbol relationship: The relationship between a specific speech sound and the corresponding letter in the alphabet for that sound. In general, the English language has a poor sound-symbol relationship. The phonetic alphabet provides an exact sound-symbol relationship.

source: The point of origin. For the generation of speech, the source is the respiratory system.

spasmodic dysphonia: Voice disorder that is caused by involuntary muscle movements in the vocal folds.

speaker: One of two individuals required for successful communication. Another name for a speaker is encoder. The term is also a component of a hearing aid that delivers an acoustic signal to the ear.

speaking rate: Speed at which a person speaks. Speaking rate is typically reported according to the number of words (or syllables) spoken per minute.

specific language impairment (SLI): Preschool child who shows difficulty with language that is not caused by a known neurological, sensory, intellectual, or emotional deficit.

speech communication: Discipline concerned with the act of speaking.

speech delay: Communication disorder in which the speaking behavior demonstrated by the individual is quantitatively (as opposed to qualitatively) different from normal.

speech reading: Deciphering of spoken language on the basis of visual cues provided by the speaker, also known as lip reading.

speech spontaneity: An aspect of speech sampling that requires the person to either speech freely or name specific words.

speech-language pathologist: Professional educated in the field of speech-language pathology.

speech-language pathology: The study of disorders that affect a person's speech, language, and swallowing behavior, including methods of assessment, treatment, and prevention.

speech recognition: Process whereby a computer learns to identify and understand discrete words and phrases—also known as automatic speech recognition or computer speech recognition.

speech sound disorder: A deviation in the production of consonants and/or vowels.

spina bifida: Serious birth abnormality in which the spinal cord is malformed during fetal development. The spinal cord lacks its usual protective skeletal and soft tissue covering.

spinal nerves: Collection of 31 pairs of nerves that enter and exit the spinal cord. The nerves provide motor, sensory, or combined input to various parts of the body.

spontaneous recovery: Natural reappearance of function following a period of lessened response. A concept associated with the recovery of communication skills shortly after a stroke.

spoonerism: The unintentional transposition of sounds within or across words that occurs when speaking.

stammering: See definition for stuttering.

standardized testing: Form of assessment in which a test is administered and scored in a consistent manner.

stapedectomy: Surgical removal of the stapes bone within the middle ear as a means of improving hearing.

stapedius: Smallest skeletal muscle of the human body whose purpose is to stabilize the stapes bone that is inserted into the oval window of the cochlea.

stapes: Innermost of the three small bones (ossicles) of the middle ear, also known as the stirrup to reflect its unique shape.

statistical learning theory: A theory that focuses on the statistical aspects of learning such as that related to the acquisition of language.

stem cell: An unspecialized cell that gives rise to a specialized cell, such as a blood cell.

Stevens, Nettie Maria: American biologist and geneticist who discovered that chromosomes determine the sex of a species.

stimulation: An aphasia treatment approach the encourages the patient to use all modalities of communication.

stoma: Surgically created opening in the surface of the body.

stops: A group of consonants that are organized according to their manner of articulation, namely the complete obstruction of forward airflow followed by a sudden release of air. The consonants /p/, /t/, and /k/ are examples of stops.

strength: The state, property, or act of being strong.

stroke: Injury to the blood vessels of the brain, usually in the form of a clot or hemorrhage.

structural: Term used to describe speech sound disorders that result from abnormalities of the mouth and vocal tract.

structure: An aspect of speech sampling that requires the person to produce speech in either a natural (home) or unnatural (clinic) environmental setting.

stuttering: Disorder in which the flow of speech is disrupted by involuntary repetitions and prolongations of sounds, syllables, words or phrases, and involuntary silent pauses or blocks—also known as stammering.

stuttering-like disfluencies: Speech disfluencies that are most indicative of a stuttering disorder. Examples of a SLD include a syllable repetition and a sound prolongation.

stuttering modification: Treatment technique in which the main goal is to stutter more easily as opposed to speaking more fluently.

stuttering severity instrument: A standardized test used to evaluate the severity of stuttering exhibited by children and adults.

subjective assessment: Approach to evaluating a communication disorder using methods of observation and questioning.

submetacentric chromosome: A chromosome whose centromere lies between its middle and its end but slightly closer to the middle.

submucous cleft: Condition in which a cleft of the palate is not visible as a result of the cleft being covered by a mucous membrane lining.

sulcus: A deep, narrow groove in tissue. Various landmarks of the cerebral cortex are demarcated on the basis of sulci.

Sullivan, Anne: Teacher and friend of Helen Keller.

substitutions: Pattern of speech misarticulation whereby the intended speech sound is replaced (substituted) by another speech sound.

swallowing center: Region in the brainstem that is involved in the coordination and regulation of essential swallowing activity.

Sweet, Henry: English linguist who made a significant contribution to the field of phonetics.

symmetrical hearing loss: A hearing loss of both areas in which the configuration and severity of the loss are identical.

syndrome: Group of symptoms that collectively characterize an abnormal condition or disease.

syntax: The study of the form of language such as grammatical rules.

syrinx: The vocal organ of a bird.

tactile communication: Form of nonverbal communication in which touching (e.g., handshaking, kissing) conveys a message from sender to receiver.

Tadoma method: Form of communication used by deaf-blind individuals to assist with comprehension of speech. The method involves placement of the hands on the speaker's face to decipher facial movements.

technology: The application of science, math, engineering, art, and other fields of knowledge to create tools and implementations deemed useful by a society.

teeth: Hard bonelike structures aligned in a row along the base of the jaw that are used for biting and chewing.

telecoil: Hearing aid device that can amplify sound waves transmitted through a telephone.

telecommunications: The science and technology of communication at a distance by electronic transmission of impulses, as by telegraph, cable, telephone, radio, or television.

telegraph: Basic communication system that is able to transmit and receive simple electric impulses.

telephone: Instrument that converts voice and other acoustic signals into a form that can be transmitted to a location where it is reconverted into an acoustic signal.

television: Electronic (and digital) apparatus that is able to receive the simultaneous transmission of images and sounds.

temperament: The manner in which a person thinks, behaves, and reacts.

Templin, Mildred: American pioneer in speech-language pathology. Known for her research in the area of phonological development.

temporal bone: A bone that forms the sides and base of the skull.

temporal lobes: Side regions of the cerebral cortex that are primarily involved in the processing of sensory input.

temporomandibular joint: A joint that connects the mandible (lower jaw) to the temporal bone of the skull.

tensor tympani: Small muscle located in the middle ear that influences the mobility of the tympanic membrane (eardrum).

teratogenic: Relating to, or causing, a malformation of an embryo or fetus.

Thelwall, John: Best known as the radical orator during the movement for parliamentary reform in Britain in the late 18th century.

Thome, A: German scholar who believed stuttering was caused by spasms of the respiratory system.

threshold: Point that must be exceeded in order to elicit a response. A person's hearing threshold represents the lowest level of loudness necessary to perceive a sound.

thrombosis: Formation of a blood clot inside a blood vessel that obstructs blood flow.

thyroarytenoid muscle: Anatomical name for the vocal folds.

thyroid cartilage: Largest of the cartilages composing the framework of the larynx. A landmark of the thyroid cartilage is a notch, also known as the Adam's apple.

tinnitus: The perception of ringing in the ears without an external cause.

Titze, Ingo: Voice scientist who has made significant contributions to vocal fold physiology and voice rehabilitation.

tongue: The fleshy moveable, muscular organ attached to the floor of the mouth. The primary organ for taste, swallowing, and speech production.

tongue advancement (or tongue carriage): Categorization of vowels according to the horizontal location of the tongue within the oral cavity.

tongue elevation (or tongue height): Categorization of vowels according to the vertical location of the tongue within the oral cavity.

tongue thrust: Forward movement of the tongue, especially in the initial stage of swallowing. An infantile swallowing pattern that should diminish with age.

tonotopic organization: Cellular structure of the inner ear whereby the frequencies represented in the cochlea are organized from high to low.

trachea: Tubelike cartilaginous structure that is a portion of the respiratory tract—also called the windpipe.

tracheoesophageal speech: Technique for speaking following laryngectomy. Air is diverted to the esophagus causing it to vibrate and create sound.

traditional approach: Term used to describe a method of treating speech sound disorders. The approach begins with teaching the sound at an isolated level and gradually progressing to the production of the same sound in conversational speech.

tragus: Projection of skin-covered cartilage in front of the ear canal.

transducer: A device that takes one form of energy and converts it into another type of energy.

transcranial magnetic stimulation: Brain stimulation technique that induces a low electrical current between two electrodes placed on the scalp.

transfer function: Transformation that is used to describe the output of a device as a function of the input of the device. Speech production involves the transformation of the original source (vocal folds) into a specific sound resulting from changes in vocal tract configuration.

transmission model: Conceptualization of communication that involves encoding (a speaker) and decoding (a listener).

traumatic brain injury: An injury that occurs when a sudden outside force causes damage to the brain.

Travis, Lee Edward: The "Father of Speech-Language Pathology in the United States." He was particularly interested in the area of stuttering.

Turner, Henry: American physician who was the first to describe a genetic condition in women caused by the absence of one of the X sex chromosomes.

Turner syndrome: Medical disorder in females as a result of an absent X (sex) chromosome.

Twain, Mark: American humorist and author whose actual name was Samuel Clemens.

twitter: Internet-based form of social messaging involving short text messages of up to 140 characters in length.

two-word combinations: Early language utterances produce by children at approximately two years of age.

tympanic membrane: Thin concave-shaped membrane that separates the outer ear canal from the middle ear —also called the eardrum.

tympanogram: The graphic display of sound reflected back from the eardrum during a tympanometry test.

tympanometer: Instrument used to measure the compliance (sometimes called admittance) of the tympanic membrane. The results of the test are displayed on a graph called a tympanogram.

tympanometry: Test performed to evaluate eardrum (tympanic membrane) mobility and middle ear functioning.

tympanoplasty: A microsurgical procedure to repair a damaged tympanic membrane.

ultrasound: Use of high-frequency sound waves to create an image of internal body structures.

unilateral cleft lip: Failure of the lip to form during fetal development on one side of the nose.

unilateral hearing loss: Type of hearing loss where one ear has normal hearing and the other ear is impaired.

universal newborn screening: Approach to the screening of hearing in newborn infants whereby all children in a setting (country, county, etc.) are evaluated.

upper respiratory tract: The cavities of the body that include the nose, mouth, and throat.

uvula: Small fleshy mass of tissue that suspends from the back of the soft palate.

validation therapy: A treatment technique used to confirm, through words and gestures, what the person with dementia says.

Van den Berg, Janwillem: Dutch scientist who proposed the myoelastic-aerodynamic theory of phonation.

Van Gogh, Vincent: Dutch painter during the 19th century.

Van Riper, Charles: American pioneer in the field of speech-language pathology. He made significant contributions to the areas of stuttering and speech sound disorders.

velopharyngeal closure: Contact between the soft palate (velum) and the back of the throat (pharynx) that normally occurs during swallowing and the production of speech.

velopharyngeal inadequacy: Malfunctioning of the physiological relationship between the soft palate (velum) and the back of the throat (pharynx), in which a lack of contact between the two structures occurs.

ventilation tube: A small tube inserted through the tympanic membrane to ventilate the middle ear and prevent fluid from accumulating. Also called a pressure equalization tube or grommet.

ventriloquism: Art of projecting voice to give the illusion of it coming from another source, such as a dummy or doll figure.

verbal communication: Basis of expressive (vocal) communication that is one way for people to communicate face-to-face.

verbalizations: Production of vocal sounds that express meaning.

vermilion border: Region of redness that surrounds the lips.

vestibular apparatus: Region of the inner ear that is important for maintaining balance and spatial orientation. Consists of the utricle, saccule, and semicircular canals.

videofluoroscopy: Motion x-ray of the body that combines traditional flouroscopy (x-ray) with video-technology.

videoflouroscopic swallowing study: The use of motion x-ray to visualize swallowing.

viral meningitis: Infection of the protective membranes surrounding the brain or spinal cord that results from a virus. This form of meningitis is quite common and is a relatively mild illness compared with bacterial meningitis.

virgules: A diagonal (/) mark that serves as a form of pronunciation. The individual phonemes of a language are usually depicted using virgules (e.g., /t/, /m/, /f/, etc.).

Visi-Pitch: Commercially available instrument designed to measure and display the vocal fundamental frequency (pitch) of spoken voice.

visual communication: The transfer of information between individuals on the basis of vision.

vocal abuse: Any behavior that strains or injures the vocal folds, thus affecting their normal functioning.

vocal folds: Two muscular bands located within the framework of the larynx that protect the trachea from the entrance of foreign matter. These muscular bands also vibrate for the generation of voice—also known as the vocal cords.

vocal function: Treatment approach to improving voice production involving increased strength and coordination of the laryngeal musculature.

vocal hygiene: The science of vocal health and steps taken to ensure proper care of the vocal mechanism.

vocal misuse: Improper speaking behavior that can lead to temporary or permanent changes to one's speaking voice.

vocal nodules: Small inflammatory or fibrous growth that develops on the vocal folds.

vocal polyp: Small swelling in the mucous membranes covering the vocal folds—also known as Reinke's edema or polypoid degeneration.

vocal tract: Anatomical cavity in animals where sound is produced.

vocalizations: Any sound produced through the action of a vocal apparatus.

vocology: The science and practice of voice rehabilitation.

voice disorder: Condition in which the natural generation of voice and voice resonance is impaired.

voice feminization: Voice therapy procedure that involves the change of voice from masculine to feminine, usually as a result of gender transformation.

voice masculinization: Voice therapy procedure that involves the change of voice from feminine to masculine, usually as a result of gender transformation.

voice quality: The subjective aspect of voice that is perceived by listeners.

voice rest: Therapy procedure that involves complete cessation of speaking (including whispering) as a means of healing the vocal folds.

voiced consonant: A consonant that is produced with vocal fold vibration such as the /z/ sound.

voiceless consonant: A consonant that is produced without vocal fold vibration, such as the /s/ sound.

Volta, Alessandro: Italian physicist who invented the voltalic pile, a forerunner of the electric battery.

von Békésy, Georg: Hungarian physiologist who received the Nobel Prize for his research on the functioning of the inner ear.

von Graefe, Karl Ferdinand: Pioneer of plastic and reconstructive surgery.

von Helmholtz, Hermann: German physicist who made important contributions in acoustics and optics.

Von Leden, Hans: Otolaryngologist who coined the term, phonosurgery, to refer to the restoration of voice using surgical techniques.

von Langenbeck, Bernard: Skilled surgeon who developed a procedure for the closure of the hard palate.

von Siebold, Carl Casper: One of the first surgeons to recognize the importance of speech therapy for individuals with cleft lip and palate.

Waldeyer, Wilhelm: German anatomist who identified the material residing within a cell nucleus that he termed, chromosome.

Wallace, Alfred: Nineteenth-century anthropologist who, together with Charles Darwin, supported the concept of natural selection.

Watson, James: Nobel Prize winner for discovering the double-helix structure of DNA. His colleague who assisted in the discovery was Francis Crick.

waveform: Graph obtained by plotting the characteristics of a sound wave against time.

Wernicke, Karl: German neurologist who deduced that the left temporal lobe region of the brain was localized for understanding language. This region became known as Wernicke's area.

Wernicke's aphasia: Language disorder that impacts the comprehension of spoken and written language, resulting from damage to the left temporal lobe (Wernicke's area)

region of the brain—also known as a form of fluent aphasia.

Wernicke's area: Region of the left cerebral temporal lobe that plays an important role in the understanding of speech and language.

whistle register: Highest register of the human voice—also known as flageolet register.

whole genome sequencing: A laboratory process whereby the genome of an individual's entire DNA is obtained.

wild boy of Aveyron: Feral child, known as Victor, who was found wandering in the woods in France. His lack of speech provided early insight to the role of the environment in learning language.

Wilson, Matthew: American Revolutionary War minister and physician who wrote a compendium of medicine called the Therapeutic Alphabet.

within-word disfluencies: Disruptions in the forward flow of speech that occur within the boundary of a single word. Examples include the repetition or prolongation of a consonant at the beginning of a word.

World Health Organization: Branch of the United Nations that is concerned with public health.

World Wide Web: The complete set of documents residing on all Internet servers at a given time that are accessible to users via a simple point-and-click system of retrieval.

written language: Form of communication that is based on the representation of language by means of a writing system.

Wundt, Wilhelm: German physiologist and psychologist who has been referred to as the "Father of Experimental Psychology."

Yearsley, James: British surgeon who advocated removal of the tonsils as a form of treatment for stuttering.

Yperman, Jehan: Medieval surgeon who developed a variety of procedures for repair of facial defects.

Zemlin, Willard R.: American speech-language pathologist who was interested in the basic anatomy and physiology of the speech and hearing mechanisms.

Zwaardemaker, Hendrik: Dutch otolaryngologist who coined the term *presbycusis.*

zygote: The cell (organism) that results from fertilization.

INDEX

G